Heart Failure in Older Adults

Editors

WILBERT S. ARONOW
ALI AHMED

HEART FAILURE CLINICS

www.heartfailure.theclinics.com

Founding Editor
JAGAT NARULA

July 2017 • Volume 13 • Number 3

ELSEVIER

1600 John F. Kennedy Boulevard • Suite 1800 • Philadelphia, Pennsylvania, 19103-2899

http://www.theclinics.com

HEART FAILURE CLINICS Volume 13, Number 3
July 2017 ISSN 1551-7136, ISBN-13: 978-0-323-53134-4

Editor: Stacy Eastman
Developmental Editor: Alison Swety

Heart Failure Clinics (ISSN 1551-7136) is published quarterly by Elsevier Inc., 360 Park Avenue South, New York, NY 10010-1710. Months of publication are January, April, July, and October. Business and editorial offices: 1600 John F. Kennedy Boulevard, Suite 1800, Philadelphia, PA 19103-2899. Periodicals postage paid at New York, NY, and additional mailing offices. Subscription prices are USD 247.00 per year for US individuals, USD 448.00 per year for US institutions, USD 100.00 per year for US students and residents, USD 288.00 per year for Canadian individuals, USD 519.00 per year for Canadian institutions, USD 309.00 per year for international individuals, USD 519.00 per year for international institutions, and USD 100.00 per year for Canadian and foreign students/residents. To receive student and resident rate, orders must be accompanied by name of affiliated institution, date of term, and the *signature* of program/residency coordinator on institution letterhead. Orders will be billed at individual rate until proof of status is received. Foreign air speed delivery is included in all *Clinics* subscription prices. All prices are subject to change without notice. **POSTMASTER:** Send address changes to *Heart Failure Clinics*, Elsevier Health Sciences Division, Subscription Customer Service, 3251 Riverport Lane, Maryland Heights, MO 63043. **Customer Service: 1-800-654-2452 (US and Canada). From outside of the US and Canada, call 314-447-8871. Fax: 314-447-8029. For print support, E-mail: JournalsCustomerService-usa@elsevier.com. For online support, E-mail: JournalsOnlineSupport-usa@elsevier.com.**

Reprints. For copies of 100 or more of articles in this publication, please contact the Commercial Reprints Department, Elsevier Inc., 360 Park Avenue South, New York, NY 10010-1710. Tel.: 212-633-3874; Fax: 212-633-3820; E-mail: reprints@elsevier.com.

Heart Failure Clinics is covered in *MEDLINE/PubMed (Index Medicus).*

Contributors

EDITORS

WILBERT S. ARONOW, MD, FACC, FAHA
Professor, Division of Cardiology, Department of Medicine, Westchester Medical Center, New York Medical College, Valhalla, New York

ALI AHMED, MD, MPH
Director, Center for Health and Aging, Veterans Affairs Medical Center, Professor of Medicine, George Washington University School of Medicine and Health Sciences, Washington, DC; Adjunct Professor of Medicine, University of Alabama at Birmingham, Birmingham, Alabama

AUTHORS

JINNETTE DAWN ABBOTT, MD
Associate Professor of Medicine, Division of Cardiovascular Medicine, The Warren Alpert Medical School of Brown University, Providence, Rhode Island

ALI AHMED, MD, MPH
Director, Center for Health and Aging, Veterans Affairs Medical Center, Professor of Medicine, George Washington University School of Medicine and Health Sciences, Washington, DC; Adjunct Professor of Medicine, University of Alabama at Birmingham, Birmingham, Alabama

HERBERT D. ARONOW, MD, MPH
Arnold T. Galkin Clinical Professor in Cardiology, Division of Cardiovascular Medicine, The Warren Alpert Medical School of Brown University, Providence, Rhode Island

WILBERT S. ARONOW, MD, FACC, FAHA
Professor, Division of Cardiology, Department of Medicine, Westchester Medical Center, New York Medical College, Valhalla, New York

CHRIS CARAANG, MD
Division of Cardiology, Department of Medicine, Westchester Medical Center, New York Medical College, Valhalla, New York

KUMAR DHARMARAJAN, MD, MBA
Section of Cardiovascular Medicine, Department of Internal Medicine, Center for Outcomes Research and Evaluation, Yale-New Haven Hospital, Yale University School of Medicine, New Haven, Connecticut

DANIEL J. DOOLEY, MD
Cardiology Fellow, Veterans Affairs Medical Center and Georgetown University/MedStar Washington Hospital Center, Washington, DC

JEROME L. FLEG, MD
Division of Cardiovascular Diseases, National Heart, Lung, and Blood Institute, Bethesda, Maryland

WILLIAM H. FRISHMAN, MD
Rosenthal Professor and Chairman, Department of Medicine, Westchester Medical Center, New York Medical College, Valhalla, New York

ALAN GASS, MD
Division of Cardiology, Department of Medicine, Westchester Medical Center, New York Medical College, Valhalla, New York

TODD W.B. GEHR, MD
Professor of Medicine, Division of Nephrology, Medical College of Virginia of Virginia Commonwealth University, Richmond, Virginia

CHHAYA AGGARWAL GUPTA, MD
Division of Cardiology, Department of Medicine, Westchester Medical Center, New York Medical College, Valhalla, New York

VEDANT A. GUPTA, MD
Division of Cardiovascular Medicine, Advanced Cardiovascular Imaging Fellow, Department of Medicine, Lexington, Kentucky

SEI IWAI, MD
Professor of Medicine, Division of Cardiology, Department of Medicine, Westchester Medical Center, New York Medical College, Valhalla, New York

JASON T. JACOBSON, MD
Associate Professor of Medicine, Division of Cardiology, Department of Medicine, Westchester Medical Center, New York Medical College, Valhalla, New York

SAHIL KHERA, MD, MPH
Division of Cardiology, Department of Medicine, Westchester Medical Center, New York Medical College, Valhalla, New York

DALANE W. KITZMAN, MD
Cardiovascular Medicine Section, Department of Internal Medicine, Wake Forest School of Medicine, Winston-Salem, North Carolina

DHAVAL KOLTE, MD, PhD
Division of Cardiovascular Medicine, The Warren Alpert Medical School of Brown University, Providence, Rhode Island

PHILLIP H. LAM, MD
Cardiology Fellow, Veterans Affairs Medical Center and Georgetown University/ MedStar Washington Hospital Center, Washington, DC

GREGG M. LANIER, MD
Division of Cardiology, Department of Medicine, Westchester Medical Center, New York Medical College, Valhalla, New York

JOHN ARTHUR McCLUNG, MD, FACP, FACC, FAHA, FASE
Professor of Clinical Medicine and Public Health, Division of Cardiology, Department of Medicine, Westchester Medical Center, New York Medical College, Valhalla, New York

NAVIN C. NANDA, MD
Echo Lab, Distinguished Professor of Medicine and Cardiovascular Disease, University of Alabama at Birmingham, Birmingham, Alabama

GURUSHER PANJRATH, MD
Associate Professor of Medicine, Director of Heart Failure and Mechanical Circulatory Support Program, George Washington University School of Medicine and Health Sciences, Washington, DC; Inova Heart and Vascular Institute, Falls Church, Virginia

JULIO A. PANZA, MD
Chief of Cardiology, Division of Cardiology, Department of Medicine, Westchester Medical Center, New York Medical College, Valhalla, New York

MICHAEL W. RICH, MD
Division of Cardiology, Department of Internal Medicine, Washington University School of Medicine, St Louis, Missouri

DOMENIC A. SICA, MD
Professor of Medicine and Pharmacology, Chairman, Clinical Pharmacology and Hypertension, Medical College of Virginia of Virginia Commonwealth University, Richmond, Virginia

STEVE SINGH, MD
Associate Chief of Staff for Education, Veterans Affairs Medical Center, Professor of Medicine, Georgetown University, Washington, DC

VINCENT L. SORRELL, MD
Anthony N. DeMaria Professor of Medicine, Associate Chief, Division of Cardiovascular Medicine, Chair, Cardiovascular Imaging, Lexington, Kentucky

GEORGE E. TAFFET, MD
Professor of Medicine, Department of Geriatrics and Cardiovascular Sciences, Baylor College of Medicine, Houston, Texas

BHARATHI UPADHYA, MD
Cardiovascular Medicine Section, Department of Internal Medicine, Wake Forest School of Medicine, Winston-Salem, North Carolina

Contents

Preface: Heart Failure in Older Adults xiii

Wilbert S. Aronow and Ali Ahmed

Epidemiology, Pathophysiology, and Prognosis of Heart Failure in Older Adults 417

Kumar Dharmarajan and Michael W. Rich

Heart failure is the quintessential cardiovascular syndrome of aging that results from common cardiovascular conditions in older adults in conjunction with age-associated changes in cardiovascular structure and function. To a large extent, heart failure is a geriatric syndrome in much the same way that dementia, falls, and frailty are geriatric syndromes. The incidence and prevalence of heart failure increase strikingly with age and make heart failure the most common reason for hospitalization among older adults. Although outcomes for older adults with heart failure have improved over time, mortality, hospitalization, and rehospitalization rates remain high.

Diagnosis and Management of Heart Failure in Older Adults 427

Gurusher Panjrath and Ali Ahmed

Aging is characterized by heterogeneity, both in health and illness. Older adults with heart failure often have preserved ejection fraction and atypical and delayed clinical manifestations. After diagnosis of heart failure is established, a cause should be sought. The patient's comorbidities may provide clues. An elevated jugular venous pressure is the most reliable clinical sign of fluid volume overload and should be carefully evaluated. Left ventricular ejection fraction must be determined to assess prognosis and guide therapy. These 5 steps, namely, diagnosis, etiologic factor, fluid volume, ejection fraction, and therapy for heart failure may be memorized by mnemonic: DEFEAT-HF.

Role of Echocardiography in the Diagnostic Assessment and Etiology of Heart Failure in Older Adults: Opacify, Quantify, and Rectify 445

Vedant A. Gupta, Navin C. Nanda, and Vincent L. Sorrell

Echocardiography allows the assessment of systolic and diastolic function and identifies many of the common causes of heart failure (HF). Patients with minimally symptomatic or unsuspected left ventricular systolic dysfunction may be identified and receive the benefits of angiotensin-converting enzyme inhibitor therapy. Echocardiography is also for assessing prognosis and can be used serially to evaluate treatment. Ventricular filling pressures, pulmonary artery pressures, and cardiac output can be sequentially determined. The authors believe that all patients with HF should receive careful assessment echocardiography. The authors believe using echocardiography is especially valuable in the elderly.

Treatment of Heart Failure with Abnormal Left Ventricular Systolic Function in Older Adults 467

Wilbert S. Aronow

Heart failure (HF) with abnormal left ventricular (LV) ejection fraction should be identified and treated. Treat hypertension with diuretics, angiotensin-converting enzyme

(ACE) inhibitors, and β-blockers. Treat myocardial ischemia with nitrates and β-blockers. Treat volume overload and HF with diuretics. Treat HF with ACE inhibitors and β-blockers. Sacubitril/valsartan may be used instead of an ACE inhibitor or ARB in chronic symptomatic HF and abnormal LV ejection fraction. Add isosorbide dinitrate/hydralazine in African Americans with class II to IV HF treated with diuretics, ACE inhibitors, and β-blockers. Exercise training is recommended. Indications for implantable cardioverter-defibrillator and cardiac resynchronization therapy are discussed.

Heart Failure with Preserved Ejection Fraction in Older Adults 485

Bharathi Upadhya and Dalane W. Kitzman

Most elderly patients, particularly women, who have heart failure, have a preserved ejection fraction. Patients with this syndrome have severe symptoms of exercise intolerance, frequent hospitalizations, and increased mortality. Despite the importance of heart failure with preserved ejection fraction (HFpEF), the understanding of its pathophysiology is incomplete, and optimal treatment remains largely undefined. Unlike the management of HFrEF, there is a paucity of large evidence-based trials demonstrating morbidity and mortality benefit for the treatment of HFpEF. An update is presented on information regarding pathophysiology, diagnosis, management, and future directions in this important and growing disorder.

Use of Diuretics in the Treatment of Heart Failure in Older Adults 503

Domenic A. Sica, Todd W.B. Gehr, and William H. Frishman

Diuretics are the most commonly prescribed class of drugs in patients with heart failure, and in the short term they remain the most effective treatment for relief from fluid congestion. This article reviews the mode of action of the various diuretic classes and the physiologic adaptations that follow and sets up the basis for their use in the treatment of volume-retaining states, particularly as applies to the elderly. In addition, the article reviews the common side effects related to diuretics.

Heart Failure Complicating Acute Mtyocardial Infarction 513

Wilbert S. Aronow

Factors predisposing the older person with acute myocardial infarction (MI) to develop heart failure (HF) include an increased prevalence of MI, multivessel coronary artery disease, decreased left ventricular (LV) contractile reserve, impairment of LV diastolic relaxation, increased hypertension, LV hypertrophy, diabetes mellitus, valvular heart disease, and renal insufficiency. HF associated with acute MI should be treated with a loop diuretic. The use of nitrates, angiotensin-converting enzyme inhibitors, angiotensin II receptor blockers, aldosterone antagonists, beta-blockers, digoxin, and positive inotropic drugs; treatment of arrhythmias and mechanical complications; and indications for use of implantable cardioverter-defibrillators and cardiac resynchronization is discussed.

The Role of Positive Inotropic Drugs in the Treatment of Older Adults with Heart Failure and Reduced Ejection Fraction 527

Daniel J. Dooley, Phillip H. Lam, Ali Ahmed, and Wilbert S. Aronow

Positive inotropic drugs have long been studied for their potential benefits in patients with heart failure and reduced ejection fraction (HFrEF). Although there has been an

to SCD, but identifies a higher risk population and may cause significant symptoms. Antiarrhythmic drugs (AAD) and catheter ablation are the mainstays for prevention of VA, but have not been shown to improve mortality. The value of implantable cardiac defibrillators (ICDs) may be influenced by patient age. This article discusses long-term treatment of VA and the use of ICDs in the elderly.

Exercise Therapy for Older Heart Failure Patients 607

Jerome L. Fleg

Both the aging process and heart failure (HF) syndrome are characterized by a dramatic reduction of aerobic capacity. Significant decreases in muscle mass and strength are also common. Few HF training studies have included meaningful numbers of older individuals, especially those greater than 80 years of age and older women with HF with reduced ejection fraction. The modest data available suggest similar benefits in older patients and excellent safety. Resistance training may provide additional benefit. Whether exercise training can reduce mortality, hospitalizations, and overall health care costs in older adults with HF awaits the outcome of adequately powered multicenter trials.

Left Ventricular Assist Device in Older Adults 619

Chris Caraang, Gregg M. Lanier, Alan Gass, Wilbert S. Aronow, and Chhaya Aggarwal Gupta

Left ventricular assist devices (LVADs) are an effective therapy for a growing and aging population in the background of limited donor supply. Selecting the proper patient involves assessment of indications, risk factors, scores for overall outcomes, assessment for right ventricular failure, and optimal timing of implantation. LVAD complications have a 5% to 10% perioperative mortality and complications of bleeding, thrombosis, stroke, infection, right ventricular failure, and device failure. As LVAD engineering technology evolves, so will the risk-prediction scores. Hence, more large-scale prospective data from multicenters will continually be required to aid in patient selection, reduce complications, and improve long-term outcomes.

End-of-Life Care in the Treatment of Heart Failure in Older Adults 633

John Arthur McClung

Heart failure presents unique challenges to the clinician who desires to provide excellent and humane care near the end of life. Accurate prediction of mortality in the individual patient is complicated by a chronic disease that is punctuated by recurrent acute episodes and sudden death. Health care providers continue to have difficulty communicating effectively with terminally ill patients and their caregivers regarding end-of-life care preferences, all of which needs to occur earlier rather than later. This article also discusses various means of providing palliative care, and specific issues regarding device therapy, cardiopulmonary resuscitation, and palliative sedation with concurrent discussion of the ethical ramifications and pitfalls of each.

HEART FAILURE CLINICS

FORTHCOMING ISSUES

October 2017
Chronobiology and Cardiovascular Diseases
Roberto Manfredini, *Editor*

January 2018
Biomarkers for Heart Failure
Toru Suzuki, *Editor*

RECENT ISSUES

April 2017
Cardio-oncology Related to Heart Failure
Daniel J. Lenihan and Douglas B. Sawyer, *Editors*

January 2017
Cardiac Resynchronization Therapy: State of the Art
Luigi Padeletti, Martina Nesti, and Giuseppe Boriani, *Editors*

October 2016
Takotsubo Syndrome
Eduardo Bossone and Raimund Erbel, *Editors*

ISSUE OF RELATED INTEREST

Clinics in Geriatric Medicine, May 2016 (Vol. 32, Issue 2)
Managing Chronic Conditions in Older Adults with Cardiovascular Disease
Michael W. Rich, Cynthia Boyd, and James T. Pacala, *Editors*
Available at: http://www.geriatric.theclinics.com

Preface
Heart Failure in Older Adults

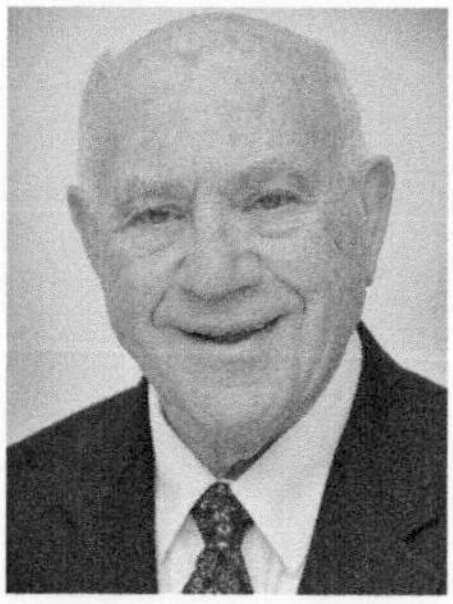

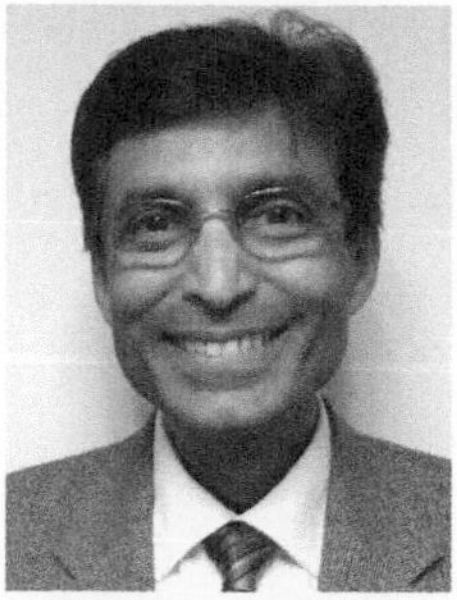

Wilbert S. Aronow, MD, FACC, FAHA Ali Ahmed, MD, MPH

Editors

An estimated 6.5 million adults in the United States have heart failure, and approximately 960,000 new cases of heart failure will occur annually in the United States. Heart failure is predominantly a disease of older persons. Approximately 80% of patients hospitalized with heart failure are older than 65 years. Heart failure is included as a contributing factor to mortality in one of every nine deaths in the United States. Approximately half of patients who develop heart failure will die within 5 years. Heart failure is also the most common cause of hospitalization and of rehospitalization within 3 months among older adults in the United States. Antecedent hypertension is present in 75% of patients who develop heart failure. Aging of the population is contributing to the epidemic of heart failure.

Much new information has accrued since Dr Aronow's previous "Heart Failure in the Elderly" issue was published in *Heart Failure Clinics* in October 2007. The current issue includes 15 articles, which are either new or markedly updated. The authors or coauthors are different from those of the previous issue in 10 of the 15 articles. The epidemiology, pathophysiology, prognosis, clinical manifestations, diagnostic assessment, cause, and role of echocardiography in the diagnostic assessment and cause of heart failure are discussed. The treatment of heart failure in older persons with a reduced ejection fraction, with a preserved ejection fraction, after acute myocardial infarction, and the use of diuretics, inotropic drugs, neurohormonal antagonists, exercise therapy, antiarrhythmic drugs, implantable cardioverter-defibrillators, cardiac resynchronization therapy, revascularization by percutaneous coronary intervention and by surgery, and left ventricular assist devices are also discussed. Finally, the last article discusses the very important topic of end-of-life care in the treatment of heart failure in older adults.

The authors who have contributed to this issue are experts in the treatment of cardiovascular disease and are dedicated to improving care and outcomes of heart failure in older adults. We extend our sincere appreciation to each of them for their excellent contributions to the articles in this issue.

Wilbert S. Aronow, MD, FACC, FAHA
Department of Medicine and Division of Cardiology
Westchester Medical Center
and New York Medical College
Valhalla, NY 10595, USA

Ali Ahmed, MD, MPH
Center for Health and Aging
Washington DC VA Medical Center
Department of Medicine
George Washington University
Washington, DC 20422, USA

E-mail addresses:
wsaronow@aol.com (W.S. Aronow)
aliahmedmdmph@gmal.com (A. Ahmed)

Heart Failure Clin 13 (2017) xiii
http://dx.doi.org/10.1016/j.hfc.2017.04.001
1551-7136/17/© 2017 Published by Elsevier Inc.

Epidemiology, Pathophysiology, and Prognosis of Heart Failure in Older Adults

Kumar Dharmarajan, MD, MBA[a,*], Michael W. Rich, MD[b]

KEYWORDS

- Heart failure • Elderly • Epidemiology • Pathophysiology • Prognosis • Mortality • Hospitalization
- Rehospitalization

KEY POINTS

- Heart failure is a common condition in older adults that results from the complex interplay of age-related diseases and age-associated physiologic changes.
- Despite recent declines in the age-adjusted incidence of heart failure, the prevalence of heart failure continues to rise due to population aging and improved treatment of both heart failure and concomitant cardiovascular conditions.
- Outcomes for older adults with heart failure have improved over time; however, mortality, hospitalization, and rehospitalization rates remain high.

INTRODUCTION

Heart failure (HF) is the quintessential cardiovascular syndrome of aging that results from age-related cardiovascular conditions and age-associated changes in cardiovascular structure and function. The incidence and prevalence of HF increase strikingly with age and make HF the most common reason for hospitalization in older adults.[1] Although outcomes of HF have improved over time, mortality, hospitalization, and rehospitalization rates remain high. Accordingly, total costs of care for persons with HF exceed $30 billion annually and are expected to rise to more than $70 billion by 2030 due to population aging and growth.[2]

This review describes the epidemiology, pathophysiology, and prognosis of HF in older adults. We present data on the incidence and prevalence of HF, including changes over time. Where data exist, we provide estimates for HF with preserved ejection fraction (HFpEF), the most common form of HF in older adults. We then describe the pathophysiology of HF in the elderly, including the

This is an updated version of an article that appeared in *Heart Failure Clinics*, Volume 3, Issue 4.
Disclosures: Dr K. Dharmarajan works under contract with the Centers for Medicare and Medicaid Services to develop and maintain performance measures and is a consultant and scientific advisory board member for Clover Health.
Funding/Support: Dr K. Dharmarajan is supported by grant K23AG048331 from the National Institute on Aging and the American Federation for Aging Research through the Paul B. Beeson Career Development Award Program. He is also supported by grant P30AG021342 via the Yale Claude D. Pepper Older Americans Independence Center.
[a] Section of Cardiovascular Medicine, Department of Internal Medicine, Center for Outcomes Research and Evaluation, Yale-New Haven Hospital, Yale University School of Medicine, 1 Church Street, Suite 200, New Haven, CT 06510, USA; [b] Division of Cardiology, Department of Internal Medicine, Washington University School of Medicine, 660 South Euclid Avenue, Campus Box 8086, St Louis, MO 63110, USA
* Corresponding author.
E-mail address: kumar.dharmarajan@yale.edu

Heart Failure Clin 13 (2017) 417–426
http://dx.doi.org/10.1016/j.hfc.2017.02.001
1551-7136/17/

contributions of age-associated physiologic changes in cardiovascular and noncardiovascular systems. Finally, we describe the prognosis of HF in older adults with regard to mortality, hospitalization, and rehospitalization.

EPIDEMIOLOGY

Identification of Heart Failure

American College of Cardiology/American Heart Association guidelines define HF as a "complex clinical syndrome that can result from any structural or functional cardiac disorder that impairs the ability of the ventricle to fill or eject blood."[3] As HF is a clinical syndrome and not a disease, many epidemiologic studies have relied on clinical diagnostic criteria for its identification.[4,5] These criteria include the Framingham criteria,[6] Boston criteria,[7] Gothenburg criteria,[8] and Cardiovascular Health Study criteria,[9] all of which have relatively similar performance characteristics for the detection of HF with high sensitivity compared with cardiologist evaluation.[10] These criteria may be less accurate for identifying acute decompensated HF[11] and do not differentiate between HF with reduced ejection fraction (HFrEF) and HFpEF. Ejection fraction criteria for distinguishing HFpEF from HFrEF have been highly variable across studies.[4]

Incidence of Heart Failure

New diagnoses of HF are common and strongly related to age. Data from the Atherosclerosis Risk in Communities Study have shown that approximately 915,000 new cases of HF occur each year in the United States.[12] Incidence rates increase with age for patients of both sexes. For example, data from the Framingham Heart Study have shown that annual rates of new HF events per 1000 person-years is 9.2 for white men 65 to 74 years of age, 22.3 for white men 75 to 84 years of age, and 43.0 for white men ≥85 years of age. Corresponding rates among white women are 4.7, 14.8, and 30.7 per 1000 person-years, respectively.[13] Similar findings relating HF incidence rates with age also have been noted among more ethnically and racially diverse populations.[14]

HF incidence varies by race, ethnicity, and socioeconomic factors. Data from the Multiethnic Study of Atherosclerosis have shown that HF incidence is highest among African American individuals, followed by Hispanic American, white American, and Chinese American individuals (incidence rates 4.6, 3.5, 2.4, and 1.0 per 1000 person-years, respectively).[12,15] Similar relationships were found in the Atherosclerosis Risk in Communities Study population, in which HF incidence rates were highest for black men, followed by black women, white men, and white women.[16] In both studies, the higher incidence of HF among African American individuals was largely explained by the greater prevalence of cardiovascular risk factors in this population. In addition, a systematic review of data from multiple countries, including the United States, Sweden, Denmark, and Scotland, found that income, educational attainment, and community factors suggestive of economic deprivation were all strongly associated with new-onset HF.[17]

The lifetime risk of developing HF is high. Data from the predominantly white Framingham Heart Study found that 1 in 5 men and women without HF at age 40 develop HF during their lifetimes.[18] A subsequent report from a more diverse study population derived from the Chicago Heart Association Detection Project and the Cardiovascular Health Study found that at age 45, lifetime risks for HF are 30% to 42% in white men, 20% to 29% in black men, 32% to 39% in white women, and 24% to 46% in black women, respectively.[19] The lower lifetime risks of HF in black men were largely due to higher competing risks for noncardiovascular death from renal failure, homicide, and other causes. Data from the international context confirm that elevated lifetime risk for HF is not restricted to the United States.[20]

With time, the incidence of HF may be declining in both North America and Europe. An examination of medical record data from Olmstead County, Minnesota, found that the age-adjusted and sex-adjusted incidence of HF declined from 315.8 per 100,000 persons in 2000 to 219.3 per 100,000 persons in 2010.[21] Similarly, an analysis of administrative data from a nationally representative sample of Medicare beneficiaries in the United States found that HF incidence declined from 32 per 1000 person-years in 1994 to 29 per 1000 person-years in 2003.[22] Both absolute and relative declines were greatest for Medicare beneficiaries aged 80 to 84 years (HF incidence declined from 57.5 to 48.4 per 1000 person-years). Similar declines in HF incidence also have been identified in Canada,[23] Scotland,[24] and Sweden.[25]

Prevalence of Heart Failure

The prevalence of HF is high and increasing over time. Recent data from the National Health and Nutrition Examination Survey (NHANES) demonstrated that approximately 5.7 million Americans have HF.[12] This number is expected to rise to at least 8 million by 2030. Factors driving the increase in HF include aging of the population, increased prevalence of specific risk factors for HF, including diabetes and obesity,[26,27] improvements in the treatment of concomitant cardiovascular conditions, and better treatment for HF itself.[2,5] Similar findings also have been noted in the international context, in which population aging and population growth continue to drive the increased prevalence of cardiovascular disease.[28]

As with HF incidence rates, the prevalence of HF increases sharply with age. Data from NHANES have shown that the proportion of adults with HF is 1.5% for men aged 40 to 59 years, 6.6% for men aged 60 to 79 years, and 10.6% for men 80 years and older.[12] Corresponding proportions among women are 1.2%, 4.8%, and 13.5%, respectively (**Fig. 1**). These data demonstrate that HF prevalence among women surpasses that of men in the oldest-old.

Heart Failure with Preserved Ejection Fraction

With time, there has been increasing interest in identifying persons with HFpEF, the predominant form of HF in older adults.[29] To date, however, there has been relatively little written about the incidence and prevalence of HFpEF. Diagnostic criteria for HFpEF, especially pertaining to left ventricular ejection fraction, have varied across studies.[5,21,29–31] In addition, administrative data are often unable to differentiate persons with HFpEF from those with HFrEF.

A recent study, however, applied validated clinical criteria[6] and specialty society definitions of HFpEF[3] to electronic health record data from Olmstead County and found that the proportion of incident HF cases due to HFpEF increased from 47.8% in 2000 to 2003, to 56.9% in 2004 to 2007, and to 52.3% in 2008 to 2010.[21] With time, there was an increase in prevalence of hypertension, diabetes mellitus, hyperlipidemia, and multiple chronic conditions at the time of HF diagnosis among persons with HFpEF. Notably, the overall incidence of both HFrEF and HFpEF decreased over time, but the decline was greater for HFrEF.

PATHOPHYSIOLOGY

The frequent development of HF in older adults relates in large part to the high prevalence of traditional cardiovascular risk factors in this population. Data from the Cardiovascular Health Study, a prospective population-based study of 5888 older adults, demonstrated that the population-attributable risk for the development of HF was 13.1% for coronary heart disease and 12.8% for a systolic blood pressure greater than 140 mm Hg.[32] These findings were confirmed in the Atherosclerosis Risk in Communities Study[26] and NHANES,[27] both of which also found that diabetes and obesity are responsible for a significant proportion of HF incidence. Even a modest reduction in these risk factors could result in large reductions in the number of persons with HF.[33]

The higher prevalence of HF in the elderly also relates to common age-associated changes in cardiovascular structure and function. These changes diminish chronotropic and inotropic responses, raise intracardiac pressures with ventricular filling, and increase afterload. As a result, the ability of the heart to respond to stress is impaired, whether that stress is physiologic (eg, exercise) or pathologic (eg, myocardial ischemia or sepsis). This decline in cardiovascular reserve is reflected in age-related reductions in peak

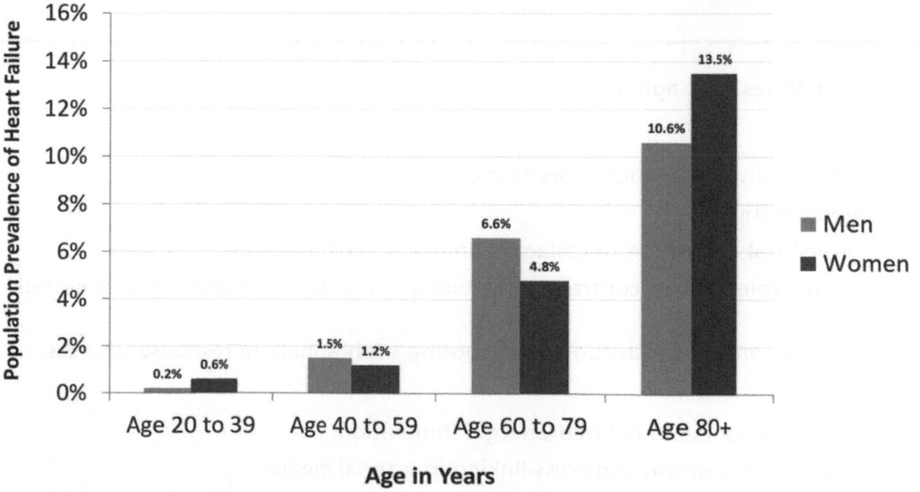

Fig. 1. Prevalence of HF in the United States by age and sex. (*Adapted from* Mozaffarian D, Benjamin EJ, Go AS, et al. Heart disease and stroke statistics-2016 update: a report from the American Heart Association. Circulation 2016;133(4):e275; with permission.)

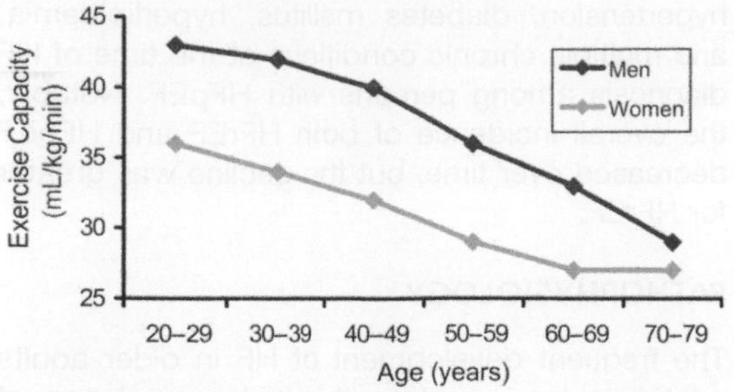

Fig. 2. Association of maximum exercise capacity with age. Maximum exercise capacity usually begins to decline between the ages of 20 and 30 years and falls approximately 10% per decade. Exercise capacity is described in terms of ml O_2/kg/min. (*From* Oxenham H, Sharpe N. Cardiovascular aging and heart failure. Eur J Heart Fail 2003;5(4):430; with permission.)

oxygen consumption (**Fig. 2**).[34] **Box 1** summarizes age-associated cardiovascular changes, 3 of which are particularly important.

First, age is associated with reduced responsiveness to beta-adrenergic stimulation. Deficits in intracellular signaling may be related to impaired G-protein coupling of receptors to adenyl cyclase, as well as to reductions in the amount and/or activation of adenyl cyclase.[35,36] These changes impair the ability of the older heart to augment cAMP in response to beta-receptor stimulation.[35] As a result, maximum heart rate (HR) declines almost linearly with age, often denoted by the formula: maximum HR = 220 − age; peak contractility also declines with age.

Second, aging alters left ventricular diastolic filling. During diastolic isovolumic relaxation and the early rapid filling period, efficiency of filling is highly dependent on active myocardial relaxation, an energy-dependent process. Aging is associated with impaired calcium release from contractile proteins and reuptake into the sarcoplasmic reticulum,[37] thereby prolonging the heart's contractile period. In contrast, efficient diastolic filling during mid and late diastole is highly dependent on the passive compliance properties of the heart. Aging is associated with myocyte hypertrophy[38] and increased interstitial deposition of collagen, amyloid, and lipofuscin, all of which increase myocardial stiffness and reduce compliance.[39,40] As a result, cardiac filling may be impaired when most needed, as in the presence of rapid atrial fibrillation or myocardial ischemia.

Third, aging leads to increased vascular stiffness. Arterial wall media in large-sized and medium-sized arteries undergo structural changes due to increased collagen content, nonenzymatic collagen cross-linking to form advanced glycation end products, and breakage of elastin fibers.[41,42] In addition, endothelium-dependent vasodilation is compromised due to diminished secretion of endothelial nitric oxide and increased signaling of angiotensin II, a potent vasopressor and mitogen.[41,43] These changes heighten afterload through increased impedance to left ventricular ejection and increase the prevalence of isolated systolic hypertension in older adults.

Cardiovascular disease and aging inevitably occur in the context of diseases and aging of other organ systems. Many of these noncardiovascular conditions and age-related changes directly contribute to the development of HF or its worsening. For example, chronic kidney disease and age-associated declines in glomerular filtration rate and renal sodium and potassium handling can increase the likelihood of acute decompensated

Box 1
Cardiovascular changes with aging

Cardiac changes

1. Diminished responsiveness to beta-adrenergic stimulation
2. Myocyte hypertrophy
3. Increased interstitial deposition of collagen, amyloid, and lipofuscin
4. Impaired calcium release from contractile proteins and reuptake into the sarcoplasmic reticulum during diastole
5. Insufficient mitochondrial production of adenosine triphosphate in response to stress

Vascular changes

1. Diminished responsiveness to beta-adrenergic stimulation
2. Increased collagen deposition and cross-linking in arterial media
3. Fragmentation of arterial elastin
4. Diminished endothelium-mediated vasodilatation

HF and adverse effects from drug treatment, including dehydration and electrolyte abnormalities.[44–46] Similarly, concomitant chronic lung disease, sleep-disordered breathing, and age-associated changes in lung function can contribute to pulmonary hypertension, diminished biventricular filling, and increased sensation of dyspnea.[47–49] More recently, it has been recognized that a large number of commonly used medications may directly contribute to the development of both chronic and acute HF.[50] The likelihood of drug-disease interactions increases with age due to the frequent presence of concomitant medical conditions and altered pharmacokinetics and pharmacodynamics associated with aging.[51–54]

PROGNOSIS

Mortality

A new diagnosis of HF is associated with a high mortality rate that exceeds that associated with many cancers.[55] A recent study of persons with new-onset HF from 2000 to 2010 in Olmstead County found mortality rates of 20.2% and 52.6% at 1 and 5 years after diagnosis, respectively.[21] One- and 5-year mortality rates increased significantly with age and were 7.4% and 24.4% for 60-year-olds and 19.5% and 54.4% for 80-year-olds, respectively. Rates of mortality were similar for persons with HFpEF and HFrEF in fully adjusted models. These data are consistent with previous research from the Framingham Heart Study,[56] a commercially managed population,[14] Medicare beneficiaries,[22] and earlier cohorts from Olmstead County[57] that also demonstrated high rates of mortality after HF diagnosis. These studies also demonstrated modest survival gains over time that largely relate to the increased use of evidence-based treatments for HFrEF.[12,58] These survival improvements may have lessened over time, however.[21]

Prognosis is worse for persons hospitalized with HF. Among US Medicare beneficiaries hospitalized with HF in 2006, mortality within 30 days and 1 year of admission was 10.8%[59] and 30.7%,[60] respectively. Mortality outcomes at 1 year demonstrate a clear relationship with age (**Fig. 3**). For example, rates of 1-year mortality in 2008 were 22.0%, 30.3%, and 42.7% for persons aged 65 to 74 years, 75 to 84 years, and 85 years and older, respectively. This figure also demonstrates that mortality outcomes after hospitalization have not improved significantly in recent years.[60] Although data describing 5-year mortality rates after hospitalization are not available for Medicare beneficiaries, research from Olmstead County found mortality rates in excess of 65% within 5 years of hospitalization.[61] Rates of mortality after hospitalization are slightly higher for patients with HFrEF compared with HFpEF[61,62] and much higher for patients discharged to a skilled nursing facility, in whom 30-day and 1-year mortality rates may exceed 14% and 50%, respectively.[63]

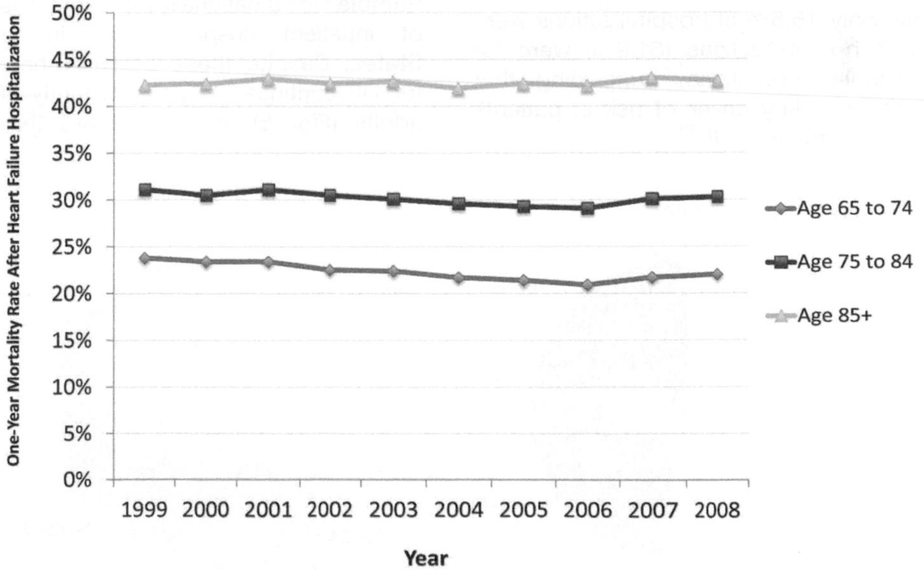

Fig. 3. Mortality within 1 year of hospitalization for HF by age in the United States, 1999 to 2008. Data reflect the national population of Medicare fee-for-service beneficiaries in the United States. Mortality rates were calculated for 1 year from the date of admission. (*Data from* Chen J, Normand SL, Wang Y, et al. National and regional trends in heart failure hospitalization and mortality rates for Medicare beneficiaries, 1998–2008. JAMA 2011;306(15):1669–78.)

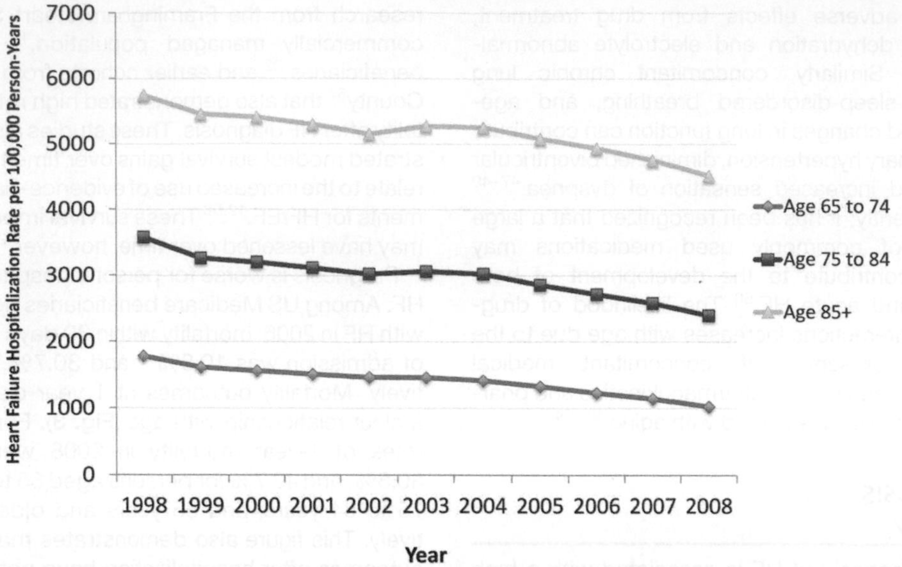

Fig. 4. HF hospitalization rates for older adults in the United States, 1998 to 2008. Data reflect the national population of Medicare fee-for-service beneficiaries in the United States. Hospitalization rates were calculated as the observed HF hospitalization rate per 100,000 person-years at risk among persons aged 65 to 74 years, 75 to 84 years, and 85 years and older. (*Data from* Chen J, Normand SL, Wang Y, et al. National and regional trends in heart failure hospitalization and mortality rates for Medicare beneficiaries, 1998–2008. JAMA 2011;306(15):1669–78.)

Hospitalization and Rehospitalization

Hospitalizations are common in patients with HF. Among those with incident HF in Olmstead County, 83% were hospitalized at least once over a mean follow-up of 4.7 years.[64] In addition, 66.9%, 53.6%, and 42.6% of patients were hospitalized at least 2, 3, and 4 times, respectively. Interestingly, only 16.5% of hospitalizations were for HF. Most hospitalizations (61.9%) were for noncardiovascular conditions, suggesting that multimorbidity is a key driver of risk in patients with HF, rather than HF itself.[52]

The risk of hospitalization for acute decompensated HF, in particular, has declined over time. Data from Medicare beneficiaries have shown that hospitalization rates for HF have decreased for older adults across age categories (**Fig. 4**). These findings have been confirmed in other data sets, including the National Inpatient Sample,[65,66] a nationally representative database of inpatient hospital stays in the United States. Despite these declines, hospitalization for HF continues to predominantly affect older adults (**Fig. 5**). In 2010, more than 70% of

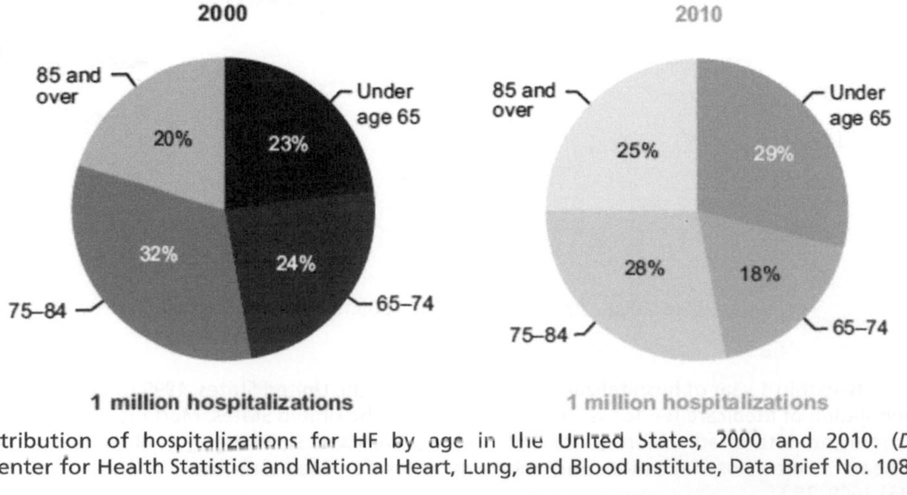

Fig. 5. Distribution of hospitalizations for HF by age in the United States, 2000 and 2010. (*Data from* National Center for Health Statistics and National Heart, Lung, and Blood Institute, Data Brief No. 108, October, 2012.)

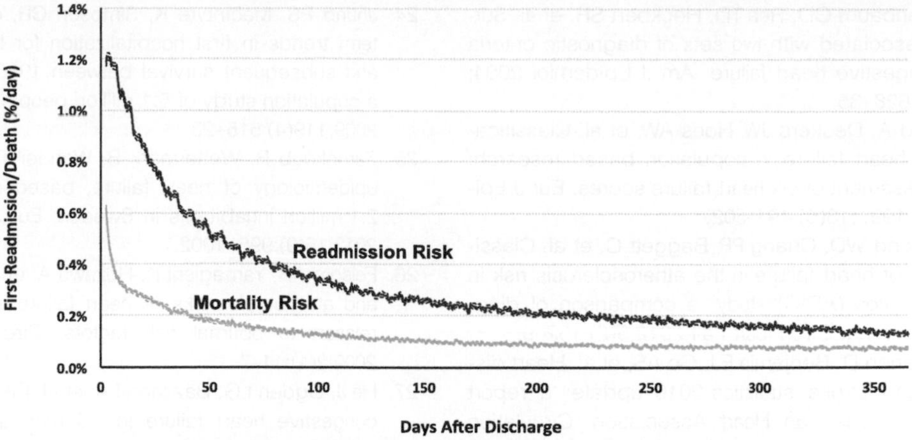

Fig. 6. Daily risk of readmission and death among older adults in the year after hospitalization for HF. Risk was calculated using hazard rates for the national population of older Medicare fee-for-service beneficiaries discharged after hospitalization for HF between 2008 and 2010. The risk of hospital readmission was calculated after incorporating the competing risk of death after hospital discharge. (*From* Dharmarajan K, Hsieh AF, Kulkarni VT, et al. Trajectories of risk after hospitalization for heart failure, acute myocardial infarction, or pneumonia: retrospective cohort study BMJ, 350 (2015), p. h 411; with permission.)

hospitalizations for HF were among adults aged 65 years and older.

Rehospitalizations are a considerable source of morbidity. Almost 25% of older adults with HF are rehospitalized within 1 month of discharge; almost 70% are rehospitalized within 1 year.[67,68] As with admissions to the hospital, readmissions after hospitalization for HF are usually not for HF and are often for noncardiovascular conditions.[67] In addition, patients remain vulnerable to major adverse events for a prolonged period after hospital discharge.[68,69] For example, it takes nearly 7 weeks for the daily risk of readmission to decline by 50% (**Fig. 6**). This period of extended vulnerability after hospitalization is not associated with increasing age,[70,71] suggesting that readmission may more strongly relate to age-independent variables, such as the quality of transitional care and complex social factors.

SUMMARY

HF is a common condition in older adults that results from the complex interplay of age-related diseases and age-associated physiologic changes. The societal burden of HF will continue to rise due to population aging, population growth, and improved treatment of HF and other cardiovascular disorders. As a result, we will be increasingly challenged to develop treatment plans and care systems that reduce the high levels of morbidity and mortality experienced by these patients, both from their HF and concomitant cardiovascular and noncardiovascular conditions.

REFERENCES

1. Agency for Healthcare Research and Quality. HCUP Statistical Brief 66: Medicare hospital stays: comparisons between the fee-for-service plan and alternative plans. 2006. Available at: https://www.hcup-us.ahrq.gov/reports/statbriefs/sb66.jsp. Accessed November 26, 2016.
2. Heidenreich PA, Albert NM, Allen LA, et al. Forecasting the impact of heart failure in the United States: a policy statement from the American Heart Association. Circ Heart Fail 2013;6(3):606–19.
3. Yancy CW, Jessup M, Bozkurt B, et al. 2013 ACCF/AHA guideline for the management of heart failure: a report of the American College of Cardiology Foundation/American Heart Association Task Force on practice guidelines. Circulation 2013;128(16):e240–327.
4. Roger VL. Epidemiology of heart failure. Circ Res 2013;113(6):646–59.
5. Dunlay SM, Roger VL. Understanding the epidemic of heart failure: past, present, and future. Curr Heart Fail Rep 2014;11(4):404–15.
6. McKee PA, Castelli WP, McNamara PM, et al. The natural history of congestive heart failure: the Framingham study. N Engl J Med 1971;285(26):1441–6.
7. Carlson KJ, Lee DC, Goroll AH, et al. An analysis of physicians' reasons for prescribing long-term digitalis therapy in outpatients. J Chronic Dis 1985;38(9):733–9.
8. Eriksson H, Caidahl K, Larsson B, et al. Cardiac and pulmonary causes of dyspnoea–validation of a scoring test for clinical-epidemiological use: the Study of Men Born in 1913. Eur Heart J 1987;8(9):1007–14.

9. Schellenbaum GD, Rea TD, Heckbert SR, et al. Survival associated with two sets of diagnostic criteria for congestive heart failure. Am J Epidemiol 2004; 160(7):628–35.
10. Mosterd A, Deckers JW, Hoes AW, et al. Classification of heart failure in population based research: an assessment of six heart failure scores. Eur J Epidemiol 1997;13(5):491–502.
11. Rosamond WD, Chang PP, Baggett C, et al. Classification of heart failure in the atherosclerosis risk in communities (ARIC) study: a comparison of diagnostic criteria. Circ Heart Fail 2012;5(2):152–9.
12. Mozaffarian D, Benjamin EJ, Go AS, et al. Heart disease and stroke statistics-2016 update: a report from the American Heart Association. Circulation 2016;133(4):e38–360.
13. National Institutes of Health. Incidence and prevalence: 2006 chart book on cardiovascular and lung diseases. Bethesda (MD): National Heart, Lung, and Blood Institute; 2006.
14. Barker WH, Mullooly JP, Getchell W. Changing incidence and survival for heart failure in a well-defined older population, 1970-1974 and 1990-1994. Circulation 2006;113(6):799–805.
15. Bahrami H, Kronmal R, Bluemke DA, et al. Differences in the incidence of congestive heart failure by ethnicity: the multi-ethnic study of atherosclerosis. Arch Intern Med 2008;168(19):2138–45.
16. Loehr LR, Rosamond WD, Chang PP, et al. Heart failure incidence and survival (from the Atherosclerosis Risk in Communities study). Am J Cardiol 2008;101(7):1016–22.
17. Hawkins NM, Jhund PS, McMurray JJ, et al. Heart failure and socioeconomic status: accumulating evidence of inequality. Eur J Heart Fail 2012;14(2):138–46.
18. Lloyd-Jones DM, Larson MG, Leip EP, et al. Lifetime risk for developing congestive heart failure: the Framingham Heart Study. Circulation 2002;106(24):3068–72.
19. Huffman MD, Berry JD, Ning H, et al. Lifetime risk for heart failure among white and black Americans: cardiovascular lifetime risk pooling project. J Am Coll Cardiol 2013;61(14):1510–7.
20. Bleumink GS, Knetsch AM, Sturkenboom MC, et al. Quantifying the heart failure epidemic: prevalence, incidence rate, lifetime risk and prognosis of heart failure The Rotterdam Study. Eur Heart J 2004; 25(18):1614–9.
21. Gerber Y, Weston SA, Redfield MM, et al. A contemporary appraisal of the heart failure epidemic in Olmsted County, Minnesota, 2000 to 2010. JAMA Intern Med 2015;175(6):996–1004.
22. Curtis LH, Whellan DJ, Hammill BG, et al. Incidence and prevalence of heart failure in elderly persons, 1994-2003. Arch Intern Med 2008;168(4):418–24.
23. Yeung DF, Boom NK, Guo H, et al. Trends in the incidence and outcomes of heart failure in Ontario, Canada: 1997 to 2007. CMAJ 2012;184(14):E765–73.
24. Jhund PS, Macintyre K, Simpson CR, et al. Long-term trends in first hospitalization for heart failure and subsequent survival between 1986 and 2003: a population study of 5.1 million people. Circulation 2009;119(4):515–23.
25. Zarrinkoub R, Wettermark B, Wandell P, et al. The epidemiology of heart failure, based on data for 2.1 million inhabitants in Sweden. Eur J Heart Fail 2013;15(9):995–1002.
26. Folsom AR, Yamagishi K, Hozawa A, et al. Absolute and attributable risks of heart failure incidence in relation to optimal risk factors. Circ Heart Fail 2009;2(1):11–7.
27. He J, Ogden LG, Bazzano LA, et al. Risk factors for congestive heart failure in US men and women: NHANES I epidemiologic follow-up study. Arch Intern Med 2001;161(7):996–1002.
28. Roth GA, Forouzanfar MH, Moran AE, et al. Demographic and epidemiologic drivers of global cardiovascular mortality. N Engl J Med 2015;372(14): 1333–41.
29. Bursi F, Weston SA, Redfield MM, et al. Systolic and diastolic heart failure in the community. JAMA 2006; 296(18):2209–16.
30. Fonarow GC, Stough WG, Abraham WT, et al. Characteristics, treatments, and outcomes of patients with preserved systolic function hospitalized for heart failure: a report from the OPTIMIZE-HF Registry. J Am Coll Cardiol 2007;50(8):768–77.
31. West R, Liang L, Fonarow GC, et al. Characterization of heart failure patients with preserved ejection fraction: a comparison between ADHERE-US registry and ADHERE-International registry. Eur J Heart Fail 2011;13(9):945–52.
32. Gottdiener JS, Arnold AM, Aurigemma GP, et al. Predictors of congestive heart failure in the elderly: the Cardiovascular Health Study. J Am Coll Cardiol 2000;35(6):1628–37.
33. Avery CL, Loehr LR, Baggett C, et al. The population burden of heart failure attributable to modifiable risk factors: the ARIC (Atherosclerosis Risk in Communities) study. J Am Coll Cardiol 2012;60(17):1640–6.
34. Oxenham H, Sharpe N. Cardiovascular aging and heart failure. Eur J Heart Fail 2003;5(4):427–34.
35. Fleg JL, Strait J. Age-associated changes in cardiovascular structure and function: a fertile milieu for future disease. Heart Fail Rev 2012;17(4–5):545–54.
36. Lakatta EG. Diminished beta-adrenergic modulation of cardiovascular function in advanced age. Cardiol Clin 1986;4(2):185–200.
37. Loffredo FS, Nikolova AP, Pancoast JR, et al. Heart failure with preserved ejection fraction: molecular pathways of the aging myocardium. Circ Res 2014;115(1):97–107.
38. Olivetti G, Melissari M, Capasso JM, et al. Cardiomyopathy of the aging human heart. Myocyte loss and reactive cellular hypertrophy. Circ Res 1991;68(6):1560–8.

39. Burgess ML, McCrea JC, Hedrick HL. Age-associated changes in cardiac matrix and integrins. Mech Ageing Dev 2001;122(15):1739–56.
40. Eghbali M, Eghbali M, Robinson TF, et al. Collagen accumulation in heart ventricles as a function of growth and aging. Cardiovasc Res 1989;23(8): 723–9.
41. Lakatta EG, Levy D. Arterial and cardiac aging: major shareholders in cardiovascular disease enterprises: part I: aging arteries: a "set up" for vascular disease. Circulation 2003;107(1):139–46.
42. Semba RD, Sun K, Schwartz AV, et al. Serum carboxymethyl-lysine, an advanced glycation end product, is associated with arterial stiffness in older adults. J Hypertens 2015;33(4):797–803 [discussion: 803].
43. Cernadas MR, Sanchez de Miguel L, Garcia-Duran M, et al. Expression of constitutive and inducible nitric oxide synthases in the vascular wall of young and aging rats. Circ Res 1998;83(3):279–86.
44. Ronco C, Haapio M, House AA, et al. Cardiorenal syndrome. J Am Coll Cardiol 2008;52(19):1527–39.
45. Ronco C, Di Lullo L. Cardiorenal syndrome. Heart Fail Clin 2014;10(2):251–80.
46. Silverberg D, Wexler D, Blum M, et al. The association between congestive heart failure and chronic renal disease. Curr Opin Nephrol Hypertens 2004; 13(2):163–70.
47. Barr RG, Bluemke DA, Ahmed FS, et al. Percent emphysema, airflow obstruction, and impaired left ventricular filling. N Engl J Med 2010;362(3):217–27.
48. Grau M, Barr RG, Lima JA, et al. Percent emphysema and right ventricular structure and function: the Multi-Ethnic Study of Atherosclerosis-Lung and Multi-Ethnic Study of Atherosclerosis-Right Ventricle Studies. Chest 2013;144(1):136–44.
49. Sajkov D, McEvoy RD. Obstructive sleep apnea and pulmonary hypertension. Prog Cardiovasc Dis 2009; 51(5):363–70.
50. Page RL 2nd, O'Bryant CL, Cheng D, et al. Drugs that may cause or exacerbate heart failure: a scientific statement from the American Heart Association. Circulation 2016;134(6):e32–69.
51. Dharmarajan K, Strait KM, Lagu T, et al. Acute decompensated heart failure is routinely treated as a cardiopulmonary syndrome. PLoS One 2013;8(10): e78222.
52. Dharmarajan K, Dunlay SM. Multimorbidity in older adults with heart failure. Clin Geriatr Med 2016; 32(2):277–89.
53. Mangoni AA, Jackson SH. Age-related changes in pharmacokinetics and pharmacodynamics: basic principles and practical applications. Br J Clin Pharmacol 2004;57(1):6–14.
54. Dharmarajan K, Strait KM, Tinetti ME, et al. Treatment for multiple acute cardiopulmonary conditions in older adults hospitalized with pneumonia, chronic obstructive pulmonary disease, or heart failure. J Am Geriatr Soc 2016;64(8):1574–82.
55. Stewart S, MacIntyre K, Hole DJ, et al. More 'malignant' than cancer? Five-year survival following a first admission for heart failure. Eur J Heart Fail 2001; 3(3):315–22.
56. Levy D, Kenchaiah S, Larson MG, et al. Long-term trends in the incidence of and survival with heart failure. N Engl J Med 2002;347(18):1397–402.
57. Roger VL, Weston SA, Redfield MM, et al. Trends in heart failure incidence and survival in a community-based population. JAMA 2004;292(3):344–50.
58. Merlo M, Pivetta A, Pinamonti B, et al. Long-term prognostic impact of therapeutic strategies in patients with idiopathic dilated cardiomyopathy: changing mortality over the last 30 years. Eur J Heart Fail 2014;16(3): 317–24.
59. Bueno H, Ross JS, Wang Y, et al. Trends in length of stay and short-term outcomes among Medicare patients hospitalized for heart failure, 1993-2006. JAMA 2010;303(21):2141–7.
60. Chen J, Normand SL, Wang Y, et al. National and regional trends in heart failure hospitalization and mortality rates for Medicare beneficiaries, 1998-2008. JAMA 2011;306(15):1669–78.
61. Owan TE, Hodge DO, Herges RM, et al. Trends in prevalence and outcome of heart failure with preserved ejection fraction. N Engl J Med 2006; 355(3):251–9.
62. Bhatia RS, Tu JV, Lee DS, et al. Outcome of heart failure with preserved ejection fraction in a population-based study. N Engl J Med 2006;355(3):260–9.
63. Allen LA, Hernandez AF, Peterson ED, et al. Discharge to a skilled nursing facility and subsequent clinical outcomes among older patients hospitalized for heart failure. Circ Heart Fail 2011;4(3): 293–300.
64. Dunlay SM, Redfield MM, Weston SA, et al. Hospitalizations after heart failure diagnosis a community perspective. J Am Coll Cardiol 2009;54(18):1695–702.
65. Chen J, Dharmarajan K, Wang Y, et al. National trends in heart failure hospital stay rates, 2001 to 2009. J Am Coll Cardiol 2013;61(10):1078–88.
66. Agarwal SK, Wruck L, Quibrera M, et al. Temporal trends in hospitalization for acute decompensated heart failure in the United States, 1998-2011. Am J Epidemiol 2016;183(5):462–70.
67. Dharmarajan K, Hsieh AF, Lin Z, et al. Diagnoses and timing of 30-day readmissions after hospitalization for heart failure, acute myocardial infarction, or pneumonia. JAMA 2013;309(4):355–63.
68. Dharmarajan K, Hsieh AF, Kulkarni VT, et al. Trajectories of risk after hospitalization for heart failure, acute myocardial infarction, or pneumonia: retrospective cohort study. BMJ 2015;350:h411.
69. Dharmarajan K. Comprehensive strategies to reduce readmissions in older patients with

cardiovascular disease. Can J Cardiol 2016;32(11): 1306–14.

70. Dharmarajan K, Hsieh A, Dreyer RP, et al. Relationship between age and trajectories of rehospitalization risk in older adults. J Am Geriatr Soc 2016; 65(2):421–6.

71. Ranasinghe I, Wang Y, Dharmarajan K, et al. Readmissions after hospitalization for heart failure, acute myocardial infarction, or pneumonia among young and middle-aged adults: a retrospective observational cohort study. PLoS Med 2014;11(9): e1001737.

Diagnosis and Management of Heart Failure in Older Adults

Gurusher Panjrath, MD[a,b], Ali Ahmed, MD, MPH[a,c,d,*]

KEYWORDS

• Heart failure • Older adults • Clinical manifestations • Diagnostic assessment • Etiologic factor

KEY POINTS

- Heart failure is a clinical diagnosis. A diagnosis of heart failure needs to be made based on medical history and clinical examination. There is no single test or procedure to rule in or rule out a diagnosis of heart failure.
- Heart failure is also a clinical syndrome. As such, after a clinical diagnosis of heart failure has been made, underlying etiologic factors for heart failure must be sought because ongoing insults from an etiologic factor such as myocardial ischemia may adversely affect prognosis.
- Heart failure symptoms are often due to fluid retention. Fluid volume status should be carefully assessed by estimating jugular venous pressure by examining both internal and external jugular veins.
- Heart failure prognosis and therapy vary by left ventricular ejection fraction, which should be measured in all heart failure patients, preferably after a clinical diagnosis has been made.
- Heart failure therapy is generally of 2 types: symptom-relieving and outcome-improving. The former applies to all heart failure patients and the latter mostly applies to heart failure and reduced ejection fraction. Recommendations from major national heart failure guidelines should be consulted and treatment of older heart failure patients must be individualized.

HEART FAILURE: A GERIATRIC SYNDROME

Heart failure (HF) is a geriatric syndrome. A disease generally has a known etiology, a known pathogenesis, and a known but variable presentation. A syndrome, on the other hand, is a set of symptoms and signs for which either the etiologic factor or the pathogenesis or both maybe unknown.[1] A geriatric syndrome, like a medical syndrome, is also characterized by a defined set of symptoms and signs but often the underlying etiologic factors are multiple and the pathogenesis may involve multiple interacting pathways (**Fig. 1**).[1]

CLINICAL PRESENTATION OF HEART FAILURE IN OLDER ADULTS

Most heart failure (HF) patients are older adults, who also suffer from multiple comorbidities and polypharmacy.[2] The management of a 78-year-old

Disclosure Statement: Dr A. Ahmed was in part supported by grants (R01-HL085561, R01-HL085561-S and R01-HL097047) from the National Heart, Lung, and Blood Institute (NHLBI). The content is solely the responsibility of the authors and does not necessarily represent the official views of the NHLBI or the National Institutes of Health.
This is an updated version of an article that appeared in *Heart Failure Clinics*, Volume 3, Issue 4.
[a] Department of Medicine, George Washington University, 2150 Pennsylvania Avenue, NW, Suite 8-416, Washington, DC 20037, USA; [b] Inova Heart and Vascular Institute, Inova Fairfax Hospital, 3300 Gallows Road, Falls Church, VA 22042, USA; [c] Center for Health and Aging, Veterans Affairs Medical Center, 50 Irving Street NW, Washington, DC 20422, USA; [d] Department of Medicine, University of Alabama at Birmingham, 933 19th Street South, CH19 201, Birmingham, AL 35294, USA
* Corresponding author. Center for Health and Aging, Washington DC VA Medical Center, 50 Irving Street Northwest, Washington, DC 20422.
E-mail addresses: aliahmedmdmph@gmail.com; gpanjrath@mfa.gwu.edu

Heart Failure Clin 13 (2017) 427–444
http://dx.doi.org/10.1016/j.hfc.2017.02.002
1551-7136/17/Published by Elsevier Inc.

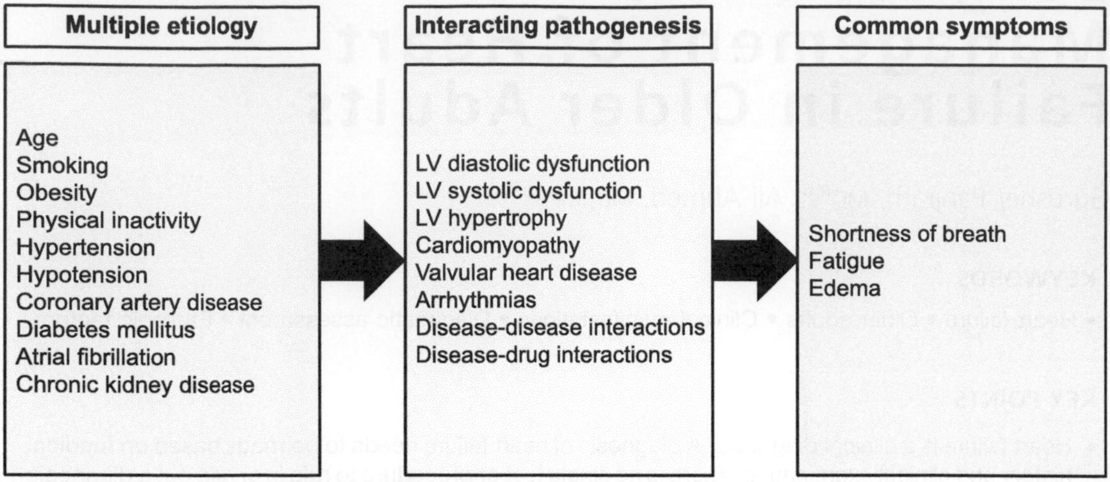

Fig. 1. Geriatric syndrome model of heart failure in older adults. LV, left ventricular. (*Adapted from* Inouye SK, Studenski S, Tinetti ME, et al. Geriatric syndromes: clinical, research, and policy implications of a core geriatric concept. J Am Geriatr Soc 2007;55:781; with permission.)

woman with HF and left ventricular ejection fraction (LVEF) greater than 55%, with hypertension, atrial fibrillation, diabetes, arthritis, chronic kidney disease, and depression, and who is taking multiple medications is more difficult than that of a 40-year-old young man with ejection fraction (EF) 25%, ischemic heart disease, and no other comorbidity. Yet, older HF patients have often been excluded from major HF trials. Thus, there is little evidence to guide management of HF in older adults.[3,4] That challenge is further compounded by the difficulty in the diagnosis and assessment of HF in older adults.[5] Older adults in general are a heterogeneous group, and as such, geriatric HF is characterized by a wide range of phenotypic heterogeneity, as illustrated in the case scenarios presented (**Table 1**). An initial assessment of HF in older adults involves a clinical diagnosis of HF, an evaluation of potential etiologic factors, an estimation of jugular venous pressure (JVP); and an evaluation of the left ventricular ejection fraction (LVEF) to guide therapy. These steps may be memorized with the mnemonic DEFEAT-HF: diagnosis, etiology, fluid volume, EF, and therapy for heart failure (**Table 2**).

DEFINITION OF HEART FAILURE

HF is a clinical syndrome that is characterized by symptoms that are manifestations of structural or functional impairment of ventricular filling or ejection of blood (see **Table 1**).[6] The cardinal manifestations of HF are dyspnea and fatigue, which may limit exercise tolerance, and fluid retention, which may lead to peripheral and pulmonary edema. Because HF is a not a primary disease, a full definition of HF needs to accompany a statement of underlying etiologic factors.

STAGES OF HEART FAILURE

Because HF is a progressive condition, clinical manifestations of HF vary depending on the stages in its natural history. Patients in stage A and stage B are asymptomatic and truly do not have clinical HF. Patients with stage A have risk factors for HF such as hypertension and coronary artery disease (CAD) but no structural myocardial disorder and no clinical HF. When stage A patients develop structural myocardial damage, such as left ventricular hypertrophy (LVH) or asymptomatic left ventricular systolic dysfunction but no clinical HF, they are referred to as stage B. Most clinical HF patients belong to stage C, with current or past symptoms. Stage D represents endstage and refractory HF and patients may require special therapy, such as durable circulatory support, cardiac transplants, or palliative care.

DESCRIPTIVE CLASSIFICATIONS OF HEART FAILURE

The most clinically relevant descriptive classification of clinical HF is based on LVEF: HF with reduced EF (HFrEF; previously known as systolic HF) and HF with preserved EF (HFpEF; previously known as diastolic HF). This classification has prognostic and therapeutic implications (see later discussion). Determination of LVEF is the first crucial step in the assessment of patients diagnosed with HF and is considered a measure of quality of care.[7,8] Other descriptive classifications of HF (see later discussion) are less clinically relevant.

Left-Sided Versus Right-Sided Heart Failure

Left-sided HF occurs when HF predominantly affects the left ventricle. Most early clinical HF patients

Table 1
Examples of clinical presentation of heart failure in older adults

Case 1	A 79-year-old man with a history of hypertension and prior acute myocardial infarction (AMI) presented at an outpatient clinic with a 6-month-old history of progressive dyspnea on exertion (DOE) and leg swelling. He had no history of dyspnea at rest, orthopnea, paroxysmal nocturnal dyspnea (PND), cough, wheezing, or chest pain. He had no emergency department (ED) visits or hospitalizations due to dyspnea. His physical examination was remarkable for mild pitting edema around his ankles and lower legs. His JVP estimated using external jugular vein (EJV) at a 30° incline was 5 cm water. He had no HJR. He had no S3 or pulmonary rales. His electrocardiogram and chest radiograph were normal. An echocardiogram showed a LVEF of 35%. He had no evidence of fluid retention and no diuretic was prescribed. He was prescribed a low-dose angiotensin-converting enzyme (ACE) inhibitor and, over the next several weeks, his symptoms, including his leg edema, improved.
Case 2	An 86-year-old woman with a history of HF with unknown EF and hypertension presented at an outpatient clinic with a 4-wk history of dyspnea and fatigue on minimal exertion (eg, turning over in bed) and orthopnea but no PND (she slept in a recliner) or chest pain. She also complained of weakness, right upper quadrant pain, nausea, loss of appetite, and severe leg swelling. She did not seek ED care, nor was she hospitalized for her symptoms. Her physical examination was remarkable for a JVP of 20 cm water (estimated using EJV in a near-seated position), a positive HJR, a right-sided S3, occasional pulmonary rales but no wheezing, an enlarged soft tender liver, and severe bilateral lower extremity edema up to mid-thigh with brown pigmentation and induration of skin, and multiple blisters over lower legs. An accentuated S2 at left fourth intercostal space suggested pulmonary hypertension, with an estimated pulmonary artery systolic pressure of 40–45 mm Hg. She had a normal electrocardiogram. A chest radiograph revealed marked cardiomegaly and pulmonary congestion. An echocardiogram later showed an EF >55%. She was on a thiazide diuretic for her hypertension, which was replaced with a loop diuretic. A week later, her symptoms were much improved.
Case 3	An 85-year-old woman with a history of hypertension and atrial fibrillation had progressive dyspnea and fatigue on exertion over the past 6 mo. She presented at the local ED with worsening dyspnea on exertion and a 2-pillow orthopnea. She reported no dyspnea at rest, PND, palpitation, or chest pain. For several days, she had ran out of her atenolol that she took for hypertension for several days. At the ED, her systolic blood pressure (BP) was 220 mm Hg. She had a few bibasilar pulmonary rales and lower extremity edema up to mid-leg. She had no S3. Her JVP was 15 cm water estimated at 50° incline using EJV with a positive HJR. An electrocardiogram was remarkable for atrial fibrillation with a ventricular rate of 170 beats/min but no evidence of ischemia. Her cardiac enzymes were normal. A chest radiograph demonstrated cardiomegaly with mild pulmonary edema. An echocardiogram later showed an EF of 55%. A diagnosis of flash pulmonary edema was made and she was treated with a loop diuretic and a beta-blocker. Her symptoms improved and she was discharged home. Despite controlled BP and heart rate, she needed long-term therapy with a low-dose loop diuretic to avoid HF symptoms.

(*continued on next page*)

Table 1 (continued)

Case 4	An 84-year-old man, with a history of hypertension and diabetes was recently hospitalized with syncope. He was physically very active and had noted mild DOE before hospitalization. He had no dyspnea at rest, orthopnea, PND, or chest pain. He had an enlarged heart by chest radiograph, an LVEF of 25% by echocardiogram but a normal coronary angiogram, He was discharged on furosemide 80 mg daily, which was later increased to 160 mg/d, due to his progressive DOE and fatigue. Over the next 2 wk, he lost over 20 pounds and his symptoms improved. He had trace leg edema. His serum creatinine was 1.5 mg/dL, and his blood urea nitrogen to creatinine ratio was normal at 15. His brain natriuretic peptide (BNP) level was elevated at 400 (normal <100) pg/ml. He was thought to have residual fluid retention and was maintained on furosemide 160 mg/d. Several weeks later, his fatigue and DOE returned. An outpatient examination was remarkable for systolic BP of 95 mm Hg and a JVP of 3 cm water. His furosemide dose was reduced to 80 mg/d. A week 2later, he gained 10 pounds and his HF symptoms improved.
Case 5	An 82-year-old woman with a history of hypertension and CAD presented with a 1-year history of dyspnea at rest, chest tightness, and dizziness presented to the local ED and was hospitalized each time. During these hospitalizations, she underwent comprehensive investigations, including an echocardiogram, a cardiac catheterization, and an MRI of brain, none of which revealed any pathologic condition. She had no DOE, orthopnea, PND, or leg swelling. Her physical examination was unremarkable with no signs of HF. Her JVP was normal at 5 cm water. However, she continued to remain symptomatic. An outpatient evaluation revealed significant loss and stress in personal and social life, and she scored positively on a geriatric depression scale. She denied sad or depressed mood. A diagnosis of somatization associated with geriatric depression was made, and she was started on a low-dose selective serotonin reuptake inhibitor (SSRI). Within several weeks, her symptoms completely resolved.

Adapted from Ahmed A. DEFEAT heart failure: clinical manifestations, diagnostic assessment, and etiology of geriatric heart failure. Heart Failure Clin 2007;3(4):389–402; with permission.

Table 2
A simple 5-step protocol for the assessment and management of chronic heart failure in older adults

D	Diagnosis	HF is a clinical diagnosis and needs to be made based on routine history and clinical examination. Symptoms and signs of HF are similar in patients with HF and reduced EF (HFrEF) and HF with preserved EF (HFpEF). There is no laboratory test to confirm or rule out a diagnosis of HF. EF should not be used to diagnose HF because more than half of all older adults with HF have HFpEF.
E	Etiology	HF is a syndrome, and as such, a diagnosis is incomplete without the identification of underlying causes. Untreated underlying etiologic factors, such as ongoing myocardial ischemia, may adversely affect prognosis.
F	Fluid volume	Fluid retention is a hallmark sign of HF and is present in nearly all newly diagnosed HF patients. Fluid retention is also a recurring problem for most patients with chronic HF. JVP in centimeters of water needs to be estimated by careful examination of both internal and external jugular venous pulsations in the middle of the neck to properly assess fluid volume status. A description of "jugular venous distension" should be avoided. Also, a description of "no fluid retention" should be avoided because some HF patients may suffer from hypovolemia, especially if overdiuresed.
E	EF	LVEF should be determined using an echocardiogram and used to assess prognosis and guide therapy.
A	and	
T	Treatment	HF therapy can be broadly categorized as symptom-relieving and outcome-improving. Because HF symptoms are indistinguishable between HFrEF and HFpEF, therapy directed to relieve HF symptoms is generally similar for both HFrEF and HFpEF. Evidence-based therapy to improve outcomes, on the other hand, is often restricted to HFrEF. Recommendations of major HF guidelines are mostly based on clinical trials in younger patients with HFrEF but most can reasonably individualized for older patients with HFrEF with the principle of start low, go slow.

Adapted from Ahmed A. Chronic heart failure in older adults. Med Clin N Am 2011;95:441; with permission.

have left-sided HF. Pure left-sided HF may result in either pulmonary congestion or systemic hypoperfusion, or both, and have associated symptoms, such as dyspnea, cough, wheezing, fatigue, hypotension, tachycardia, confusion, syncope, delirium, and oliguria, pulmonary rales, and left-sided third heart sound (S3). As HF progresses, left-sided HF eventually leads to right-sided HF.[9] The presence of low right ventricular EF is associated with poor outcomes in patients with HFrEF.[10,11]

Right-sided HF occurs when HF predominantly affects the right ventricle. Common symptoms and signs of right-sided HF are often due to systemic congestion, resulting in dyspnea, fatigue, leg swelling, nausea, vomiting, epigastric and upper abdominal pain, elevated JVP, hepatojugular reflux (HJR), hepatomegaly, right-sided S3, prominent pulmonic component of the second heart sound (S2), and dependent edema. Little is known about the parameters of right ventricular function and dysfunction, and the cellular and molecular basis of right-sided HF.[12] Common causes of right HF include pulmonary conditions (cor pulmonale) and left HF.

Thus, most advanced HF patients have both left-sided and right-sided HF, as noted in case 2. However, symptoms and signs related to biventricular HF may also been seen in most patients with early HF who often present with dyspnea on exertion (DOE) and leg edema (case 1).

Backward Versus Forward Heart Failure

The concept of backward failure was first proposed by James Hope in 1832. He suggested that congestion in HF was due to backward pressure in the venous and capillary system as a result of the failing heart's inability to pump forward.[13] This notion is supported in that most left HF are associated with some degree of right HF.[9,14] However, it was later demonstrated that congestion in HF often precedes increase in pressure in the venous and capillary systems and is due to decreased renal blood flow directly associated with forward failure.[15,16] Diminished renal blood flow has later been shown to be associated with the activation of the renin-angiotensin-aldosterone system in HF.[17] Most HF patients have clinical manifestations of both backward and forward HF (cases 1–4). HF may not be clinically distinguished as forward or backward, and such distinctions probably have no diagnostic, therapeutic or prognostic implications.

High-Output Versus Low-Output Heart Failure

Most older HF patients have low-output HF (cases 1–4). High-output HF, characterized by high cardiac output, although rare in older adults, may be associated with hyperdynamic conditions such as severe anemia, thyrotoxicosis, and arteriovenous fistula, including those used for hemodialysis.[18–20] Although anemia may cause exacerbation of HF symptoms, it rarely causes high-output HF in the absence of other cardiac disease and/or severe anemia (hemoglobin <5 gm/dl).[14,21] Thyrotoxicosis alone also rarely causes high-output HF. Clinical features of high-output and low-output HF may be indistinguishable. However, high-output HF patients may have warm extremities. Assessment of all new HF patients should include laboratory tests for anemia, kidney function, and thyroid function.[21–23]

Acute Versus Chronic Heart Failure

The concept of acute and chronic HF is used in 2 different contexts: severity (mild to moderate vs severe) and onset (sudden vs gradual) of symptoms. Most chronic HF patients undergo acute exacerbations of symptoms from time to time (cases 2 and 4). More than two-thirds of all hospitalized HF patients have known chronic HF.[24] Decompensation of chronic HF may be due to noncompliance with drugs, salt or fluid, acute myocardial ischemia, severe hypertension, or natural disease progression. In many of these patients, symptoms are severe and require ED visit or hospitalization for acute management. HF is associated with over 1 million hospitalizations in the United States and is the main reason for hospitalization for persons 65 years and older.[25,26] This is despite that fact that older HF patients often attribute their HF symptoms to aging and thus delay care, even when symptoms are severe (case 2). Clinical manifestations of ambulatory chronic HF and hospitalized acute HF are generally similar but may be more severe in the latter group.

Clinical manifestations of HF may be sudden, as after a large acute myocardial infarction with or without valve damage, typically leading to HFrEF, and in severe systolic hypertension with flash pulmonary edema, often leading to HFpEF (case 3).[27,28] HF may also present acutely with syncope (case 4). Clinical manifestations of HF may be gradual in the presence of chronic myocardial ischemia and less severe hypertension. Acute exacerbations due to noncompliance are also generally gradual in onset. Both sudden and gradual onset of symptoms may occur in the setting of incident or prevalent HF.

DIAGNOSTIC ASSESSMENT OF HEART FAILURE IN OLDER ADULTS

The diagnostic assessment of HF in older adults should begin with a clinical diagnosis of HF, followed by the establishment of potential underlying causes of HF. Evaluation of JVP is an essential part of the diagnostic process. JVP should also be evaluated during subsequent visits to assess HF control status. Once a clinical diagnosis is made, EF should be measured using an echocardiogram. These key steps may be memorized by the mnemonic DEFEAT: diagnosis, etiology, fluid volume, EF, and treatment.

CLINICAL DIAGNOSIS OF HEART FAILURE

HF is a clinical diagnosis and a diagnosis of HF should be established preferably before an echocardiogram is ordered. This is especially important in patients with limited (case 1) or atypical (case 4) clinical manifestations of HF. In these patients, a normal LVEF may bias diagnostic assessment. For example, case 1 only had DOE and edema, both nonspecific symptoms, and case 4 had syncopal episode, which is an atypical HF symptom (**Table 3**). If a diagnosis of HF is not already made, a normal LVEF may increase the risk of a false-negative diagnosis, leading to worsening of symptoms, possible emergency room visits or hospitalizations, and delays in diagnosis and therapy. However, when a classic constellation of symptoms and signs of HF is present, and a clinical diagnosis of HF can be established without difficulty (cases 2 and 3), a normal LVEF does not make the clinician question the diagnosis but instead helps classify HF as HFpEF.

Functional, physiologic, and psychological heterogeneity of older adults should be taken into consideration when evaluating clinical manifestations in the diagnostic assessment of HF. DOE is a nonspecific symptom. However, that was the basis of a presumptive clinical diagnosis of HF for case 1. He was a very active man who refused to restrict his activities due to his DOE, which could not be explained otherwise by another illness. In addition, his DOE was accompanied by new-onset leg edema and he had several risk factors for HF. All these pointed toward a clinical diagnosis of HF. This would be difficult if he was obese, deconditioned, or had chronic obstructive pulmonary disease (COPD) (see **Table 3**). Case 5 had dyspnea at rest but no DOE, which is almost always due to nonorganic causes. Further questioning also revealed that about a year ago she

Table 3
Diagnosis and etiologic factors of heart failure in older adults

	Cases					
	1	**2**	**3**	**4**	**5**	**Comments**
DOE	**Yes**	**Yes**	**Yes**	**Yes**	No	Case 1 had DOE without other associated symptoms and signs, and a clinical diagnosis of HF could not be made. He had low EF but because of his DOE he could not be diagnosed to have asymptomatic LV systolic dysfunction. So, his low EF in the context of DOE helped make a diagnosis of HF.
Orthopnea	No	**Yes**	**Yes**	No	No	Case 2 slept in in recliner to avoid orthopnea. Use of multiple pillows or sleep in a recliner, or use blocks or bricks to raise the head of bed to avoid orthopnea may be used as markers of orthopnea.
PND	No	**Yes**	No	No	No	Case 2 slept in in recliner to avoid orthopnea and thus may also have avoided PND.
Dyspnea at rest	No	**Yes**	No	No	**Yes**	Case 2 had near-class IV symptoms. Case 5 had dyspnea at rest but not on exertion, unlikely to be HF.
Fatigue	Yes	**Yes**	**Yes**	No	No	Often experienced when patients do things at their own pace.
Dizziness	No	No	No	**Yes**	**Yes**	Not a typical HF symptom. Likely due to hypotension (case 4) or somatization (case 5).
Syncope	No	No	No	**Yes**	No	Atypical. Likely due to hypotension (case 4). A risk factor for sudden cardiac death.
Chest pain	No	No	No	No	No	Uncommon as an HF symptom.
Cough	No	No	No	No	No	Rare. May follow dyspnea or PND but may also precede dyspnea.
Swelling of foot or leg	**Yes**	**Yes**	**Yes**	**Yes**	No	When onset of leg swelling is simultaneous with DOE, as in case 1, it may be more suggestive of HF than having different onsets.
GI symptoms	No	**Yes**	No	No	No	Rare in chronic HF. May suggest congestive hepatopathy. Maybe accompanied by right upper quadrant pain and tenderness, and some mild abnormalities of liver function.
COPD	No	No	No	No	No	Differentiating dyspnea of HF from that of COPD may be difficult. Important to carefully estimate JVP to assess fluid balance.
Deconditioning	No	**Yes**	No	No	No	May manifest as DOE and fatigue but often there is no orthopnea, PND, leg edema.
Depression	No	No	No	No	**Yes**	May manifest as somatization, as in case 4. Physiologically implausible symptoms, such as dyspnea at rest without DOE, should raise suspicion
HF risk factors	**Yes**	**Yes**	**Yes**	**Yes**	**Yes**	Often present as morbidities in older patients with HF.
JVP	5	20	15	3	5	Almost always present during initial presentation and acute exacerbation of HF but chronic stable patients may have normal JVP, and may even be low if overdiuresed.

(*continued on next page*)

Table 3
(continued)

	Cases					
	1	**2**	**3**	**4**	**5**	**Comments**
Jugular waveforms	?	?	?	?	?	Not needed to estimate JVP or make a diagnosis of HF. Familiarity with the double undulation of the jugular venous pulsation may help distinguish it from carotid pulsation.
Third heart sound	No	**Yes**	No	No	No	Often present but not necessary to establish a diagnosis of HF.
Pulmonary rales	No	**Yes**	**Yes**	No	No	Rare in chronic HF due to efficient pulmonary lymphatic system in these patients.
HJR	No	**Yes**	**Yes**	No	No	It helps identify the position and patency of EJV in neck. When present in those with normal JVP it may indicate early fluid retention.
LE edema	**Yes**	**Yes**	**Yes**	Yes	No	Pitting edema despite normal JVP may indicate chronic venous insufficiency. It is also accompanied by skin discoloration and stasis dermatitis.
Cardiomegaly	No	**Yes**	**Yes**	**Yes**	No	Cardiomegaly by chest radiograph may help support a clinical diagnosis of HF
Pulmonary venous congestion	No	**Yes**	No	No	No	Uncommon in chronic HF but when present in radiograph may support diagnosis
Pulmonary edema	No	No	**Yes**	No	No	Rare in chronic HF. May occur in acute decompensation.
Pleural effusion	No	No	No	No	No	Not uncommon, usually bilateral.
BNP	Not done	Not done	Not done	400	No	Elevated BNP and NT-pro-BNP levels may support the diagnosis of HF. HF is unlikely if BNP <100 pg/mL and NT-pro-BNP <300 pg/mL. Role in older adults is less clear. Rarely needed for diagnosis and management. Case 4 had elevated BNP when he was dry and that may have led to overdiuresis and hypovolemia.
LVEF	35%	55%	55%	25%	55%	A low EF may support a diagnosis of HF when clinical presentation is atypical or insufficient as in case 1. A normal EF should not be used to rule out a diagnosis of HF.
Response to diuretics	NA	**Yes**	**Yes**	**Yes**	NA	A therapeutic response to diuretic may help confirm the diagnosis of HF when clinical presentation is atypical or insufficient.
ED visit	No	No	**Yes**	No	**Yes**	Older adults often attribute HF symptoms to aging thus delaying diagnosis and therapy that may increase their risk of ED visit and hospital admission.
Hospitalization	No	No	No	**Yes**	**Yes**	Charts from prior hospital admissions for HF maybe help in the diagnosis, especially in patients whose symptoms and signs are compensated.

Case 1: no clinical evidence of HF and the diagnosis was facilitated by low EF.
Case 2: a classic textbook presentation of HF.
Case 3: flash pulmonary edema, ongoing symptoms, and need for diuretic therapy.
Case 4: HF symptoms, low EF, and diuretic response.
Case 5: no HF, symptoms were likely somatization associated with depression.
Abbreviations: BNP, brain natriuretic peptide; COPD, chronic obstructive pulmonary disease; GI, gastrointestinal; LE, lower extremity; NA, not applicable; NT-pro-BNP, N-terminal probrain natriuretic peptide.

lost her husband of many years and moved to a new home close to her children. She was diagnosed with depression and therapy with antidepressant completely resolved her symptoms (see **Table 3**).

In case 4, a diagnosis of HF was almost missed due to his atypical presentation (syncope) and would probably have been delayed if he had normal LVEF. Brain natriuretic peptide (BNP) may be useful when a clinical diagnosis of HF is uncertain, especially when other competing causes of dyspnea, such as COPD or obesity, exist. However, too much reliance on BNP should be discouraged (see **Table 3**).[29] As illustrated in case 4, after his furosemide was increased, he became euvolemic and asymptomatic. However, his BNP remained relatively high and he was continued on the same dose of furosemide. Subsequent overdiuresis led to hypovolemia, hypoperfusion, and recurrence of symptoms. After his furosemide dose was decreased, he gained about 10 pounds over the next week, and his symptoms improved. Biomarkers maybe useful in the diagnosis of HF when the clinical presentation is complicated or less clear. N-terminal probrain natriuretic peptide (NT-pro-BNP) is elevated in most patients with HF. However, the cutoff values may differ among older HF patients and tend to be higher with age and renal dysfunction, which is common in the older HF patient. Biomarkers may be used at the time of diagnosis for determination of prognosis and to guide therapy. However, biomarker-guided therapy for HF has not been shown to be associated with better clinical outcomes or quality of life when compared with therapy guided by clinical symptoms and signs of HF (**Table 4**).[30]

DETERMINATION OF ETIOLOGIC FACTORS OF HEART FAILURE

HF is multifactorial in older patients. Aging results in biochemical and structural changes in the myocardium and predisposes to systolic, as well as diastolic, impairment in the older patient. An etiologic factor for HF must be established for all HF patients. HF in older adults may be associated with multiple etiologic factors (**Fig. 1**). Often, the historic role of an etiologic factor may not be ascertained but the presence of a risk factor as comorbidity suggests a potential etiologic role. When no etiologic factors can be found, primary care physicians should consider referring new geriatric HF patients to cardiologists for evaluation of underlying etiologic factors, such as myocardial ischemia and familial and/or infiltrative cardiomyopathy, which if present may cause continued myocardial damage. For example, case 1 underwent a nuclear stress test that showed mild myocardial ischemia, which possibly played an etiologic role, along with hypertension, in his HF, and was referred for cardiology consultation. Case 4 had a long history of hypertension and diabetes, 2 known predictors of HF in older adults (see **Table 3**).[31] He had a normal coronary angiogram. However, microvascular dysfunction, in the absence of epicardial CAD, has also been shown to cause HF.[32,33]

Hypertension and CAD are the 2 most common causes of HF in all ages, including older adults.[31,34] In the Cardiovascular Health Study, 5888 community-dwelling older adults (65 years and older, mean age 73 years) without HF at baseline were followed for a median of 5.5 years and 597 developed new-onset HF. Individuals with CAD or hypertension had 87% and 36%, respectively, higher risk of incident HF. However, due to high prevalence of hypertension (41% vs 17% for CAD), the population-attributable risk for CAD and hypertension were similar (both 13%). Thus, if CAD and hypertension were removed as risk factors, each would prevent HF in about 13% of the population. Relative risks of other risk factors were: diabetes (78%), serum creatinine 1.4 mg/dL or more (81%), LVH by electrocardiogram (129%), low LVEF (180%), and atrial fibrillation (106%).[31] However, because the prevalence of these conditions was low, their population-attributable risks were also low (8% for diabetes and 2% for atrial fibrillation, and others in between).

Presence of these risk factors may often be determined from history and other tests. It is important to identify the presence of these comorbidities, whether they are causally associated with HF or not. The presence of most of these comorbidities is associated with poor outcomes in HF and thus should be managed according to established guidelines. With the exception of CAD, primary care physicians should be able to identify and manage most of these comorbidities. However, because many older adults might have silent ischemia, which may cause further myocardial damage and disease progression, all HF patients with CAD should be referred to cardiologists for appropriate assessment and treatment of ischemic heart disease.

DETERMINATION OF FLUID VOLUME STATUS

JVP is expected to be elevated in patients presenting with HF for the first time and a normal JVP rules out clinical HF. JVP may be low in a patient with chronic HF and may be a marker of volume depletion and overdiuresis. Thus, fluid volume needs to

Table 4
Symptoms and signs of heart failure in older adults

Dyspnea	DOE or exertional fatigue, with or without some degree of lower extremity swelling, is generally the most common early symptom of HF (cases 1 and 3). With progression of disease, especially in the absence of appropriate treatment, DOE or fatigue gradually become more severe and appears with decreasing exertion (case 2), and eventually at rest. Older adults often attribute their DOE or fatigue on exertion to aging and respond to their early symptoms by restricting their physical activities, thus delaying clinical manifestations and diagnosis. It is important to take that into consideration while inquiring about DOE from an older adult (see **Table 2**). When a patient presents with dyspnea at rest, it is important to determine its duration and if it was preceded by DOE. Dyspnea at rest without DOE is almost never organic in cause and may represent somatization in older adults.[85]
Orthopnea	Orthopnea is a relatively specific symptom for HF in older adults (see **Table 2**).[5,86] Orthopnea is particularly helpful if associated with edema (may help distinguish from rare orthopnea due to pulmonary causes). It is usually occurs soon after lying down and is also relieved promptly by sitting or standing up. However, orthopnea is relatively infrequent symptom in older adults with HF and may not be reported until fluid overload is severe, as in cases 2 and 3.[87,88] Many older adults may sleep in a chair or a recliner to avoid orthopnea and may not voluntarily report that unless specifically asked.
PND	PND is a more specific HF symptom.[5,86] Dyspnea in PND may occur 2–3 h after onset of sleep, and causes patients to wake up from sleep with dyspnea, which may be followed by cough and/or wheezing. Relief starts with sitting up but complete relief of symptoms may take about 30 min. Patients sleeping with multiple pillows or on a recliner to avoid orthopnea may not experience PND. When PND is due to COPD, cough maybe the early and predominant symptom. However, PND is relatively infrequent in older adults.[87,88]
LE edema	Edema is a relatively nonspecific symptom. It is estimated that 5 L of extra fluid must accumulate before edema become clinically manifest.[14] Edema is generally dependent and progressive if untreated. Edema associated with HF is always symmetric and pitting. Chronic venous insufficiency is common in older adults and may cause pitting edema. Unilateral edema may be caused by cellulitis, past trauma or surgery, deep vein thrombosis, or arthritis. Chronic severe edema may lead to skin changes, including erythema, brown pigmentation, and induration. Leg edema alone should not be used to assess fluid volume status.
Other symptoms	Other less common and atypical symptoms of HF in older adults include fatigue, syncope, angina, nocturia, oliguria, and changes in mental status. Weight gain almost always accompanies symptomatic HF but is rarely reported as a symptom by older HF patients. However, if educated by their doctors about the importance of daily weight, most older HF patients are likely to monitor and report. This may, however, confounded by loss of appetite and early satiety, which in turn may result in weight loss and failure to thrive.
JVP	An elevated JVP is the most specific sign of fluid overload in HF and is the most important physical examination in the initial and subsequent examinations of an older HF patient.[89] External jugular veins (EJV) maybe more easily seen than internal jugular vein (IJV) in older adults with chronic HF and maybe used judiciously to estimate JVP. Using EJV and the right technique, JVP can be estimated in 90%–95% of all HF patients.
HJR	HJR reflects inability of the right ventricles to respond to increased venous return, which is caused by pressure over an abdomen in which the veins may already be congested with blood.[90] HJR is considered positive if the JVP rises by 2–3 cm and remains elevated for about 10 s when sustained pressure is applied to the mid-abdomen area. In 1 study, a positive HJR predicted right atrial pressure >9 mm Hg with high sensitivity (100%) and specificity (85%).[91] A positive HJR in the presence of high JVP confirms fluid overload.[90,91] A positive HJR in the presence of normal or low JVP may indicate mild residual fluid overload (may be baseline for some HF patients).
Other signs	An fourth heart sound (S4) may be common in older HF patients. Ascites and pleural effusion are nonspecific signs and must be coordinated with other symptoms and signs.

Adapted from Ahmed A. DEFEAT heart failure: clinical manifestations, diagnostic assessment, and etiology of geriatric heart failure. Heart Failure Clin 2007;4:389–402; with permission.

be routinely assessed in all HF patients to achieve an euvolemic state to reduce symptoms and hospital admission and readmission. Careful estimation of JVP may allow accurate assessment of fluid balance in almost all older patients with HF (**Figs. 2** and **3**, **Table 5**). Ideally, JVP should be estimated using the internal jugular vein (IJV). The IJV, which lies deep in the neck behind the sternocleidomastoid muscle, is not visible in the neck and its pulsation is transmitted to the surface through the neck muscles. Thus, the transmitted IJV pulsation may be confused with the transmitted carotid pulsation. Generally speaking, unlike carotid pulsation, the low-pressure jugular pulsation cannot be palpated. In addition, jugular pulsation is distinguished from the carotid pulsation by its double waveforms and its response to respiration and HJR maneuver. IJV pulsation is better seen in the upper medial part of the neck when the head is turned to the opposite side. However, IJV pulsation may not be easily visible in patients with chronic HF. The external jugular vein (EJV) is superficial and its contour is visible like that of the veins on the dorsum of the hand. EJV pulsation is more visible than the IJV pulsation, and maybe reliably used to estimate JVP.[35] EJV pulsation is best seen with the head in the neutral position because when head is turned to the other side the taut neck skin may obliterate the superficial EJV, making the pulsation disappear. Because EJV is superficial, it may be blocked by internally (thrombosed valves) or externally (subcutaneous scarring). Thus, a distended EJV without a visible pulsation is useless for the estimation of JVP. When both IJV and EJV pulsations are visible, IJV should be used to estimate JVP. When EJV on both sides of the neck have different heights, the lower should be used.

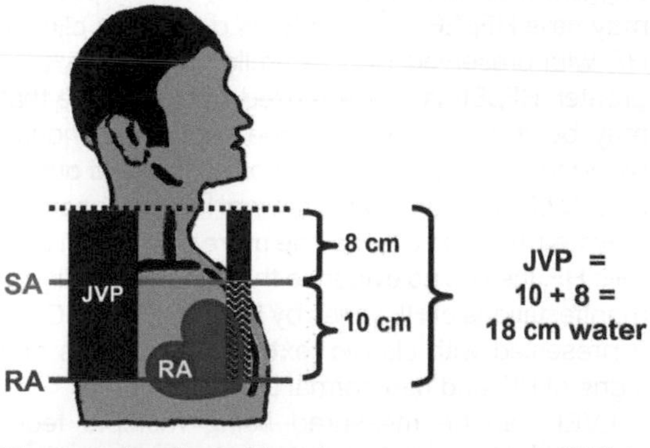

Fig. 2. Estimation of jugular venous pressure (JVP) in centimeters (cm) of water. First, estimate the distance between the sternal angle (SA) and the top of the jugular venous pulsation (marked by the horizontal dotted blue line) in cm (8 cm in the example above). Then, estimate the distances between right atrium (RA) and SA (10 cm in the example above, but would vary depending on the body position as shown in **Fig. 3**). Finally, add these two numbers to get the estimated JVP (18 cm water in the example above). (*Adapted from* Ahmed A. Chronic heart failure in older adults. Med Clin N Am 2011;95:439–61; with permission.)

Proper estimation of JVP requires both training and practice. The textbook rule that the head of the bed or examination table must be at 30° or 45° of incline has no relevance to the proper estimation of JVP. The key in JVP estimation is to make the top of the EJV or IJV pulsation visible in the middle of the neck so that its vertical distance from right atrium (RA) can be estimated. Because the RA to top of jugular pulsation vertical distance cannot be directly measured, the sternal angle (SA) is used as a landmark to measure SA to top of jugular pulsation vertical distance (see **Fig. 2**). The SA to top of jugular pulsation distance is then added to the RA to SA position-specific distance to obtain the estimated JVP (**Fig. 2**). When the JVP is low, the top of the jugular pulsation in neck is at a lower level than SA, and as such the SA to top of jugular pulsation distance is negative (ie, less than the RA to SA distance), and should be subtracted from the RA to SA position-specific distance to obtain the estimated JVP.

The process of estimating the vertical distance from the SA to top of IJV or EJV pulsation is rather simple and requires careful adjustment of the incline of examination table or bed so that the top of the pulsation is visible in the middle of the neck (see **Fig. 3**). For example, the top of the jugular pulsation for a patient with low JVP is only visible in a supine position (0° incline; see **Fig. 3**). In contrast, the top of the jugular pulsation for a patient with very high JVP is only visible in a sitting position (90° incline; see **Fig. 3** and **Table 6**). It is important to remember that the SA to top of IJV or EJV pulsation distance is vertical. Thus, in patients with low JVP when the patient is in a supine position, the SA to top of IJV or EJV pulsation distance is generally negative because the anterior chest wall is at a higher level than the neck. As such, the top of IJV or EJV pulsation is vertically below the imaginary horizontal line passing through the SA. This is important because when the JVP is low, the negative SA to top of jugular pulsation distance should be subtracted from the RA to SA distance to obtain the estimated JVP. The textbook assumption of a 5 cm RA to SA distance in all positions may underestimate the JVP. Estimates based on computerized tomography scans of chest suggest that the RA to SA distance is about 5 cm in supine position, 8 cm at 30°, and 10 cm at 45° or higher inclines.[36] Thus, the RA to SA to be used to estimate JVP needs to be position-specific (see **Fig. 3**).

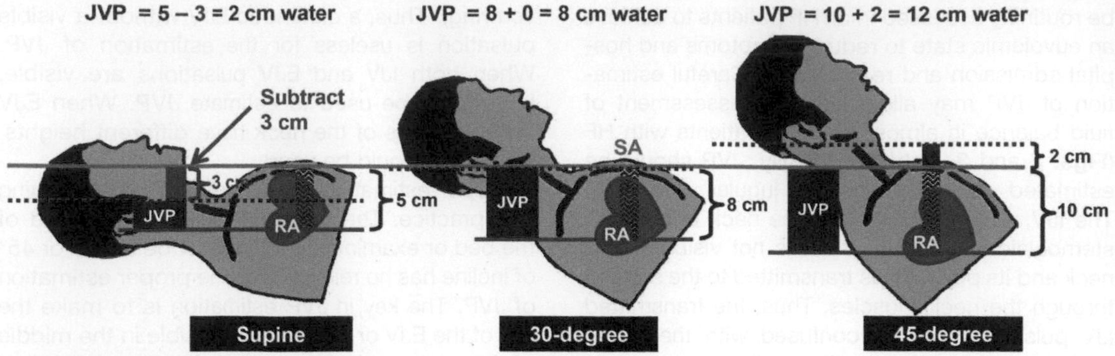

Fig. 3. Estimation of jugular venous pressure (JVP, marked by the vertical blue bars) in centimeters (cm) of water. First, identify the top of the external jugular venous pulsation in the middle of the neck (the blue line in neck) by adjusting the patient's position. Second, estimate the distance between the sternal angle (SA, marked by the dark brown line), and the top of venous pulsation (marked by the horizontal dotted blue lines). Third, estimate the distance from right atrium (RA, marked by the red line) to SA (note that this distance would vary with the body position). Finally, add these two numbers, the "SA to the top of the jugular venous pulsation distance" and the "RA to SA distance", to obtain JVP in cm water. Please note that when JVP is low as it in the left panel, the top of jugular pulsation is only visible in the middle of the neck when the patient is in the supine position. Because in this position, the top of the jugular pulsation is below the SA, the JVP is estimated by subtracting the "SA to the top of the jugular venous pulsation distance" from the "RA to SA distance. (*Adapted from* Ahmed A. Chronic Heart Failure in Older Adults. Med Clin N Am 2011;95:439–61; with permission.)

Recent weight may also be used to assess fluid volume status. Weight gain or loss in the range of 2 to 3 pounds in 2 to 3 days is almost always due to fluid overload or diuresis. If educated and encouraged to do so, most patients who have HF will monitor and report daily weight. Assessment, achievement, and maintenance of euvolemia ensure proper physical functioning, which is particularly important in older adults because they are likely to decondition quickly. Physical activity and exercise reduce deconditioning, improve quality of life, and also may reduce mortality in HF.[37–39] If not properly assessed by clinicians, however, older patients who have HF may not report DOE and other exertional symptoms. Instead, they might restrict their activities in response to those symptoms and become deconditioned.

DETERMINATION OF LEFT VENTRICULAR EJECTION FRACTION

Once a diagnosis of HF is established, every patient who has HF should have an echocardiographic determination of LVEF. In patients who have HFrEF, there is no need to repeat the procedure unless indicated by major changes in clinical conditions. LVEF should be checked periodically in patients who have HFpEF because these patients may eventually develop HFrEF.[40,41]

HFrEF is defined as clinical HF with reduced EF. Varying EF cutoffs ranging between 35% and 45% have been used to define HFrEF.[42–48] Recent American College of Cardiology/American Heart Association (ACC/AHA) guidelines define systolic HF as LVEF 40% or less.[6] HFrEF is typically characterized by a large thin-walled ventricle that is weak and unable to eject enough blood to produce a normal cardiac output (**Table 6**). Over the past 2 decades, most randomized clinical trials in HF were restricted to HFrEF.[42–50] It is also the predominant type of HF among younger adults.[51] However, epidemiologic data from the past several decades suggest that as many as 50% of all HF patients may have HFpEF.[52–57] HFpEF is defined as clinical HF with preserved EF, generally 45% to 55% or greater. HFpEF is characterized by a ventricle that may be small or stiff, and does not have enough blood to pump to produce a normal cardiac output (see **Table 6**). Even though several HF signs, namely elevated JVP and S3, may be more frequent in systolic HF, there is no evidence that the overall clinical manifestations of HF varies by LVEF.[21,22,58–60] Case 2 presented with classic textbook symptoms and signs of HF, and had normal LVEF.

LVEF can be measured using multiple techniques.[61] However, transthoracic 2-dimensional echocardiography with Doppler imaging is usually preferred. This is widely available, safe, and noninvasive with little or no patient discomfort, and provides excellent images of not only the heart but also the great vessels and paracardiac structures.[62] Assessment of LVEF is important because it is of crucial therapeutic and prognostic significance.[21,22,58,60] However, LVEF should not be assessed until after a clinical diagnosis has been made or clinical suspicion exists.

Table 5
Estimation of jugular venous pressure in older adults with heart failure

	Cases					
	1	**2**	**3**	**4**	**5**	**Comments**
IJV used to estimate JVP?	No	No	No	Yes	No	Transmitted IJV pulsation is most ideal for reliable estimation of JVP but not easily visible in older adults with chronic HF.
EJV used to estimate JVP?	Yes	Yes	Yes	Yes	Yes	EJV contour is visible and its pulsation is more easily visible; a reliable source for JVP estimation.
HJR	No	Yes	Yes	No	No	Not needed for JVP estimation; useful to check for patency of EJV.
Incline needed to make top of jugular pulsation visible in neck	0°	90°	30°	0°	0°	The head of the examination table or bed must be adjusted to make the top of the IJV or EJV pulsation visible in the middle of the neck.
Estimated distance from RA to SA (cm)	5	10	8	5	5	The RA to SA distance is rather fixed and is incline-specific (5, 8, and 10 cm at 0°, 30°, and ≥45° incline).[36]
Estimated distance from SA to jugular pulsation top (cm)	0	10	7	−2	0	The SA to top of jugular pulsation distance is vertical, not horizontal. This is especially important to remember in patients with low JVP (Case 5) who should be in a supine or near-supine position.
Estimated JVP (cm water)	5	20	15	3	5	5–8 cm water normal for most, and up to 10 for some HF patients. A lower JVP may indicate over-diuresis.
How JVP (cm water) was estimated	5 + 0 = 5	10 + 10 = 20	8 + 7 = 15	5–2 = 3	5 + 0 = 5	The vertical SA to top of jugular pulsation distance is added to the incline-specific RA to SA distance to estimate JVP; however, it must be **subtracted** from the RA to SA distance when JVP is low (Case 5).

Abbreviations: RA, right atrium; SA, sternal angle.

Table 6
A simplified example demonstrating how patients with heart failure with reduced ejection fraction and with heart failure preserved ejection fraction have similar symptoms and signs

	End-Diastolic Volume (mL)	LVEF (%)	Left Ventricular Stroke Volume (mL)	Heart Rate (Beats per min)	Cardiac Output (liters per min)	Symptoms
Normal	150	55	75	72	5.4	None
HFrEF	200	25	50	72	3.6	Dyspnea, fatigue, edema
HFpEF	100	55	50	72	3.6	Dyspnea, fatigue, edema

Adapted from Ahmed A. DEFEAT heart failure: clinical manifestations, diagnostic assessment, and etiology of geriatric heart failure. Heart Failure Clin 2007;4:391; with permission.

Most diastolic HF patients have significant abnormalities in active and passive relaxation.[55,63] However, it is not essential to determine diastolic abnormalities to make a clinical diagnosis of HFpEF.[56] Doppler studies of velocity of transmitral blood flow can determine ventricular filling patterns. In HFpEF, the peak transmitral E velocity (represents early filling during active ventricular relaxation) is decreased, whereas there is a relative increase in the peak A velocity (due to a compensatory increase in atrial contraction in late diastole). Thus, the E/A ratio is decreased, and even reversed to less than 1 in diastolic HF.[23,55,64] However, E/A ratio may also be decreased with normal aging[65] and may be normalized with progressive diastolic HF (pseudonormalization).[66,67] However, mitral annular tissue Doppler imaging can distinguish normal from pseudonormal filling patterns and, if combined with transmitral flow Doppler imaging and clinical history, can accurately determine severity of diastolic abnormalities.[55,66,67] There is evidence that severity of diastolic dysfunction may be associated with increased mortality.[55]

OTHER DIAGNOSTIC ASSESSMENTS

Initial evaluation for HF should also include a 12-lead electrocardiogram, a chest radiograph, and a laboratory workup, including serum electrolytes, renal function, liver function, thyroid function, lipid profile, complete cell count, fasting blood glucose, and hemoglobin A1C. All newly diagnosed patients who have HF should be screened for depression using a 15-item Geriatric Depression Scale. Functional status should be ascertained using New York Heart Association (NYHA) functional class. Higher NYHA class is associated with poor outcomes.[68,69]

TREATMENT OF HEART FAILURE

Therapy for older HF patients is similar to that for younger adults but needs to be initiated and titrated with caution following the principle of geriatric pharmacotherapy: start low, go slow! Evidence-based therapy is primarily guided by LVEF and is restricted for patients with HFrEF. These patients should be treated with an angiotensin-converting enzyme (ACE) inhibitor or an angiotensin receptor blocker unless contraindicated.[70] Chronic kidney disease is common in HF and should not be considered a contraindication to these drugs.[71,72] Older HFrEF patients should be treated with approved beta-blockers.[70] There is no need to wait to initiate beta-blockers until a target dose of ACE inhibitor has been achieved. Low-dose digoxin should be used for patients with HFrEF who are symptomatic despite therapy with an ACE inhibitor and a beta-blocker.[73] Aldosterone antagonists should be used in advanced symptomatic HF patients with normal potassium and normal renal function. There is little evidence that these drugs improve outcomes in HFpEF.[74–82] Diuretics are essential for the management of fluid overload in both HFrEF and HFpEF. However, there are little or no data on the long-term safety and these drugs should be in the lowest dose needed to keep patients euvolemic and asymptomatic.[83] Hypokalemia should be avoided and corrected.[84] Decisions to use device-based therapies should be individualized based on patients' functional status and preference.

SUMMARY

Clinical manifestation of HF in older adults may be atypical and diagnostic assessment might be delayed. Assessment of HF in older adults may be made simple by following a simple 5-step process, DEFEAT-HF: diagnosis, etiology, fluid status, EF, and treatment of HF. A thorough history and a careful physical examination should allow proper clinical diagnosis of HF in most cases. An effort to identify an underlying cause for HF must be made. All patients who have HF should be assessed carefully for volume status to achieve euvolemia. LVEF must be determined in all patients with a clinical diagnosis of HF to assess prognosis and guide therapy. All HF patients should be treated with evidence-based therapies according to the recommendations of a major national HF guideline. Older HF patients offer unique challenges in diagnosis and management. A careful consideration and evaluation of comorbidities may afford tailored approaches for management of these patients and contributes toward improving quality of care and outcomes.

REFERENCES

1. Inouye SK, Studenski S, Tinetti ME, et al. Geriatric syndromes: clinical, research, and policy implications of a core geriatric concept. J Am Geriatr Soc 2007;55:780–91.
2. Aronow WS. Epidemiology, pathophysiology, prognosis, and treatment of systolic and diastolic heart failure. Cardiol Rev 2006;14:108–24.
3. Aronow WS. Drug treatment of systolic and of diastolic heart failure in elderly persons. J Gerontol A Biol Sci Med Sci 2005;60:1597–605.
4. Ahmed A. American College of Cardiology/American Heart Association chronic heart failure evaluation and management guidelines: Relevance to the geriatric practice. J Am Geriatr Soc 2003;51:123–6.
5. Ahmed A, Allman RM, Aronow WS, et al. Diagnosis of heart failure in older adults: predictive value of dyspnea at rest. Arch Gerontol Geriatr 2004;38:297–307.
6. Yancy CW, Jessup M, Bozkurt B, et al. 2016 ACC/AHA/HFSA focused update on new pharmacological therapy for heart failure: an update of the 2013 ACCF/AHA Guideline for the management of heart failure: a report of the American College of Cardiology/American Heart Association Task Force on Clinical Practice Guidelines and the Heart Failure Society of America. J Am Coll Cardiol 2016;68:1476–88.
7. Centers for Medicare & Medicaid Services. Overview of specifications of measures displayed on hospital compare as of December 15, 2005. 2006. Available at: http://www.cms.hhs.gov/HospitalQualityInits/10_HospitalQualityMeasures.asp#TopOfPage. Accessed June 3, 2006.
8. Joint Commission on Accreditation of Healthcare Organizations. A comprehensive review of development and testin for national implementation of hospital core measures. 2006. Available at: http://www.jointcommission.org/NR/exeres/5A8BFA1C-B844-4A9A-86B2-F16DBE0E20C7.htm. Accessed June 3, 2006.
9. Desai RV, Meyer P, Ahmed MI, et al. Relationship between left and right ventricular ejection fractions in chronic advanced systolic heart failure: insights from the BEST trial. Eur J Heart Fail 2011;13:392–7.
10. Meyer P, Filippatos GS, Ahmed MI, et al. Effects of right ventricular ejection fraction on outcomes in chronic systolic heart failure. Circulation 2010;121:252–8.
11. Meyer P, Desai RV, Mujib M, et al. Right ventricular ejection fraction <20% is an independent predictor of mortality but not of hospitalization in older systolic heart failure patients. Int J Cardiol 2012;155:120–5.
12. The National Heart, Lung, and Blood Institute., Working group on cellular and molecular mechanisms of right heart failure: Executive summary. October 6–7, 2005. Available at: http://www.nhlbi.nih.gov/meetings/workshops/right-heart.htm. Accessed June 3, 2006.
13. Cosentino AM. The congested state in renal failure: a historical and diagnostic perspective. Semin Dial 1999;12:307–10.
14. Perloff JK, Braunwald E. Physical examination of the heart and circulation. In: Braunwald E, editor. Heart disease: a text book of cardiovascular medicine, vol. 1, 5th edition. Philadelphia: W. B. Saunders Company; 1997. p. 15–52.
15. Warren JV, Stead EA Jr. Fluid dynamics in chronic congestive heart failure. Arch Intern Med 1944;73:138–47.
16. Merrill AJ. Edema and decreased renal blood flow in patients with chronic congestive heart failure: evidence of "forward failure" as the primary cause of edema. J Clin Invest 1946;25:389–400.
17. Francis GS, Goldsmith SR, Levine TB, et al. The neurohumoral axis in congestive heart failure. Ann Intern Med 1984;101:370–7.
18. Ingram CW, Satler LF, Rackley CE. Progressive heart failure secondary to a high output state. Chest 1987;92:1117–8.
19. Froeschl M, Haddad H, Commons AS, et al. Thyrotoxicosis-an uncommon cause of heart failure. Cardiovasc Pathol 2005;14:24–7.
20. Ahearn DJ, Maher JF. Heart failure as a complication of hemodialysis arteriovenous fistula. Ann Intern Med 1972;77:201–4.
21. Hunt SA, Abraham WT, Chin MH, et al. ACC/AHA 2005 guideline update for the diagnosis and management of chronic heart failure in the adult: a report of the American College of Cardiology/American Heart Association Task Force on practice guidelines (writing committee to update the 2001 guidelines for the evaluation and management of heart failure): developed in collaboration with the American College of Chest Physicians and the International

Society for Heart and Lung Transplantation: endorsed by the Heart Rhythm Society. Circulation 2005;112:e154–235.
22. Adams K, Lindenfeld J, Arnold J, et al. Executive summary: HFSA 2006 comprehensive heart failure practice guideline. J Card Fail 2006;12:10–38.
23. Swedberg K, Cleland J, Dargie H, et al. Guidelines for the diagnosis and treatment of chronic heart failure: executive summary (update 2005): the task force for the diagnosis and treatment of chronic heart failure of the European Society of Cardiology. Eur Heart J 2005;26:1115–40.
24. Gheorghiade M, Zannad F, Sopko G, et al. Acute heart failure syndromes: current state and framework for future research. Circulation 2005;112: 3958–68.
25. Haldeman GA, Croft JB, Giles WH, et al. Hospitalization of patients with heart failure: National Hospital Discharge Survey, 1985 to 1995. Am Heart J 1999; 137:352–60.
26. Thom T, Haase N, Rosamond W, et al. Heart disease and stroke statistics-2006 update: a report from the American Heart Association Statistics committee and stroke statistics subcommittee. Circulation 2006;113:e85–151.
27. Nieminen MS, Bohm M, Cowie MR, et al. Executive summary of the guidelines on the diagnosis and treatment of acute heart failure: the task force on acute heart failure of the European Society of Cardiology. Eur Heart J 2005;26:384–416.
28. Kramer K, Kirkman P, Kitzman D, et al. Flash pulmonary edema: association with hypertension and reoccurrence despite coronary revascularization. Am Heart J 2000;140:451–5.
29. Aronow WS. Brain natriuretic peptide in heart failure. J Am Geriatr Soc 2006;54:368–9 [author reply: 369].
30. Pfisterer M, Buser P, Rickli H, et al. BNP-guided vs symptom-guided heart failure therapy: the Trial of intensified vs standard medical therapy in elderly patients with congestive heart failure (TIME-CHF) randomized trial. JAMA 2009;301: 383–92.
31. Gottdiener JS, Arnold AM, Aurigemma GP, et al. Predictors of congestive heart failure in the elderly: the Cardiovascular Health Study. J Am Coll Cardiol 2000;35:1628–37.
32. Rajappan K, Rimoldi OE, Dutka DP, et al. Mechanisms of coronary microcirculatory dysfunction in patients with aortic stenosis and angiographically normal coronary arteries. Circulation 2002;105: 470–6.
33. Cecchi F, Olivotto I, Gistri R, et al. Coronary microvascular dysfunction and prognosis in hypertrophic cardiomyopathy. N Engl J Med 2003;349: 1027–35.
34. Kannel WB. Vital epidemiologic clues in heart failure. J Clin Epidemiol 2000;53:229–35.
35. Vinayak AG, Levitt J, Gehlbach B, et al. Usefulness of the external jugular vein examination in detecting abnormal central venous pressure in critically ill patients. Arch Intern Med 2006;166:2132–7.
36. Seth R, Magner P, Matzinger F, et al. How far is the sternal angle from the mid-right atrium? J Gen Intern Med 2002;17:852–6.
37. Coats AJ, Adamopoulos S, Radaelli A, et al. Controlled trial of physical training in chronic heart failure. Exercise performance, hemodynamics, ventilation, and autonomic function. Circulation 1992;85: 2119–31.
38. Ko JK, McKelvie RS. The role of exercise training for patients with heart failure. Eura Medicophys. 2005; 41:35–47.
39. Tenenbaum A, Freimark D, Ahron E, et al. Long-term versus intermediate-term supervised exercise training in advanced heart failure: effects on exercise tolerance and mortality. Int J Cardiol 2006; 113(3):364–70.
40. Cahill JM, Ryan E, Travers B, et al. Progression of preserved systolic function heart failure to systolic dysfunction – a natural history study. Int J Cardiol 2006;106:95–102.
41. Yu CM, Lin H, Yang H, et al. Progression of systolic abnormalities in patients with "isolated" diastolic heart failure and diastolic dysfunction. Circulation 2002;105:1195–201.
42. The SOLVD Investigators. Effect of enalapril on survival in patients with reduced left ventricular ejection fractions and congestive heart failure. N Engl J Med 1991;325:293–302.
43. Pfeffer MA, Braunwald E, Moye LA, et al. Effect of captopril on mortality and morbidity in patients with left ventricular dysfunction after myocardial infarction. Results of the survival and ventricular enlargement trial. The SAVE Investigators. N Engl J Med 1992;327:669–77.
44. The Digitalis Investigation Group. The effect of digoxin on mortality and morbidity in patients with heart failure. N Engl J Med 1997;336:525–33.
45. Packer M, Bristow MR, Cohn JN, et al. The effect of carvedilol on morbidity and mortality in patients with chronic heart failure. U.S. Carvedilol Heart Failure Study Group. N Engl J Med 1996;334: 1349–55.
46. MERIT-HF Study Group. Effect of metoprolol CR/XL in chronic heart failure: Metoprolol CR/XL randomised intervention trial in congestive heart failure (MERIT-HF). Lancet 1999;353:2001–7.
47. Pitt B, Zannad F, Remme WJ, et al. The effect of spironolactone on morbidity and mortality in patients with severe heart failure. Randomized Aldactone Evaluation Study Investigators. N Engl J Med 1999;341:709–17.

48. Pitt B, Poole-Wilson PA, Segal R, et al. Effect of losartan compared with captopril on mortality in patients with symptomatic heart failure: randomised trial–the Losartan Heart Failure Survival Study ELITE II. Lancet. 2000;355:1582–7.
49. Zannad F, McMurray JJ, Krum H, et al. Eplerenone in patients with systolic heart failure and mild symptoms. N Engl J Med 2011;364:11–21.
50. McMurray JJ, Packer M, Desai AS, et al. Angiotensin-neprilysin inhibition versus enalapril in heart failure. N Engl J Med 2014;371:993–1004.
51. Hogg K, Swedberg K, McMurray J. Heart failure with preserved left ventricular systolic function; epidemiology, clinical characteristics, and prognosis. J Am Coll Cardiol 2004;43:317–27.
52. Vasan RS, Larson MG, Benjamin EJ, et al. Congestive heart failure in subjects with normal versus reduced left ventricular ejection fraction: prevalence and mortality in a population-based cohort. J Am Coll Cardiol 1999;33:1948–55.
53. Gottdiener JS, McClelland RL, Marshall R, et al. Outcome of congestive heart failure in elderly persons: influence of left ventricular systolic function. The Cardiovascular Health Study. Ann Intern Med 2002;137:631–9.
54. Senni M, Redfield MM. Heart failure with preserved systolic function. A different natural history? J Am Coll Cardiol 2001;38:1277–82.
55. Redfield MM, Jacobsen SJ, Burnett JC Jr, et al. Burden of systolic and diastolic ventricular dysfunction in the community: appreciating the scope of the heart failure epidemic. JAMA 2003;289:194–202.
56. Zile MR, Gaasch WH, Carroll JD, et al. Heart failure with a normal ejection fraction: is measurement of diastolic function necessary to make the diagnosis of diastolic heart failure? Circulation 2001;104:779–82.
57. Kitzman DW, Little WC, Brubaker PH, et al. Pathophysiological characterization of isolated diastolic heart failure in comparison to systolic heart failure. JAMA 2002;288:2144–50.
58. Ahmed A, Roseman JM, Duxbury AS, et al. Correlates and outcomes of preserved left ventricular systolic function among older adults hospitalized with heart failure. Am Heart J 2002;144:365–72.
59. Ahmed A, Nanda NC, Weaver MT, et al. Clinical correlates of isolated left ventricular diastolic dysfunction among hospitalized older heart failure patients. Am J Geriatr Cardiol 2003;12:82–9.
60. Ahmed A. Association of diastolic dysfunction and outcomes in ambulatory older adults with chronic heart failure. J Gerontol A Biol Sci Med Sci 2005;60:1339–44.
61. Radford MJ, Arnold JM, Bennett SJ, et al. ACC/AHA key data elements and definitions for measuring the clinical management and outcomes of patients with chronic heart failure: a report of the American College of Cardiology/American Heart Association Task Force on Clinical Data Standards (Writing Committee to Develop Heart Failure Clinical Data Standards): developed in collaboration with the American College of Chest Physicians and the International Society for Heart and Lung Transplantation: endorsed by the Heart Failure Society of America. Circulation 2005;112:1888–916.
62. Cheitlin MD, Armstrong WF, Aurigemma GP, et al. ACC/AHA/ASE 2003 guideline update for the clinical application of echocardiography: summary article: a report of the American College of Cardiology/American Heart Association Task Force on Practice Guidelines (ACC/AHA/ASE Committee to Update the 1997 Guidelines for the Clinical Application of Echocardiography). Circulation 2003;108:1146–62.
63. Zile MR, Baicu CF, Gaasch WH. Diastolic heart failure–abnormalities in active relaxation and passive stiffness of the left ventricle. N Engl J Med 2004;350:1953–9.
64. Thomas JD, Choong CY, Flachskampf FA, et al. Analysis of the early transmitral Doppler velocity curve: effect of primary physiologic changes and compensatory preload adjustment. J Am Coll Cardiol 1990;16:644–55.
65. Fleg JL, Shapiro EP, O'Connor F, et al. Left ventricular diastolic filling performance in older male athletes. JAMA 1995;273:1371–5.
66. Nagueh SF, Middleton KJ, Kopelen HA, et al. Doppler tissue imaging: a noninvasive technique for evaluation of left ventricular relaxation and estimation of filling pressures. J Am Coll Cardiol 1997;30:1527–33.
67. Sohn DW, Chai IH, Lee DJ, et al. Assessment of mitral annulus velocity by Doppler tissue imaging in the evaluation of left ventricular diastolic function. J Am Coll Cardiol 1997;30:474–80.
68. Ahmed A, Aronow WS, Fleg JL. Higher New York Heart Association classes and increased mortality and hospitalization in patients with heart failure and preserved left ventricular function. Am Heart J 2006;151:444–50.
69. Scrutinio D, Lagioia R, Ricci A, et al. Prediction of mortality in mild to moderately symptomatic patients with left ventricular dysfunction. The role of the New York Heart Association classification, cardiopulmonary exercise testing, two-dimensional echocardiography and Holter monitoring. Eur Heart J 1994;15:1089–95.
70. Yancy CW, Jessup M, Bozkurt B, et al. 2013 ACCF/AHA guideline for the management of heart failure: a report of the American College of Cardiology Foundation/American Heart Association Task Force on Practice Guidelines. J Am Coll Cardiol 2013;62:e147–239.
71. Ahmed A. Use of angiotensin-converting enzyme inhibitors in patients with heart failure and renal insufficiency: how concerned should we be by the rise

in serum creatinine? J Am Geriatr Soc 2002;50: 1297–300.
72. Ahmed A, Fonarow GC, Zhang Y, et al. Renin-angiotensin inhibition in systolic heart failure and chronic kidney disease. Am J Med 2012;125:399–410.
73. Ahmed A, Rich MW, Love TE, et al. Digoxin and reduction in mortality and hospitalization in heart failure: a comprehensive post hoc analysis of the DIG trial. Eur Heart J 2006;27:178–86.
74. Yusuf S, Pfeffer MA, Swedberg K, et al. Effects of candesartan in patients with chronic heart failure and preserved left-ventricular ejection fraction: the CHARM-Preserved Trial. Lancet. 2003;362:777–81.
75. Massie BM, Carson PE, McMurray JJ, et al. Irbesartan in patients with heart failure and preserved ejection fraction. N Engl J Med 2008;359:2456–67.
76. Cleland JG, Tendera M, Adamus J, et al. The perindopril in elderly people with chronic heart failure (PEP-CHF) study. Eur Heart J 2006;27:2338–45.
77. Ahmed A, Rich MW, Fleg JL, et al. Effects of digoxin on morbidity and mortality in diastolic heart failure: the ancillary digitalis investigation group trial. Circulation 2006;114:397–403.
78. Pitt B, Pfeffer MA, Assmann SF, et al. Spironolactone for heart failure with preserved ejection fraction. N Engl J Med 2014;370:1383–92.
79. Mujib M, Patel K, Fonarow GC, et al. Angiotensin-converting enzyme inhibitors and outcomes in heart failure and preserved ejection fraction. Am J Med 2013;126:401–10.
80. Patel K, Fonarow GC, Kitzman DW, et al. Angiotensin receptor blockers and outcomes in real-world older patients with heart failure and preserved ejection fraction: a propensity-matched inception cohort clinical effectiveness study. Eur J Heart Fail 2012;14: 1179–88.
81. Patel K, Fonarow GC, Kitzman DW, et al. Aldosterone antagonists and outcomes in real-world older patients with heart failure and preserved ejection fraction. JACC Heart Fail 2013;1:40–7.
82. Patel K, Fonarow GC, Ekundayo OJ, et al. Beta-blockers in older patients with heart failure and preserved ejection fraction: class, dosage, and outcomes. Int J Cardiol 2014;173:393–401.
83. Ahmed A, Husain A, Love TE, et al. Heart failure, chronic diuretic use, and increase in mortality and hospitalization: an observational study using propensity score methods. Eur Heart J 2006;27: 1431–9.
84. Ahmed A, Zannad F, Love TE, et al. A propensity-matched study of the association of low serum potassium levels and mortality in chronic heart failure. Eur Heart J 2007;28:1334–43.
85. Ahmed A, Yaffe MJ, Thornton PL, et al. Depression in older adults: the case of an 82-year-old woman with dizziness. J Am Geriatr Soc 2006;54:187–8.
86. Wang CS, FitzGerald JM, Schulzer M, et al. Does this dyspneic patient in the emergency department have congestive heart failure? JAMA 2005;294: 1944–56.
87. Ahmed A, Allman RM, Kiefe CI, et al. Association of consultation between generalists and cardiologists with quality and outcomes of heart failure care. Am Heart J 2003;145:1086–93.
88. Mueller C, Scholer A, Laule-Kilian K, et al. Use of B-type natriuretic peptide in the evaluation and management of acute dyspnea. N Engl J Med 2004; 350:647–54.
89. Butman SM, Ewy GA, Standen JR, et al. Bedside cardiovascular examination in patients with severe chronic heart failure: importance of rest or inducible jugular venous distension. J Am Coll Cardiol 1993; 22:968–74.
90. Ducas J, Magder S, McGregor M. Validity of the hepatojugular reflux as a clinical test for congestive heart failure. Am J Cardiol 1983;52:1299–303.
91. Sochowski RA, Dubbin JD, Naqvi SZ. Clinical and hemodynamic assessment of the hepatojugular reflux. Am J Cardiol 1990;66:1002–6.

Role of Echocardiography in the Diagnostic Assessment and Etiology of Heart Failure in Older Adults

Opacify, Quantify, and Rectify

Vedant A. Gupta, MD[a], Navin C. Nanda, MD[b], Vincent L. Sorrell, MD[c,*]

KEYWORDS

- Heart failure • Echocardiography • Contrast • Three-dimensional echocardiography
- Speckle tracking • Doppler • Resynchronization

KEY POINTS

- Heart failure (HF) is the number one (and growing) cardiovascular disease worldwide and is becoming epidemic in the elderly population.
- Echocardiography is a critical diagnostic tool for the initial and serial evaluation of these patients.
- The major type of HF in the elderly is HF with "preserved" ejection fraction.
- Echocardiography provides a highly accurate, noninvasive means to quantify the left ventricular (and right ventricular) morphology, volume, and function.
- Understanding the strengths and limitations of echocardiography is critical to using this tool to its greatest capabilities.

Heart failure (HF) has continued to be the number one cause of cardiovascular hospitalization in older adults, affecting more than 10% of those aged 80 to 89 years in the United States.[1] This disease is common, disabling (up to 60% of patients requiring help with self-care), and especially deadly in the elderly population. Hypertension and coronary artery disease are the leading causes of HF. A precise diagnosis of the cardiac pathology is paramount for adequate treatment, and echocardiography offers an evaluation that is comprehensive, noninvasive, and relatively inexpensive. With an organized approach using 2-dimensional echocardiography (2DE) and Doppler echocardiography, clinicians can determine the systolic and diastolic left ventricular (LV) performance; determine right ventricular (RV) performance, estimate the cardiac output, pulmonary artery, and ventricular filling pressures; and identify surgically correctable valve disease. The major limitation of echocardiography has been patient-specific factors that lead to suboptimal acoustic windows. However, the use of intravenous contrast can opacify the LV cavity and enhance

This is an updated version of an article that appeared in *Heart Failure Clinics*, Volume 3, Issue 4.
Disclosure Statement: No relevant disclosures or potential conflicts of interest.
[a] Division of Cardiovascular Medicine, Department of Medicine, University of Kentucky, 900 South Limestone, 320 C.T. Wethington Building, Lexington, KY 40536, USA; [b] Echo Lab, University of Alabama at Birmingham, SW/S102, 619 19th Street South, Birmingham, AL 35249, USA; [c] Cardiovascular Imaging, Division of Cardiovascular Medicine, Department of Medicine, University of Kentucky, 900 South Limestone, 320 C.T. Wethington Building, Lexington, KY 40536, USA
* Corresponding author.
E-mail address: v.sorrell@uky.edu

Heart Failure Clin 13 (2017) 445–466
http://dx.doi.org/10.1016/j.hfc.2017.02.003
1551-7136/17/

the endocardial border in these patients. Real-time 3-dimensional echocardiography (3DE) provides unprecedented volume data to quantify the LV. More recently, assessment of myocardial mechanics with strain and strain rate assessment (using primarily 2D speckle tracking, but also tissue Doppler echocardiography [TDE]) allows for the assessment of subclinical LV dysfunction. Furthermore, echocardiography can also provide therapeutic guidance. Imaging data about myocardial velocity and strain, derived from TDE, provide extremely fine details about the regional variations in myocardial synchrony and predict responders to cardiac resynchronization therapy (CRT). Thus, echocardiographic tools provide the basis for determining when to attempt to rectify the LV dysfunction with strategically placed, biventricular pacemaker leads.

Although HF remains a clinical diagnosis, echocardiography assists in determining the etiology, systolic and diastolic function, and hemodynamic state, and the echocardiographic profile of elderly HF patients is different than younger HF patients.[2] To understand the echocardiographic assessment, it is important to understand how the cardiovascular system changes with age. Since our previous report on this subject, new guidelines have been published and incorporated, offering more insight into the measurement of diastolic function, RV function, and valvular heart disease.[3] Furthermore, the article has been reorganized to allow for a more focused discussion of each aspect of the echocardiogram.

With advancing age, subclinical fibrosis leads to decreased ventricular compliance with a subsequent prolongation in the rate of myocardial contraction and relaxation. This abnormality in relaxation may account for the higher prevalence of normal LV systolic function seen in elderly patients with HF, where approximately 50% of patients older than 80 years have normal or near-normal systolic function (defined as a LV ejection fraction [LVEF] >40%).[4] The clinical findings in systolic and diastolic HF are indistinguishable, making the history and physical examination inadequate for estimating LV function. Although HF patients with a diastolic blood pressure of approximately 105 mm Hg and no jugular venous distention have been shown to have a normal LV systolic EF with a positive predictive value of 100%, this combination of findings is uncommon.[5] Most other historical variables (age, symptom duration, hypertension, ischemia) and clinical variables (S3 gallop, edema, cardiomegaly, pulmonary or peripheral edema) are not significantly different in HF patients with normal or abnormal LVEF.[6] A systematic and comprehensive echocardiography should be performed in all patients with new-onset or worsening HF symptoms and provides critical information to assist in the subsequent management of the patient.

LEFT VENTRICULAR SYSTOLIC FUNCTION

Symptoms or exercise tolerance have a limited predictable relationship to the LVEF; however, prognosis does correlate with LVEF. Some patients are asymptomatic with an LVEF of less than 20%, whereas others are moribund with an LVEF of greater than 30%. In general, survival is shorter in patients with lower LVEF.[7,8] The differentiation of normal versus reduced LV systolic function is not only vitally important for subsequent treatment considerations, but it also impacts prognosis. In 1 study, the single best predictor of mortality in elderly patients with HF (and associated coronary artery disease) was the EF.[9] This prospective evaluation revealed that 47% of all elderly patients with congestive HF had normal LV systolic function. Despite having coronary heart disease, 41% of these patients still had normal systolic function. Survival rates in this group were 78% at 1 year, 62% at 2 years, and 44% at 4 years. In contrast, survival rates for patients with reduced LV systolic function were only 53% at 1 year, 29% at 2 years, and 15% at 4 years. In the Vasodilator Heart Failure Trial, patients with congestive HF and normal EFs had an average annual mortality rate of 8%, but those with abnormal EFs had an annual mortality rate of 19%.[10] Thus, echocardiography can assist in determining prognosis (**Table 1**). The LV end-diastolic volume (EDV) index often exceeds 100 mL/m^2 (the upper limit of normal is approximately 70 mL/m^2). LV size is another critical predictor of outcome and an LF EDV index of greater than 120 mL/m^2 predicts a worse outcome for HF patients.[11] end-systolic volume (ESV) index of 45 mL/m^2 identifies patients with a poor outcome.[12]

ANATOMIC FINDINGS (1-, 2-, AND 3-DIMENSIONAL ECHOCARDIOGRAPHY)

Echocardiography is ideal for assessing LV function, and this has become the most common reason for performing the study. Echocardiography can accurately resolve the endocardial borders throughout the cardiac cycle in multiple well-defined anatomic planes. With M-mode, the fractional shortening ([LV diastolic diameter − LV systolic diameter]/LV diastolic diameter) can be used as a rapid method for estimating LV systolic performance. With 2DE, inspection of the initial

Table 1
Studies using echocardiography to predict survival of elderly patients with HF

Population	Echocardiographic Data	Survival After 1 y (%)	After 2 y (%)
Elderly with HF[7]	Normal LVEF	78	62
	Reduced LVEF	53	29
Vasodilator HF study[8]	Normal LVEF	92	—
	Reduced LVEF	81	—
HF, ICD, mean EF 29% (n = 84)[11]	Grade ≥ III	72	—
	Grade < III	38	—
Chronic HF (n = 173)[44]	Grade I or II DD	94	—
	Grade III DD	81	—
	Grade IV DD	45	—
CM (76% CAD; n = 144)[45]	Grade III	—	89
	Grade IV	—	63
DSE (elderly HF)[46]	Grade III (rev w/Dob)	79	—
	Grade IV (fix with Dob)	49	—
98% male (n = 4000)[47]	IVC >50% collapse	95	—
	IVC <50% collapse	67	—
Class II, III HF[48]	RVEF >35%	—	93
	RVEF 25%–35%	—	77
	RVEF <25%	—	59

Abbreviations: CAD, coronary artery disease; CM, cardiomyopathy; DD, diastolic dysfunction; DSE, dobutamine stress echo; EF, ejection fraction; fix w/Dob, restrictive filling pattern remains unchanged with dobutamine; HF, heart failure; ICD, implantable cardioverter defibrillator; IVC, inferior vena cava; LVEF, left ventricular ejection fraction; rev w/Dob, restrictive filling pattern improves with dobutamine; RVEF, right ventricular ejection fraction.

parasternal long axis view will often correctly identify patients with either normal or severely reduced LVEF (**Fig. 1**).

Additional views are required for accuracy. Using validated geometric equations, 2DE can determine the LVEF, stroke volume (SV) and cardiac output. By calculating the LV EDV and ESV, the SV is readily derived (SV = EDV − ESV). In the absence of significant valvular regurgitation, cardiac output is estimated as the product of the SV and heart rate. Furthermore, the EF can then be calculated (EF = SV/EDV). For determining LV volumes, 2DE offers considerable advantages over M-mode methods and should be used for quantitative assessment. Even in the presence of wall motion abnormalities, 2DE provides excellent correlation with angiographic techniques.[13] Current ultrasound systems include software that can calculate volumes based on hand-traced regions of interest (**Fig. 2**). Images with good technical quality are necessary and have been improved by the development of second harmonic imaging.[14] When LV border delineation remains suboptimal, intracardiac contrast agents should be used. These agents cross the pulmonary circuit after intravenous injection and opacify the LV cavity for several cardiac cycles (**Fig. 3**).[15] The use of intravenous injection of contrast further improves the accuracy and reproducibility of LV volumes when compared with cardiac MRI as the gold standard.[16] Additionally, most vendors have software that allows the LV chamber to be traced automatically on line using real-time, automated border detection, thus providing beat-to-beat estimates of EDV, ESV, and LVEF.[17] The 3DE techniques have evolved from the necessity to integrate multiple 2D imaging planes to generate a 3D reconstruction, to the intelligent acquisition of near–real-time volume data (**Fig. 4**). This allows 3DE to produce LVEF values similar to other imaging reference standards and offers incremental benefit over 2D techniques with improved accuracy and reproducibility.[18] In addition, 3DE has been investigated as a tool to quantify LV dyssynchrony in patients being considered for CRT (**Fig. 5**).

Volumetric assessment of LV size and function is important when possible (diagnostic quality images); however, a unique issue arises in the elderly. The normal ranges for volumes often vary with ages, and are derived from large, population-based studies of normal patients. However, of the 5 large databases used, 3 did not enroll any patients above the age of 75, and the other 2 had median ages of 47 and 52 years.[19] In fact, the nomograms in the American Society of Echocardiography guidelines go up to 80 years of age for men and 75 years of age for women. Most

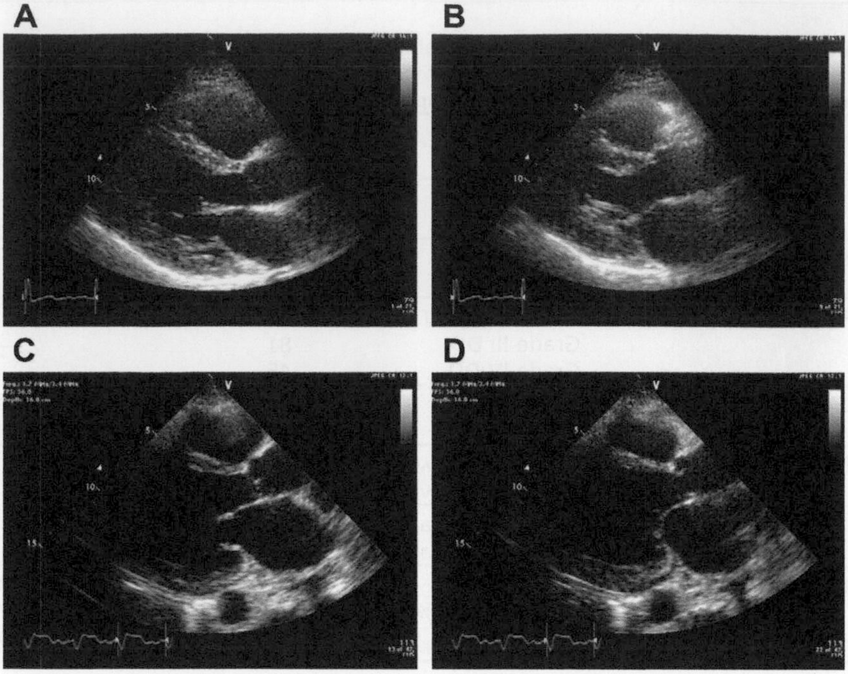

Fig. 1. Parasternal long axis 2-dimensional echocardiography (2DE) view in diastole (*A*) and systole (*B*) in an elderly female with New York Heart Association (NYHA) functional class III heart failure symptoms. The normal left ventricular ejection fraction (LVEF) is immediately evident and raises the likelihood of diastolic dysfunction, or transient systolic dysfunction from ischemia or arrhythmias. In contrast, the parasternal long axis 2DE view in diastole (*C*) and systole (*D*) in another elderly female with NYHA functional class II symptoms immediately displays a dilated cardiomyopathy with a reduced LVEF.

clinicians apply the normal range for younger patients to the elderly, but with limited evidence.

In addition to providing a quantitative assessment of EF, many echocardiography laboratories visually estimate this important parameter. In experienced hands, visual estimates are associated with a standard error of approximately 11%, which compares favorably with quantitative echocardiographic methods (10%) and radionuclide angiographic methods (7%).[20] Despite experience, visual estimates are only accurate when the LV function is either normal or severely reduced. When the LV function is intermediate or indeterminate, 2D or 3D quantitative techniques should be used.

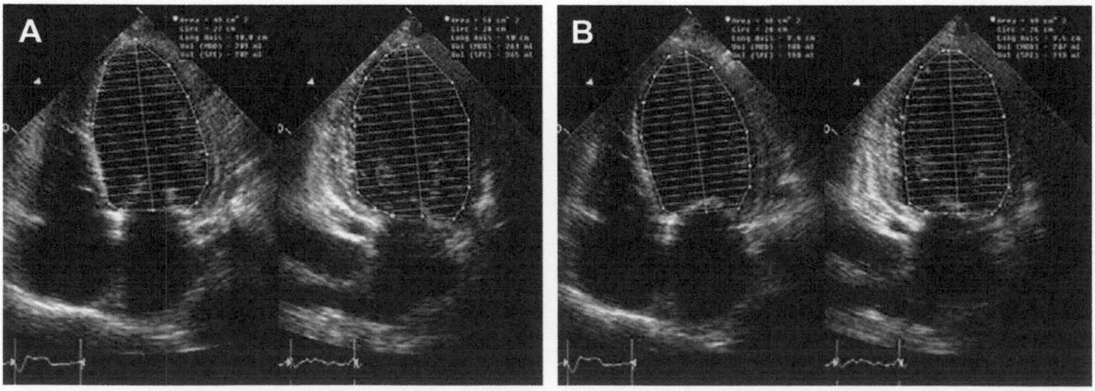

Fig. 2. Apical 4-chamber (*left*) and 2-chamber (*right*) views in diastole (*A*) and systole (*B*) with the manual endocardial borders traced allowing the computer to determine the left ventricular (LV) volumes using the modified Simpson's method-of-discs rule. The 2 views are averaged to create diastolic (LV_d) and systolic (LV_s) volumes and the LV ejection fraction: $(LV_d - LV_s)/LV_d$ or (231 mL − 198 mL)/231 mL = 14%.

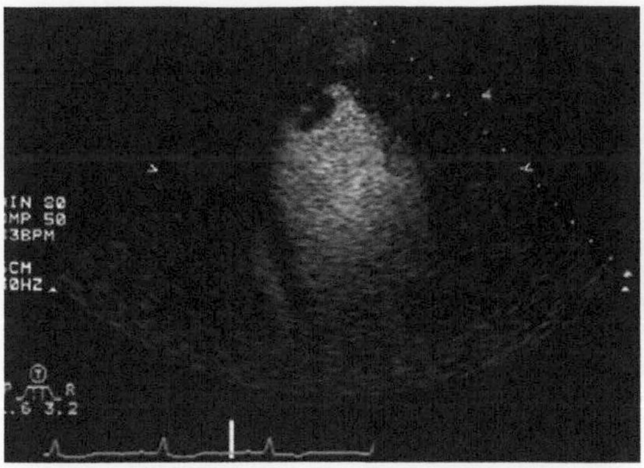

Fig. 3. Apical 4-chamber view after the injection of a 1-mL bolus of activated perflutren. The cavity is enhanced and brighter than the relatively darker myocardium. A thrombus is also seen as a filling defect in the left ventricular apex.

One of the largest areas of growth in both the investigation and the clinical application of echocardiography in HF is identification of subclinical systolic dysfunction. The natural history of structural and functional changes of the left ventricle in this patient population is poorly reported. In 38 patients (mean age 72 years) with HF and preserved systolic function (LVEF >45%), repeat echocardiography in 3 months confirmed that 21% had either global (n = 6) or regional (n = 3) LV dysfunction with an LVEF of less than 45%.[21] None of these patients had a change in their clinical status, further emphasizing that subclinical LV systolic dysfunction is common.

The term "strain" refers to an object's fractional or percentage change from its original, unstressed, dimension (eg, a change in length corrected for the original length).[22] It reflects deformation of a structure and, when applied to the myocardium, strain directly describes the contraction–relaxation pattern. Strain can be calculated in several dimensions: longitudinal, circumferential, or radial. The strain rate is the rate of this deformation. The use of strain and strain rate imaging (also known as myocardial deformation imaging) has allowed for better quantification of subclinical dysfunction. Original iterations of strain echocardiography used tissue Doppler, but more recently this has evolved to 2D-based speckle tracking methods. Speckle tracking has had an added benefit of being independent of the angle of acquisition, as well as translational motion. Regression analysis and then integration of the raw velocity data produces measures of instantaneous strain. Using strain echocardiography, an individual's myocardial mechanics can be determined and longitudinal, radial, and torsional motion can be quantified. Global longitudinal strain has been studied extensively in younger populations, and has been shown to be associated with worse prognosis in many subsets of patients with HF with preserved ejection fraction (HFpEF).[23] Although normative ranges for regional longitudinal strain have been investigated, the clinical application to the assessment of regional function has not been well-established. Also, radial and torsional motion in HF populations requires further investigation. These findings have been well-studied to assess for myocardial dyssynchrony and to predict a successful response to CRT (**Fig. 6**). These parameters have also been used to detect early, preclinical diseases of the myocardium.[24]

Similar to issues with LV volumes, strain imaging of the LV requires some special considerations in the elderly. Specifically, strain and strain rates in

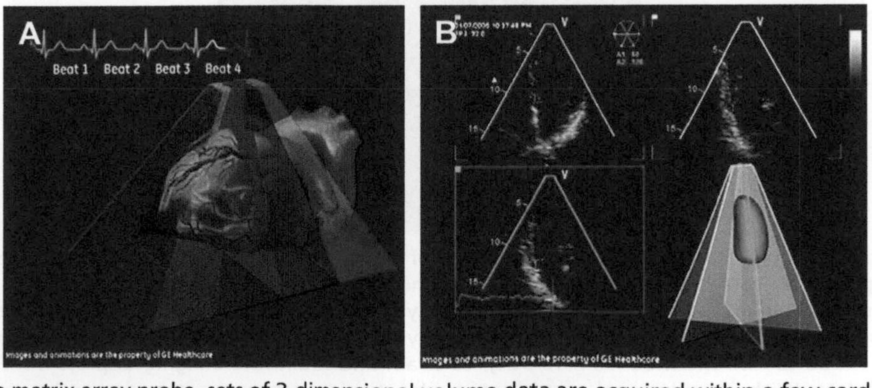

Fig. 4. With a matrix array probe, sets of 3-dimensional volume data are acquired within a few cardiac cycles (*A*). Four individual 15 degree sectors of volume data are stacked together and stored as a single image, allowing optimal assessment of cardiac volumes. With triplane imaging (*B*), the apical 2-, 3-, and 4-chamber views can be displayed simultaneously to allow volume assessment via the modified Simpson method. (*Courtesy of* GE Healthcare, Chalfont St. Giles, United Kingdom; with permission.)

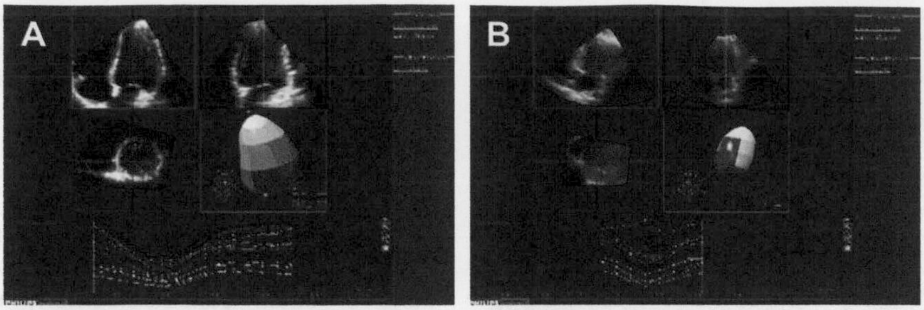

Fig. 5. Sets of 3-dimensional volume data enable the creation of a volume-rendered image and regional time/volume curves. In a normal left ventricle, these 17-segment curves reach end-systole at nearly the same time (*A*), but in a patient with left ventricular dyssynchrony, these curves are chaotic (*B*). (*Courtesy of* Philips Medical Systems, New York, NY; with permission.)

healthy elderly populations are lower than in healthy younger populations.[25] As such, applying normal ranges for younger adults to the elderly would overestimate subclinical systolic dysfunction. Further investigation is needed to identify an appropriate diagnostic cutoff for strain rate in elderly patients with HF.

LEFT VENTRICULAR DIASTOLIC FUNCTION

As mentioned, subclinical fibrosis leads to decreased LV compliance and increases the time needed for LV contraction and relaxation. As such, the prevalence of HFpEF is higher in elderly patients than in younger HF cohorts.[2] A significant

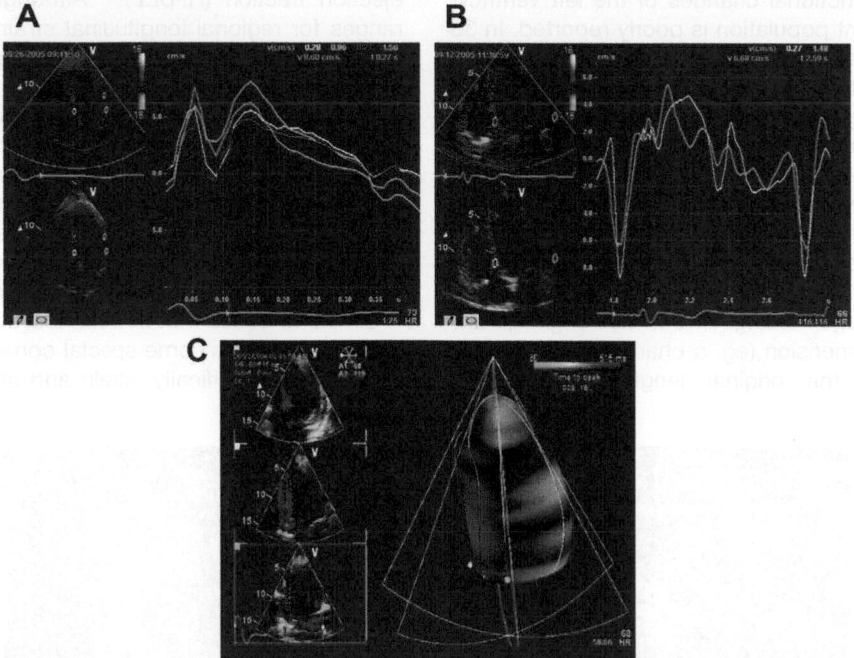

Fig. 6. Parametric color map and quantitative display of the tissue Doppler echocardiography-obtained tissue velocity imaging in a normal elderly patient (*A*). Note the overlapping velocity contours from the basal septal, mid-septal, and lateral walls, confirming left ventricular synchrony. In an elderly patient with a dilated cardiomyopathy, the basal septal (*yellow*) and lateral (*blue*) velocity curves do not overlap and are dyssynchronous (*B*). The same display mode can be switched from velocity, to strain and strain-rate imaging displays from the same acquired set of data. With 3-dimensional acquisition modes, tissue synchronous imaging can be used to provide a 3-dimensional model with thresholds for normal (*green* or *yellow*) or delayed (*red*) time-to-peak velocity graphically displayed (*C*). This elderly heart failure patient has an left bundle branch block pattern electrocardiogram, a left ventricular ejection fraction of less than 30%, and is a candidate for cardiac resynchronization therapy (see text for details).

proportion of HFpEF patient have abnormalities in diastolic filling with an increase in LV end-diastolic pressure. Although diastolic dysfunction is common in HFpEF, an echocardiographic assessment of diastolic function is important in confirming the diagnosis.[26] No noninvasive technique can directly measure diastolic function, but Doppler echocardiography uses diastolic filling parameters to infer diastolic function parameters. Importantly, any process that impairs the systolic function of the myocardium affects diastolic function as well. The various physiologic factors that affect mitral inflow velocities have been studied in experimental settings, allowing the individual contributions of each to be considered.[27] These experiments have shown that (1) elevated left atrial pressure causes an increased acceleration rate, a shortened isovolumic relaxation time (IVRT), and increased peak velocities, (2) slowing relaxation causes a delay in filling, and lower peak velocities and acceleration, (3) increasing ventricular stiffness blunts the E-wave velocity, and (4) reducing systolic function causes a similar effect as increasing stiffness. Transmitral flow incorporates early filling (E wave), passive filling (diastasis), and atrial contraction (A wave). The initial systolic forward flow (S1 wave) in pulmonary veins occurs because of atrial relaxation (x-descent) and a second systolic flow (S2) is the result of the descent of the base of the left ventricle during contraction. A late forward flow enters the left atrium during ventricular diastole (D wave) and is roughly timed with the mitral E wave. In most cases, a careful assessment of the transmitral, tissue Doppler and pulmonary venous flow patterns, combined with Valsalva maneuver, can provide an accurate estimate of diastolic performance.

Previous guideline documents on assessing diastolic function focused on 4 grades of diastolic dysfunction largely determined by the mitral inflow pattern on pulsed wave Doppler echocardiography at the leaflet tips of the mitral valve. Adjunct findings were then incorporated to support the grading. The first grade of diastolic dysfunction was identified by reduction in LV filling during the early diastolic filling period (termed E-A reversal). However, healthy elderly patients were noted to frequently have E-A reversal, and this led to some confusion about the classification of these patients. This confusion has largely been addressed in the newest iterations of the diastolic dysfunction guidelines.[28] Now, multiple findings are needed to first qualify as having diastolic dysfunction before grading and grading is focused on the identification of left atrial pressure (and in the absence of significant mitral valve disease, the LV end-diastolic pressure). The newest guidelines have also increased the role of tissue Doppler imaging (TDI, also referred to as DTI), estimation of left atrial pressure (primarily using E/e'), and downstream hemodynamic consequences of elevated LV end diastolic pressure (increase in left atrial size and increases in pulmonary pressures).

Simple pattern recognition allows the identification of 3 common abnormal pulsed-wave Doppler patterns of mitral valve inflow: an LV "relaxation abnormality" pattern (mild, grade I), a "pseudonormal" pattern (moderate, grade II), and a "restrictive physiology" pattern (severe, grade III [reversible] or grade IV [fixed]).[29] Two predominant mitral inflow patterns exist: (1) impaired LV relaxation (grade I) and (2) restrictive LV filling (grade III or IV; **Fig. 7**). As mentioned, grade I diastolic dysfunction includes a reduced E wave and increased A wave, with resultant reversal of the normal E/A ratio. However, such a pattern is also noted in patients with normal aging (or reduced left atrial pressure). Therefore, this pattern in isolation should be interpreted with caution. Other echocardiographic findings that support a grade

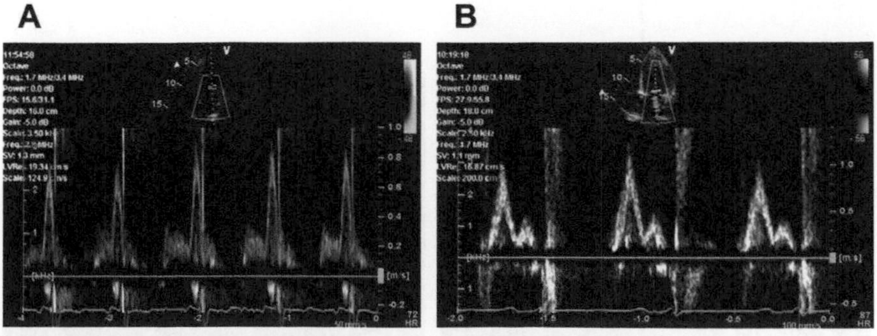

Fig. 7. Mitral inflow pulsed-wave spectral Doppler envelope in an elderly patient with heart failure who has grade I diastolic dysfunction (*A*) and another patient with grade III diastolic dysfunction (*B*). Although both patients had identical symptoms and left ventricular ejection fractions, the patient represented in (*A*) has a better prognosis than the patient in (*B*).

I pattern include prolongation of the IVRT (>90 ms) and deceleration time of the E wave (>240 ms). The pulmonary vein diastolic (PV-D) wave parallels the mitral E wave and is decreased with an associated increase in the pulmonary vein systolic (PV-S) wave (ratio of systolic pulmonary vein inflow velocity [S] to diastolic pulmonary vein inflow velocity [D] [(S/D ratio) >1.1]).

Despite the limitations of echocardiography for evaluating lesser degrees of diastolic dysfunction, the presence of a "restrictive" mitral inflow filling pattern (grade III) is fairly specific for the combination of reduced ventricular compliance and elevated left atrial filling pressure. The reduction in ventricular compliance may be owing to a primary abnormality of diastolic performance or secondary-to-marked systolic dysfunction. Additional Doppler alterations associated with severe diastolic dysfunction include reduced deceleration time (<160 ms), reduced IVRT (<70 ms), reduced S/D ratio (usually <0.6), and an increased atrial reversal velocity (>35 cm/s). When this restrictive filling pattern is persistent despite aggressive medical therapy or fixed and unaltered during Valsalva maneuver (E/A ratio change <0.5), then this pattern is advanced to grade IV (**Fig. 8**).[30] With normal aging, grade I patterns are common and the filling pressure of the left ventricle is usually normal owing to the brief presystolic increase in pressure induced by atrial contraction being compensated by the normal pressure prevailing during the remainder of diastole. Age-associated nomograms have been developed to identify acceptable values for different age groups.[31] For individuals over 60 year old, the following "extreme values" (2 standard errors above the normal mean value) may be used as a reference guide: E/A ratio of less than 0.60, deceleration time of greater than 260 ms, atrial reversal pulmonary vein velocity of greater than 43 cm/s, and an IVRT greater than 101 ms (**Box 1**). These "extreme values" are unlikely be exceeded in normal aging and may be useful for evaluating the elderly patient with HF. The most difficult mitral inflow pattern to understand is grade II, the so-called "pseudonormal" filling pattern. This pattern resembles a normal pattern but is actually in transition between delayed relaxation (grade I) and restriction (grades III or IV).

It should be standard practice to perform a Valsalva maneuver during echocardiography when a "normal" pattern is detected in an elderly patient (**Fig. 9**). If the mitral pattern is due to mildly elevated filling pressure, this maneuver will briefly lower that pressure and transiently convert this pattern to one of delayed relaxation (grade I).[32] TDE is an important adjunct for the clarification of this "pseudonormal" pattern and is simple to acquire, relative to pulmonary vein flow analysis. This technique is similar to the use of Doppler ultrasound imaging to assess blood flow, but with a focus on the lower velocity frequency shifts of myocardial tissue motion. By providing a quantitative representation of the motion of the longitudinal axis of myocardial contraction and relaxation, TDE provides a new method of analyzing the extent and timing of diastolic wall motion.[33] It is important to have patients hold their breath during TDE recordings to minimize artifacts from cardiac translation, because this technique is exquisitely sensitive to small alterations in cardiac motion. The TDE-derived mitral annular velocity measured at the septal or lateral mitral annulus in the apical 4-chamber view reflects changes in the long axis dimension of the left ventricle. The velocity of diastolic movement of the mitral annulus away from the cardiac apex has 2 peaks roughly corresponding with the E and A waves of Doppler transmitral flow. For clarification, these low velocities are referred to as e' and a' to be distinguished from the higher velocity E and A waves of mitral inflow. The transition from normal to pathologic

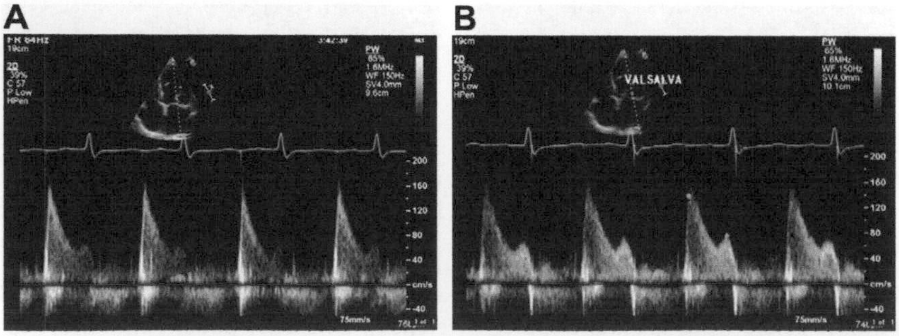

Fig. 8. Grade III or IV mitral inflow (restrictive filling pattern) is displayed by the high-velocity E wave, high E/A ratio, and short deceleration time (*A*). However, a Valsalva maneuver is required to confirm that this is grade IV (E/A ratio change during Valsalva <0.5) and the prognosis is significantly worse than grade III (*B*).

Box 1
Echocardiographic classification of left ventricular diastolic function (and LAP)

I. For patients with normal LVEF (and structurally normal hearts)

Abnormal diastolic function is present when most of the following parameters are met:

- Average E/e' >14
- Septal e' <7 cm/s
- Lateral e' <10 cm/s
- Maximal tricuspid regurgitation velocity >2.8m/s
- LAVI >34 mL/m^2

II. For patients with reduced LVEF (and structurally abnormal hearts)

Grade I diastolic dysfunction (normal LAP)

- E/A ratio $\leq$0.8 and E $\leq$50 cm/s
- Majority of above parameters are negative

Grade II diastolic dysfunction (increased LAP)

- E/A ratio between 0.8 and 2.0
- Majority of above parameters are positive

Grade III diastolic dysfunction (increased LAP)

- E/A ratio $\geq$2.0

Note: When there are too few parameters to measure or there is a mixed pattern of findings, the following additional parameters may be of value and are considered abnormal:

- E deceleration time >240 ms (suggests grade I) or <160 ms (suggests grade III)
- E/A ratio during Valsalva maneuver changes by 50% (suggests grades II or III)
- Pulmonary vein S/D ratio <1.0 (suggests grade II) or less than 0.6 (suggests grade III)
- Pulmonary vein systolic fraction of <40% (suggests increased LAP)
- Pulmonary vein atrial reversal wave >35 ms (suggests increased LAP)
- Pulmonary vein atrial reversal wave >30 ms longer than A wave (increased LAP)

Abbreviations: LAP, left atrial pressure; LAVI, left atrial volume index; LVEF, left ventricular ejection fraction.

myocardial velocities is distinct and consistent and, unlike the mitral inflow transition, it does not progress through a "pseudonormal" stage (**Fig. 10**). Also, the ratio of the E/e' has been repeatedly confirmed as a valid measure of left atrial pressure. The major strength is that ratios of less than 8 and greater than 15 (>12 if using the higher velocity lateral wall e') can confidently

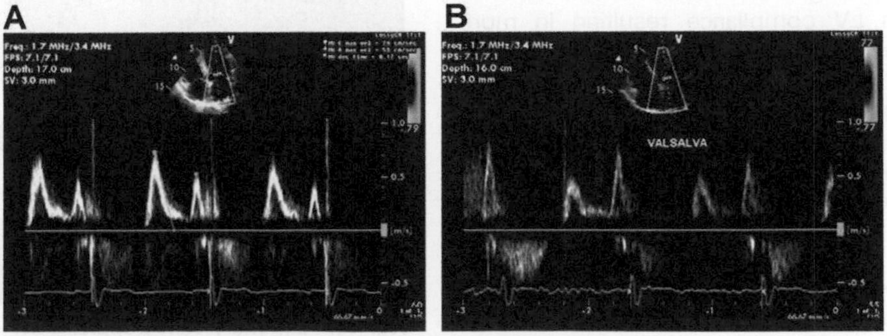

Fig. 9. Grade II (pseudonormal) mitral inflow Doppler filling pattern may be misinterpreted as a normal filling pattern (*A*). The late low-velocity slowing of the E wave is a clue to grade II diastolic dysfunction, but this is shown dramatically with the Valsalva maneuver, which reverses the E/A ratio to an obvious grade I pattern (*B*).

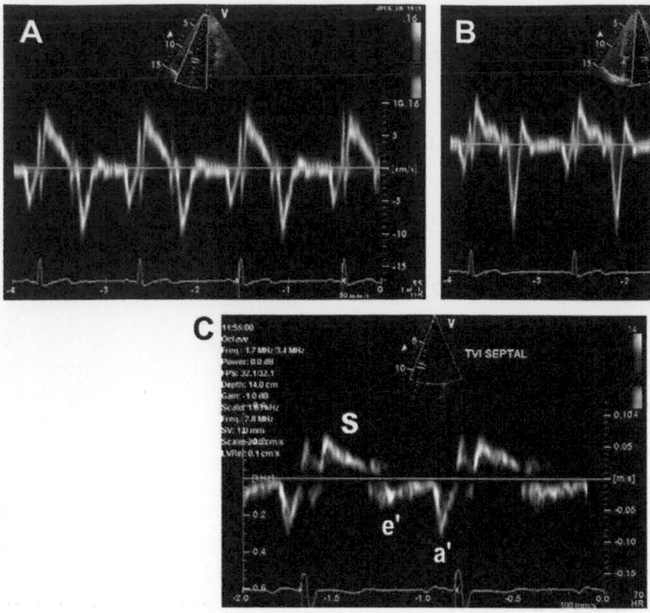

Fig. 10. Tissue Doppler echocardiography (TDE) image obtained at the mitral annulus in a normal patient. (*A*) Medial annulus. (*B*) Lateral annulus. (*C*) TDE display in an elderly patient with class II heart failure symptoms and a "normal appearing" mitral Doppler filling pattern. With an early TDE (e') velocity much lower than the late TDE velocity (a'), the patient is certain to have grade-II diastolic dysfunction. S, systolic wave; TVI, time velocity integral.

separate normal from elevated filling pressures. Interrogating the pattern of pulmonary vein flow is both feasible and helpful, especially when the tissue Doppler findings are inadequate or unreliable.

The pulmonary vein is assessed by using color Doppler guidance to assist in placing a pulsed Doppler sample volume in the right upper pulmonary vein, located along the atrial septum (apical 4-chamber view). Three distinct waves are seen: the PV-S, PV-D, and atrial reversal waves (**Fig. 11**). Often, the sample volume must be repositioned more distally to optimize the atrial reversal Doppler velocity envelope. Also, in healthy older adults, the systolic fraction of pulmonary venous forward flow is greater than 50% owing to a decrease in LV compliance resulting in more vigorous atrial contraction and enhanced atrial relaxation.[34] However, during faster heart rates, diastole shortens and the presystolic increase in pressure is one of the mechanisms of exercise intolerance associated with aging. Another limitation of current methods for evaluating diastolic filling is that they have been well-validated in sinus rhythm only. Many elderly patients have atrial fibrillation with variable cardiac cycle lengths and no organized atrial contraction. More studies are needed to optimize the assessment of diastolic function in patients with atrial fibrillation. However, the peak acceleration rate of the E wave seems to correlate well with the LV filling pressure.[35] Also, it seems that the deceleration time of the mitral valve inflow and the E/e' ratio remains prognostic.[36] The pulmonary artery systolic pressure is readily determined by the peak velocity of tricuspid regurgitation on Doppler echocardiography. Also, Doppler echocardiography detects some degree of pulmonary regurgitation on most echocardiographic examinations. This is usually of minimal hemodynamic significance and is often secondary to

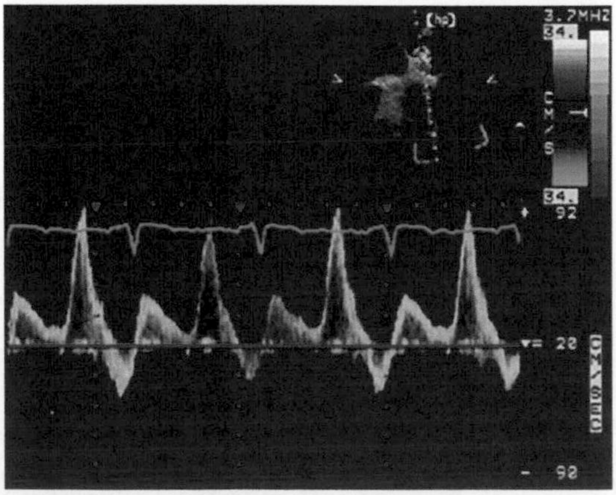

Fig. 11. Pulmonary vein Doppler flow display in an elderly patient with heart failure symptoms. The S/D ratio of less than 0.6 is consistent with elevated left atrial pressure.

pulmonary hypertension, but it provides a wonderful opportunity for determining the diastolic pressure of the pulmonary artery.

A pulmonary regurgitation end-diastolic velocity of greater than 110 cm/s (equivalent to 5 mm Hg) predicts an overall worse cardiac prognosis, higher New York Heart Association functional class, higher brain natriuretic peptide, and poorer exercise tolerance, than in patients with a pulmonary regurgitation end-diastolic velocity of less than 5 mm Hg.[37] This is equivalent to the prognostic capabilities of a tricuspid regurgitation gradient of greater than 30 mm Hg and may be used in place of the tricuspid regurgitation when this is not present. This pulmonary regurgitation end-diastolic velocity correlates with the pulmonary artery wedge pressure, regardless of the etiology of HF or severity of tricuspid regurgitation and can be used to assess changes in LV filling pressures resulting from therapy.[38]

Color M-mode imaging is another technique that allows determination of LV filling pressure and is predictive of in-hospital HF and short-term survival after a myocardial infarction.[39–41] When the ratio of the mitral inflow peak E-wave velocity to flow propagation velocity (E/V_p), as determined by the color M-mode, is greater than 1.5, then long-term survival after a myocardial infarction is unlikely. A V_p of less than 45 cm/s is itself a predictor of worse outcomes and a V_p of less than 40 cm/s correlates with an increased left atrial pressure (**Fig. 12**).

Doppler echocardiography provides a useful tool for assessing diastolic function in elderly patients. Because no absolute variables are available

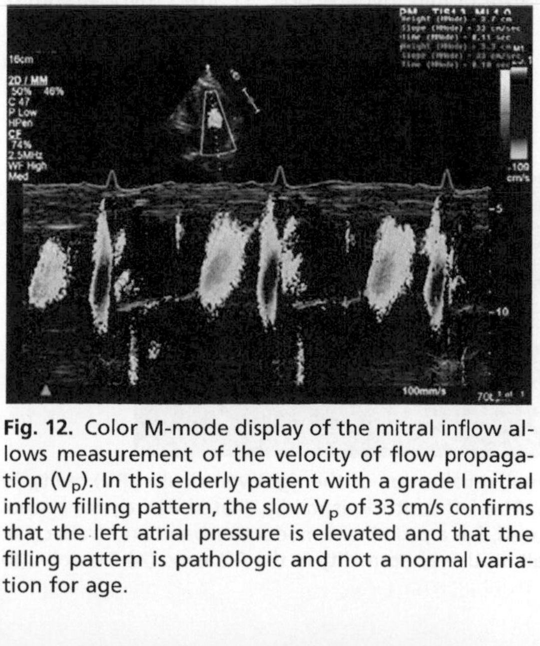

Fig. 12. Color M-mode display of the mitral inflow allows measurement of the velocity of flow propagation (V_p). In this elderly patient with a grade I mitral inflow filling pattern, the slow V_p of 33 cm/s confirms that the left atrial pressure is elevated and that the filling pattern is pathologic and not a normal variation for age.

to categorize patients into mild, moderate, or severe diastolic dysfunction, all available measurements must be evaluated to minimize interpretive error. Normal aging alters these parameters and the aforementioned extreme values are provided in an effort to minimize false diagnoses. Death from HF or an appropriate implantable cardioverter defibrillator shock was evaluated in 84 patients with chronic HF and a mean LVEF of 29%.[42] Of those 84 patients, 22 (26%) had experienced an event by the time of the 1-year follow-up. Seven of those 22 died. In comparison with the patients who did not have an event, those 22 patients had longer QRS durations (169 vs 146 ms), higher mitral E/e' ratios (16.0 vs 12.8), and a more frequent filling pattern (44% vs 9%). Multivariate regression analysis identified a restrictive filling pattern as the only independent predictor of an event (hazard ratio, 3.65) and the event-free survival rate was 38% versus 72% compared with those without a restrictive filling pattern. Echocardiography and catheterization were performed in elderly patients (mean age, 64 years) and a multiple regression model of all echocardiographic variables showed that the addition of the E/e' ratio to the clinical history and LVEF provided incremental prognostic information.[43] An E/e' ratio of greater than 15 identified those with a higher risk of new-onset or recurrent HF. The presence of a restrictive filling pattern has significant prognostic implications. In patients with dilated cardiomyopathy (DCM), this pattern is more predictive of the development of severe symptoms than are indices of systolic function. In patients with amyloidosis, restrictive filling is associated with poor 1-year survival.[44,45]

The prognostic value of abnormal mitral flow velocity may be enhanced by assessing changes in this parameter during alterations in loading conditions. This was illustrated in a report of 173 patients with chronic HF. The report measured the outcomes at 17 months in 4 subgroups that were distinguished by differences in changes in mitral valve flow velocity observed during nitroprusside infusion (resulting in a reversible or nonreversible restrictive pattern) and passive leg lifting (resulting in a stable or unstable nonrestrictive pattern).[46] In this study, the event rate of cardiac death or urgent transplantation worsened progressively from a stable nonrestrictive pattern (6%), to a reversible restrictive pattern (19%), to an unstable nonrestrictive pattern (33%), and finally to an irreversible restrictive pattern (55%). In 144 patients with HF (76% with coronary artery disease), an initial restrictive pattern that resolved by 6 months of optimal medical therapy had a lower cardiac mortality (11% vs 37%) at 2 years than those without

Doppler improvements. This reversible restrictive filling pattern (grade III) has consistently proven superior for survival relative to a fixed restrictive filling pattern (grade IV).[47]

The Valsalva maneuver is a simple, bedside technique to deliver similar prognostic value and should be performed in all elderly HF patients with a restrictive filling pattern. The effect of dobutamine stress on a restrictive pattern also seems to have prognostic value and a restrictive LV filling at rest, which reverts to a nonrestrictive pattern during dobutamine infusion, has a markedly improved survival (79% vs 49%) over a fixed pattern. Persistence of the restrictive pattern was associated with a marked increase in left atrial pressure and a markedly attenuated inotropic response.[48] During stress echocardiography, this mitral inflow pattern should be sought for its incremental prognostic capability.

SPECIFIC CARDIOMYOPATHIES

Determining the etiology of HF is paramount to developing an adequate treatment regimen. In addition to numerous myocardial diseases, the clinical findings of HF may be due to such diverse causes as unsuspected valvar stenosis or regurgitation, chronic pulmonary disease, or pericardial constraint. One-dimensional (M-mode) echocardiography and 2DE provide excellent spatial resolution to evaluate the anatomy of the myocardium and cardiac valves. Each of the 4 major World Health Organization classifications of cardiomyopathies can be reasonably categorized with echocardiography.[49] DCM, a primary myocardial disease, is usually idiopathic and creates a spherically enlarged LV with normal or thin-walled muscle and reduced LVEF. Although late-stage DCM is easy to recognize, DCM is often difficult to detect in its early stages. Early anatomic echocardiography features that may precede a detectable drop in LV systolic function include a decrease in the descent of the cardiac base, an increase in sphericity, and an increase in ESV index, which seems to be sensitive to changes in global contractility.[50–52] A hypertrophic cardiomyopathy is a primary cardiomyopathy that results in a markedly thickened LV myocardial wall with normal LV contractility until very late in the disease process. This late presentation is not uncommon in the elderly population. A restrictive cardiomyopathy is an unusual classification in that it requires one to combine Doppler information with the usual 2D cardiac appearance of normal or small LV cavity and markedly dilated left and right atria. DCM and hypertrophic cardiomyopathy both have a notoriously grave outcome. Arrhythmogenic RV cardiomyopathy (dysplasia) is difficult to detect in the early concealed phase, but once fully developed results in a dilated, dysfunctional right ventricle with a normal left ventricle (**Fig. 13**). This is a diagnosis of exclusion and should not be considered if significant pulmonary hypertension exists. Other characteristic features of this rare cardiomyopathy include focal aneurysms or thinning at the "triangle of dysplasia," which includes the RV inflow, the RV outflow and the RV apex.[53] Although echocardiography is rarely able to establish the exact cause of myocardial pathology, some diseases have characteristic echocardiographic features that increase their likelihood. Regional wall motion abnormalities typically occur in patients with underlying coronary artery disease, but are also present in patients with advanced DCM. However, an area of normal myocardial thickening with abrupt transition to an area of thin, hyperechoic, scarred myocardium is more characteristic of an ischemic cardiomyopathy. For serial comparisons of regional wall motion assessment and greater consistency among all

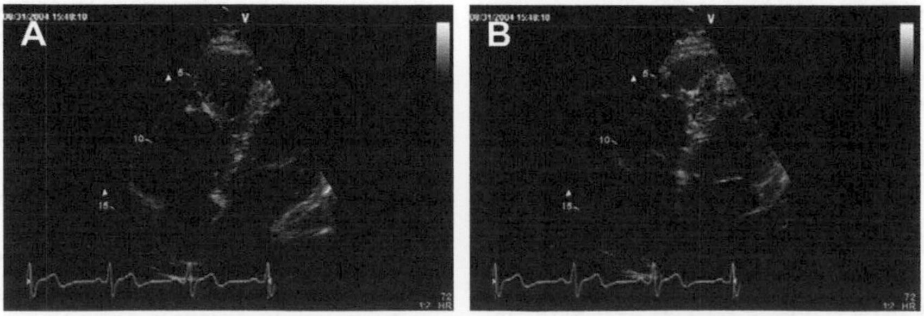

Fig. 13. Apical 4-chamber view, tilted rightward for maximal visualization of the right ventricular (RV) cavity, in an elderly man with known arryhthmogenic RV dysplasia. The left ventricle is mildly dilated and dysfunctional (common in late stages), but the RV cavity is markedly dilated, has a prominent moderator band and trabeculae in the absence of pulmonary hypertension, and a focal wall motion abnormality in the RV apex. (*A*) Diastole. (*B*) Systole.

imaging modalities, a 17-segment myocardial model should be used.[54] A sparkled appearance within the myocardium is said to be highly predictive of amyloidosis, but the authors believe that any cause of LV hypertrophy may have this appearance with modern ultrasound transducers. When dramatic and accompanied by other echocardiographic features of amyloidosis, such as a pericardial effusion and myocardial, valvar, and atrial septal thickening, this diagnosis becomes more likely. Occurring in patients with a travel or immigration history from South and Central American countries, the finding of a segmental cardiomyopathy, without coronary artery disease, raises the possibility of Chagas' disease. The most common abnormality is an apical aneurysm that, unlike coronary disease, spares the interventricular septum.[55] As this disease progresses, the echocardiographic appearance may mimic DCM.

LV noncompaction is an uncommon cause of a DCM that results from intrauterine arrest of compaction of the loose interwoven meshwork that makes up the fetal myocardial primordium. This disorder should be suspected when unexpectedly heavy LV trabeculation is noted, particularly toward the apex. This disease entity has only recently been identified in elderly populations and the diagnosis is aided with the use of contrast, with or without 3DE (**Fig. 14**).[56] Normal-appearing LV size and function associated with an enlarged RV cavity, reduced RV function, and an elevated pulmonary artery pressure raise the suspicion of pulmonary artery thromboemboli or primary lung disease (**Fig. 15**).[57,58] If the RV free wall (best seen with subcostal imaging) is not thickened (<5 mm), then chronic elevation of the pulmonary artery pressure is unlikely, further reducing the etiology to a more acute diagnosis.

VALVULAR HEART DISEASE

Aortic valve disease is extremely common in the elderly and ranges from calcific degeneration (aortic sclerosis) to severe, critical aortic stenosis. Furthermore, with the development of transcatheter aortic valve implantation or replacement has further reinforced the need for timely and comprehensive assessment of the aortic valve given available interventions for patients who are not deemed surgical candidates. Despite a detailed and careful physical examination, the severity of aortic stenosis is often in doubt, especially in the elderly.[59] Combined with conventional Doppler, 2DE is well-suited to investigate the severity of aortic stenosis. Assessment of valve morphology with 2DE and 3DE is important to assess for a primary valve leaflet morphology and excursion. As important as valve structure is, the hallmark of echocardiographic evaluation for aortic stenosis is the hemodynamic assessment. Primary outcome data were initially associated with peak velocity across the aortic valve.[60] The modified Bernoulli equation converts measured velocities to mean and peak pressure gradients, and the continuity equation provides an estimate of the aortic valve area.

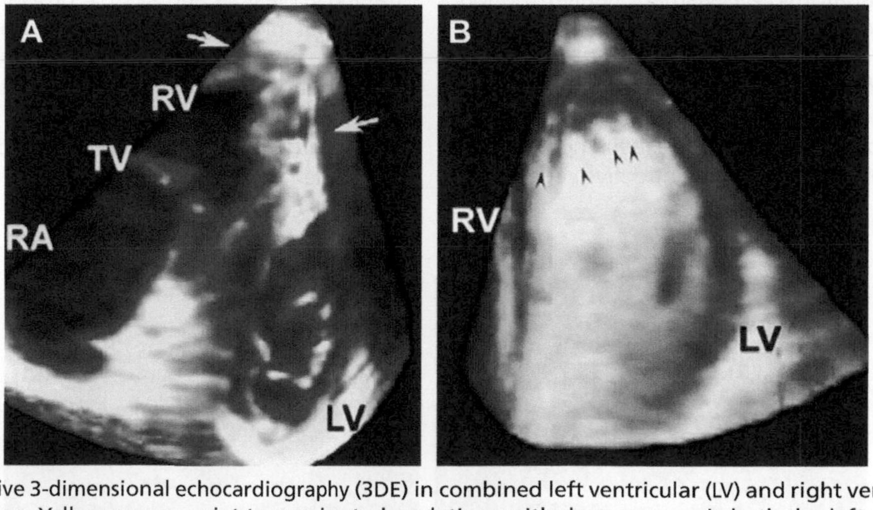

Fig. 14. (*A*) Live 3-dimensional echocardiography (3DE) in combined left ventricular (LV) and right ventricular (RV) noncompaction. Yellow arrows point to massive trabeculations with deep recesses in both the left ventricle and the right ventricle with the diagnosis of isolated noncompaction of the left ventricle (and *right ventricle*). (*B*) Live 3DE contrast study using activated perflutren microspheres showing filling of intertrabecular recesses with the contrast agent (*black arrows*). RA, right atrium; TV, tricuspid valve. (*From* Bodiwala K, Miller AP, Nanda NC, et al. Live three-dimensional transthoracic echocardiographic assessment of ventricular non-compaction. Echocardiography 2005;22:615; with permission.)

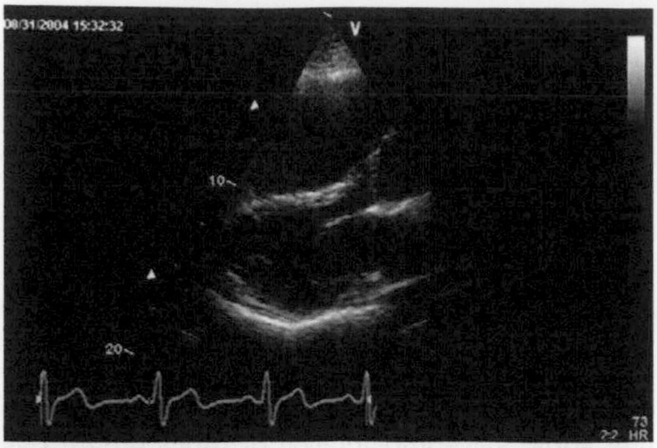

Fig. 15. Parasternal long axis 2-dimensional echocardiography (2DE) view in an elderly male with New York Heart Association functional class III heart failure symptoms. The diagnosis of cor pulmonale is immediately suggested by the massive right ventricle on this initial 2DE view.

Color flow Doppler imaging can assist in obtaining an accurate estimate of the aortic valve area.[61] When the transthoracic echocardiographic findings are uncertain, transesophageal echocardiography or stress echocardiography can provide additional insight into the severity of the valve lesion.[62,63] Also, real-time 3DE enables direct visualization and measurement of the stenotic aortic valve opening. Real-time 3DE may be more accurate than 2DE with Doppler.[64] In addition to assessing for aortic stenosis, it is also essential to assess for regurgitant lesions, either occurring concurrently with aortic stenosis or in isolation. The severity of aortic regurgitation involves incorporation of anatomic assessment (leaflet motion, flail leaflet, or malcoaptation) and hemodynamic assessment from color flow and continuous wave Doppler echocardiography (pressure half-time and deceleration time). This can be incorporated with other quantitative assessments (such as vena contracta, jet height, effective regurgitant orifice area).[65] In assessing hemodynamic parameters, it is important to note vital signs (specifically heart rate and blood pressure) for appropriate interpretation of hemodynamic parameters.

Mitral valve disease may also result in the clinical presentation of HF. Mitral regurgitation (MR) is nearly universal when the LVEF is reduced and the left ventricle is enlarged. With mitral annular dilatation, coaptation of the valve is compromised and secondary, central MR occurs. The 2D appearance of the valve is often normal and the degree of MR is rarely severe until late in the disease progression. When LV dysfunction is secondary to MR, the 2D appearance of the mitral valve is universally abnormal. In this situation, the degree of MR is often severe, and the direction of the regurgitant jet is commonly eccentric (directed away from a prolapsing or flail leaflet, or toward a restricted or scarred leaflet). Quantifying the degree of MR is vitally important when considering surgery and real-time 3DE supplements 2DE and color Doppler in the assessment of MR severity.[66–68] If possible, severe MR should be repaired early to minimize progression of LV systolic dysfunction. In rare cases, this repair provides a surgical cure for HF.[69]

RIGHT VENTRICLE

The right ventricle is notoriously difficult to completely analyze owing to its complex, nongeometric shape and a high degree of normal variability in shape and regional motion. Using the apical 4-chamber view, simple endocardial tracing in diastole and systole provides a reliable, albeit not highly accurate, estimate of systolic function, expressed as a percentage of fractional area change (**Fig. 16**). Although not specifically investigated in elderly individuals, a fractional area change of greater than 32% (35% is easier to remember) has been found in normal

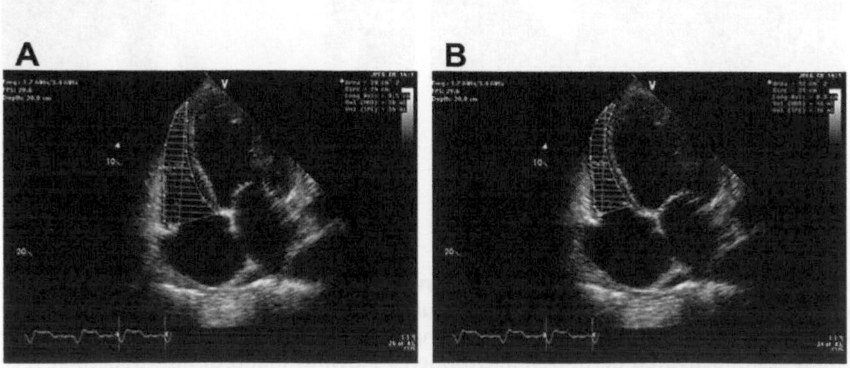

Fig. 16. Apical 4-chamber view tilted rightward allows the assessment of the right ventricular (RV) function using the fractional area change (FAC) method of tracing the endocardial borders in diastole (*A*) and systole (*B*). FAC = (RV diastole − RV systole)/RV diastole = (38–16)/38 = 57%.

controls.[53] A useful and easily obtained measurement of RV function is the tricuspid annular plane systolic excursion (descent of the base). In 1 report, an excursion of 14 mm added significant prognostic information to other clinical and echocardiographic findings in DCM.[70] Other measures of normal RV systolic function include tissue Doppler imaging (S' >10 cm/s), RV myocardial performance index (right index of myocardial performance <0.40 by pulsed wave Doppler echocardiography or right index of myocardial performance <0.55 by tissue Doppler), and RVEF by 3DE of greater than 44%.[71] Similar to LV assessment, most normative values were studied in younger healthier populations with either subset of elderly patients or extrapolation of data.

A dilated inferior vena cava without collapse during inspiration is associated with worse survival in men independent of a history of HF, other comorbidities, ventricular function, and pulmonary artery pressure (**Fig. 17**). A reduction in diameter of less than 50% of the inferior vena cava in response to "sniffing" is not only a predictor of increased right atrial pressure, but a predictor of survival. In a series of more than 4000 consecutive outpatient echocardiograms (98% men), survival rates were influenced strongly by the inferior vena cava appearance. In patients with an inspiratory collapse of their inferior vena cava, the survival

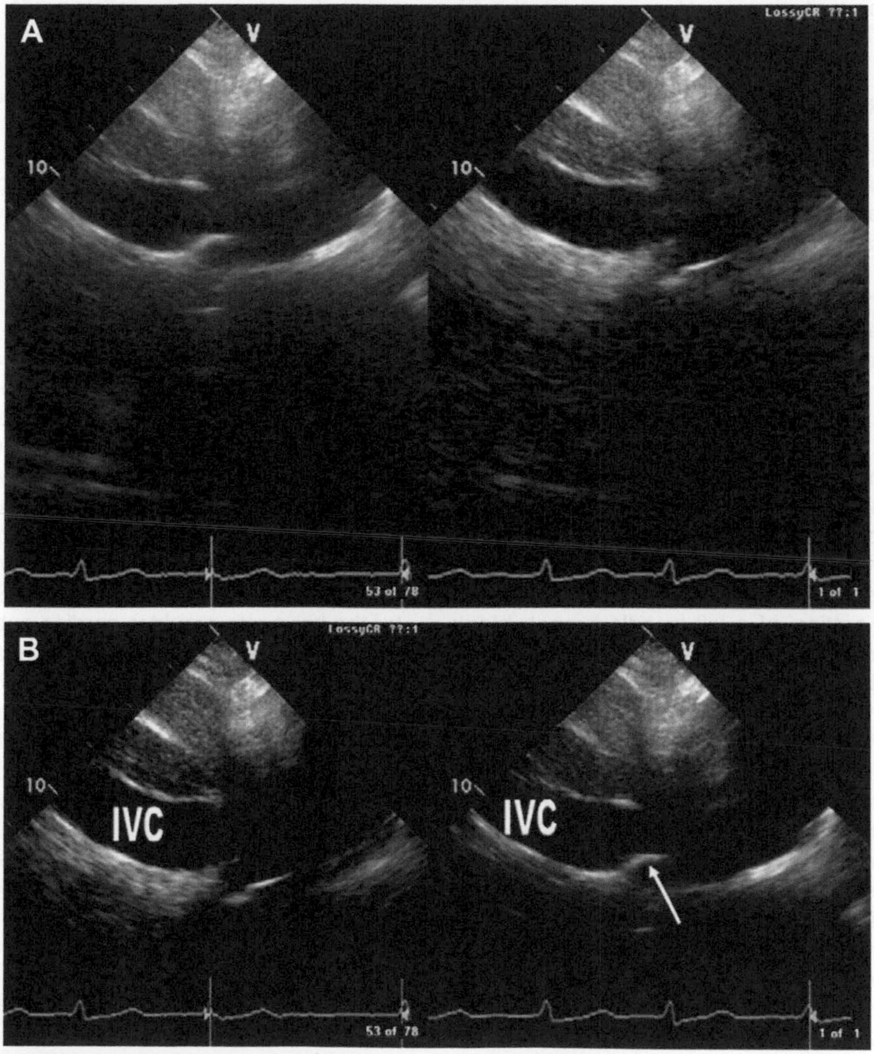

Fig. 17. Subcostal 2-dimensional echocardiography image of the inferior vena cava in an elderly female with class III heart failure (*A*). The inferior vena cava (IVC) is dilated at held expiration (*left*) and does not collapse with inspiration (*right*). This confirms elevated right atrial pressure and is associated with a poor prognosis. Note the diaphragm motion during sniffing (*white arrow* in *B*).

rates were 99% after 90 days and 95% after 1 year, as compared with 89% after 90 days and 67% after 1 year for those with less than 50% collapse.[72] RV systolic dysfunction also may contribute to prognosis in patients with HF.[73] Echocardiographic measurements of reduced RV function include a reduction in RVEF fraction, RV enlargement, and tricuspid regurgitation. In patients with class II or III HF, the RVEF was an independent predictor of 1- and 2-year survival and event-free cardiac survival. At 2 years, the event-free survival rates from cardiovascular mortality and urgent transplantation was 93% for those with an RVEF of 35%; 77% for those with an RVEF of greater than 25% but less than 35%; and 59% for those with an RVEF of less than 25%. In addition to the RVEF, the severity of tricuspid regurgitation is also associated with prognosis.[74]

CARDIAC RESYNCHRONIZATION THERAPY

The most significant recent advance in systolic HF treatment has been achieved with the placement of strategically positioned biventricular pacemaker leads to create an improved pattern of myocardial contraction. This process is CRT. Numerous trials have shown improved outcomes. The effect of CRT in elderly patients has also been shown to be beneficial. In 170 consecutive patients with clinical and echocardiographic improvements after CRT at 6 months, survival at 2 years was similar in patients older than 70 years compared with those patients younger than 70 years.[75] The echocardiography community has known for years that the placement of an RV pacemaker is associated with an abnormal, paradoxic distal septal motion owing to preactivation at the site of the RV apical lead. In the setting of a left bundle branch block pattern electrocardiograph, the native septum has a variable degree of paradoxic motion that can be witnessed with 2DE or 3DE. The more abnormal the left bundle branch block pattern, the more abnormal is the 2DE motion. It is intuitive that this dyssynchronous pattern of contraction could be improved by placing a pacemaker lead in the lateral wall and causing preactivation of this relatively delayed myocardial segment. In essence, this is what CRT does. Although echocardiographic findings can often predict responders of CRT, echocardiography is not a perfect tool. However, it can reliably predict nonresponders by recognizing lateral wall scars. These nonresponders will improve contraction with pacing and therefore should not undergo attempted CRT. Furthermore, echocardiography is the basis for CRT because, in theory, a patient with an EF of 36% would not benefit from CRT, but a patient with an EF of 34% would. This is further justification of the need for quantification of LVEF. To more precisely identify regions of myocardial dyssynchrony, numerous techniques are available, but none have proven superior over the others. Certainly, one of the simplest, most reproducible methods is 3DE (see **Fig. 5**). This method is criticized for having a low temporal resolution. Others have carefully analyzed the subtle gray-scale relationships of 2DE, known as speckle tracking, as a means to improve on this temporal resolution issue and have shown early success.[76] Finally, dobutamine infusion has a role in elderly patients with LV systolic dysfunction. If the global dysfunction improves with a low dose, then the left ventricle is viable and worthy of continued investigation for an ischemic etiology. If it does not improve, then there is no reason to pursue this line of investigation. If improvement occurs at a low dose and is sustained at higher, target doses, then a nonischemic etiology should be considered. If the low-dose improvement worsens again at higher doses, then ischemia is suggested and revascularization should be advised.

HEMODYNAMIC ASSESSMENT

Hemodynamic Data (Conventional and Tissue Doppler)

Pulsed or continuous wave Doppler echocardiography quickly and accurately estimates cardiac output. By placing the sample volume within the LV outflow tract, the Doppler envelope can be obtained and traced to provide the time velocity integral. This "stroke distance" is then multiplied by the LV outflow tract area (LV outflow tract diameter^2 $\times$ 0.785) to obtain the SV. The SV multiplied by the heart rate provides cardiac output.[77] Using continuous wave Doppler, the cardiac output is determined by multiplying the time velocity integral by the diameter of the sinotubular junction (in the absence of aortic stenosis). The validity of the cardiac output has been shown even in the presence of a low-output state or significant tricuspid regurgitation.[78] A global index of myocardial performance that combines both systolic and diastolic parameters has been described for both the right and left ventricles, but the clinical usefulness of this index in older patients with congestive HF has not yet been well-validated.[79,80]

In summary, through an extensive use of Doppler techniques, one can obtain comprehensive hemodynamic data at bedside,[81] which can be used to provide valuable diagnostic and prognostic information in the elderly patient with known or suspected HF. The human and economic burden of HF increases with aging. Only during the past decade have surveys incorporated echocardiography to confirm structural heart disease in people with nonspecific symptoms. Multiple studies have confirmed that the incidence of structural heart disease exceeds the clinical findings.[82–86] In one such cross-sectional observational study of more than 2000 elderly people (60–86 years old), prevalence rates of clinical HF, and LV systolic dysfunction (LVEF <50%) were studied.[87] These investigators confirmed that clinical HF increased with advancing age with a 4.4-fold increase from early 1960s to early 1980s. LV systolic dysfunction occurred more commonly than clinical HF, suggesting that symptoms only reveal the tip of the iceberg. Although 21.1% had structural heart disease, only 6.3% had clinical HF. Moreover, of the 5.9% of participants with LV systolic dysfunction, 59% were in the preclinical stage of disease.

In another study, investigators reported a 6% to 10% prevalence of clinical HF in patients over the age of 65.[88] In this study, HF status was ascertained using clinical scores that have a poor sensitivity and specificity for structural heart disease. Because secondary preventive measures have been shown to be effective for patients with preclinical LV systolic dysfunction, these preclinical disease states must be identified. Targeted screening programs of high-risk people (such as older age groups) should be evaluated for their cost effectiveness and echocardiography is the ideal tool for this purpose. Just as systolic dysfunction is frequently preclinical, diastolic dysfunction, even when moderate to severe, may be asymptomatic.

In a community-based survey of more than 2000 subjects, 28% had diastolic dysfunction (7.3% moderate to severe), despite only 1% with symptoms.[82] In addition to diastolic dysfunction, transient LV systolic dysfunction, as seen with myocardial ischemia, may also present as congestive HF with normal, resting LV systolic function. A regional wall motion abnormality, often subtle at rest, may be the only echocardiographic finding. Therefore, in patients with severe HF symptoms, normal wall motion and normal or mildly abnormal diastolic function, myocardial ischemia should be suspected and consideration given for the performance of stress echocardiography. By measuring the degree of LV thickening and the diameter of the LV cavity, the ventricular mass/volume ratio can be obtained and may facilitate the separation of patients likely to have myocardial ischemia, despite similar degrees of diastolic dysfunction and exercise intolerance. Patients with a low ratio (<1.8), indicating less myocardial mass, are more likely to have coronary artery disease with up to 80% having severe coronary artery stenosis.[77] Conversely, in patients with a ventricular mass/volume ratio of greater than 1.8, the etiology is more often progressive LV hypertrophy owing to hypertension, and these patients are less likely to have coronary artery disease (**Fig. 18**). This assessment allows therapy to be aimed properly at either LV hypertrophy regression or, more specifically, the improvement of myocardial ischemia. In addition to the LVEF, the size and shape of the left ventricle, as well as the Doppler findings, may predict the development and severity of congestive HF symptoms.

In a substudy of the Studies of Left Ventricular Dysfunction-95, 311 patients with symptomatic LV dysfunction (treatment arm) and 258 patients with asymptomatic LV dysfunction (prevention arm) were evaluated.[89] Compared with patients without symptoms, symptomatic patients had larger LV end-diastolic diameters and LV ESVs,

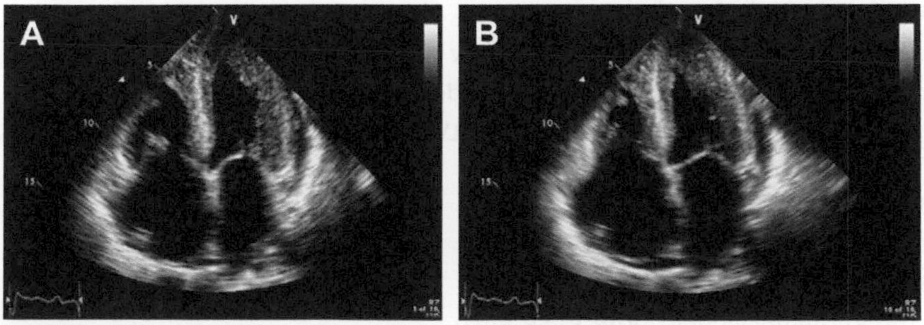

Fig. 18. Apical 4-chamber view (*A*) diastole (*B*) systole in a 61-year-old woman with progressive heart failure symptoms. The left ventricular (LV) and right ventricular (RV) myocardial walls are thickened, the size of the LV cavity is normal, and the LV mass/volume ratio is greater than 1.8, decreasing the likelihood that the etiology of LV systolic dysfunction is coronary artery disease. This patient had cardiac amyloidosis, which was suggested by the thickened valves and atrial septum, small pericardial effusion, and the restrictive 2-dimensional echocardiography and mitral Doppler inflow.

higher sphericity indexes (a measure of the "roundness" of the LV), and a higher E/A ratio. These patients also had a greater incidence of ventricular dysrhythmias. These data suggest that both diastolic properties and the degree of ventricular remodeling affect the clinical status of patients with LV dysfunction, and that echocardiography provides useful information in this assessment. Few studies have investigated the use and impact of echocardiography in the management of congestive HF. In 1 such study, the management and clinical outcome of patients with congestive HF were classified according to whether or not an echocardiogram was performed.[90] Although limited by its retrospective design, this study revealed that patients who did not receive an echocardiogram had decreased survival, increased morbidity, and underuse of angiotensin-converting enzyme inhibitor therapy. With the aid of echocardiography, the elderly patient with HF can be skillfully treated, assessed for treatment response, referred for surgery when indicated, and counseled regarding prognosis. Without knowledge of LV systolic and diastolic function, an angiotensin-converting enzyme inhibitor, digoxin, and diuretics may be used inappropriately in the 40% to 50% of elderly patients who have a normal LV systolic function. Furthermore, the unfortunate patient with unsuspected, surgically correctable, valvular heart disease would go untreated and remain at risk for progressive, irreversible myocardial damage.

SUMMARY

Echocardiography allows the assessment of systolic and diastolic function and identifies many of the common causes of HF. Patients with minimally symptomatic or unsuspected LV systolic dysfunction may be identified and receive the benefits of angiotensin-converting enzyme inhibitor therapy. Echocardiography is also useful for assessing the prognosis and can be used serially to evaluate the effectiveness of treatment. Ventricular filling

Box 2
Echocardiographic approach to the elderly patient with heart failure

Step 1. Visually estimate the LV systolic function

- If completely normal (LVEF >60%), proceed to step 2;
- If low normal or mildly reduced (LVEF = 40%–60%), proceed to step 3;
- If moderately or severely reduced (LVEF <40%), proceed to step 4.

Step 2. Evaluate LV structure (and consider assessment of myocardial mechanics)

- Evaluate relative LV wall thickness and calculate LV mass index
  - Categorize into normal, hypertrophy, or remodeling
- Measure the global longitudinal strain
- If both are normal, measure diastolic function (for HFpEF; structurally normal algorithm)
- Carefully evaluate the RV function and assess pulmonary pressures
- Consider stress echocardiography

Step 3. Quantify LV systolic function

- Use 2D and/or 3D volumetric method to quantify the LVEF
- Use LV contrast agent if 2 apical segments not adequately visualized
- If LVEF is <52% (male) or 54% (female), measure LV diastolic function using the structurally abnormal algorithm
- Carefully evaluate the RV function

Step 4. Hemodynamic and prognostic assessment

- Report the estimated LV filling pressures (LAP)
- Evaluate the RV hemodynamics (RAP, RVSP, PAD)
- Look for marked LV dyssynchrony and if QRS wide, consider CRT candidacy

Abbreviations: CRT, cardiac resynchronization therapy; HFpEF, heart failure with "preserved" ejection fraction; LAP, left atrial pressure; LV, left ventricular; LVEF, left ventricular ejection fraction; PAD, pulmonary artery diastolic pressure; RAP, right atrial pressure; RV, right ventricular; RVSP, right ventricular systolic pressure.

pressures, pulmonary artery pressures, and cardiac output can be determined sequentially. The authors believe that all patients with HF should undergo careful assessment with 2DE, M-mode echocardiography, and Doppler echocardiography (with strategic use of contrast and 3DE where available; **Box 2**). Furthermore, the authors believe the use of echocardiography is especially valuable in the elderly who have the poorest prognosis and are more likely to have HF with a normal LVEF or a reduced LVEF and no clinical symptoms.

REFERENCES

1. Kannel WB, Belanger AJ. Epidemiology of heart failure. Am Heart J 1991;121:951–7.
2. Komajda M, Hanon O, Hochadel M, et al. Contemporary management of octogenarians hospitalized for heart failure in Europe: Euro Heart Failure Survey II. Eur Heart J 2009;30:478–86.
3. Sorrell VL, Nanda NC. Role of echocardiography in the diagnostic assessment and etiology of heart failure in the elderly – opacify, quantify and rectify. Heart Fail Clin 2007;3:403–22.
4. Bonow RO, Udelson JE. Left ventricular diastolic dysfunction as a cause of congestive heart failure: mechanisms and management. Ann Intern Med 1992;117:502–10.
5. Ihlen H, Amlie JP, Dale J, et al. Determination of cardiac output by Doppler echocardiography. Br Heart J 1984;51:54.
6. Ghali JK, Kadakia S, Cooper RS, et al. Bedside diagnosis of preserved versus impaired left ventricular systolic function in heart failure. Am J Cardiol 1992;67:1002–6.
7. Wong M, Staszewsky L, Latini R, et al. Severity of left ventricular remodeling defines outcomes and response to therapy in heart failure: Valsartan Heart Failure Trial (Val-HeFT) echocardiographic data. J Am Coll Cardiol 2004;43:2022.
8. Quinones MA, Greenberg BH, Kopelen HA, et al. Echocardiographic predictors of clinical outcome in patients with left ventricular dysfunction enrolled in the SOLVD registry and trials: significance of left ventricular hypertrophy. J Am Coll Cardiol 2000;35:1237.
9. Aronow WS, Ahn C, Kronzon I. Prognosis of congestive heart failure in elderly patients with normal versus abnormal left ventricular systolic function associated with coronary artery disease. Am J Cardiol 1990;66:1257–9.
10. Cohn JN, Johnson G. Heart failure with normal ejection fraction. The V-HeFT study. Veterans Administration Cooperative Study Group. Circulation 1980;81(2 suppl):III-48-53.
11. Grayburn PA, Appleton CP, DeMaria AN, et al. Echocardiographic predictors of morbidity and mortality in patients with advanced heart failure: the Beta-blocker Evaluation of Survival Trial (BEST). J Am Coll Cardiol 2005;45:1064.
12. White HD, Norris RM, Brown MA, et al. Left ventricular end-systolic volume as the major determinant of survival after recovery from myocardial infarction. Circulation 1987;76:44.
13. Parisi AF, Moyihan PF, Folland ED, et al. Approaches to determination of left ventricular volumes and ejection fraction by real-time two dimensional echocardiography. Clin Cardiol 1979;2:257.
14. Caidahl K, Kazzam E, Lidberg J, et al. New concept in echocardiography: harmonic imaging of tissue without use of a contrast agent. Lancet 1998;352:1264–70.
15. Senior R. Role of contrast echocardiography for the assessment of left ventricular function. Echocardiography 1999;16:747–52.
16. Malm S, Frigstad S, Sagberg E, et al. Accurate and reproducible measurement of left ventricular volume and ejection fraction by contrast echocardiography: a comparison with magnetic resonance imaging. J Am Coll Cardiol 2004;44:1030–5.
17. Vandenberg BF, Rath LS, Stuhlmuller P, et al. Estimation of left ventricular cavity area with an on-line, semi-automated echocardiographic edge detection system. Circulation 1992;86:159–66.
18. Corsi C, Lang RM, Veronesi F, et al. Volumetric quantification of global and regional left ventricular function from real-time three-dimensional echocardiographic images. Circulation 2005;112:1161.
19. Lang RM, Badano LP, Mor-Avi V, et al. Recommendations for cardiac chamber quantification by echocardiography in adults: an update from the American Society of Echocardiography and the European Association of Cardiovascular Imaging. J Am Soc Echocardiogr 2015;28:1–39.
20. Marcus ML, Skorton DJ, Schelbert HR, et al, editors. Cardiac imaging: a companion to Braunwald's heart disease. 3rd edition. Philadelphia: W.B. Saunders; 1991. p. 377.
21. Cahill JM, Ryan E, Travers B, et al. Progression of preserved systolic function heart failure to systolic dysfunction: a natural history study. Int J Cardiol 2006;106:95–102.
22. Sorrell VL, Reeves WC. Noninvasive right and left heart catheterization: taking the echo lab beyond an image-only laboratory. Echocardiography 2001;18:31–41.
23. Mor-Avi V, Lang RM, Badano LP, et al. Current and evolving techniques for the quantitative evaluation of cardiac mechanics: ASE/EAE consensus statement on methodology and indications. J Am Soc Echocardiogr 2011;24:277–313.
24. Marwick TH. Measurement of strain and strain rate by echocardiography: ready for prime time? J Am Coll Cardiol 2006;47:1313.

25. Xia JZ, Xia JY, Li G, et al. Left ventricular strain examination of different aged adults with 3D speckle tracking echocardiography. Echocardiography 2014;31:335–9.
26. Zile MR, Gaasch WH, Carroll JD, et al. Heart failure with a normal ejection fraction: is measurement of diastolic function necessary to make the diagnosis of diastolic heart failure? Circulation 2001;104:779.
27. Thomas JD, Weyman AE. Echocardiographic Doppler evaluation of left ventricular diastolic function: physics and physiology. Circulation 1991; 84:977.
28. Nagueh SF, Smiseth OA, Appleton CP, et al. Recommendations for the evaluation of left ventricular diastolic function by echocardiography: an update from the American Society of Echocardiography and the European Society of Cardiovascular Imaging. J Am Soc Echocardiogr 2016;29:277–314.
29. Nishimura RA, Tajik AJ. Evaluation of diastolic filling of the left ventricle in health and disease: Doppler echocardiography is the clinician's Rosetta stone. J Am Coll Cardiol 1997;30:8–18.
30. Pinamonti B, Zecchin M, Di Lenarda A, et al. Persistence of restrictive left ventricular filling pattern in dilated cardiomyopathy: an ominous prognostic sign. J Am Coll Cardiol 1997;29:604–12.
31. Oh JK, Seward JB, Tajik AJ. The echo manual. 2nd edition. Philadelphia: Lippincott Raven; 1999. p. 53.
32. Dumesnil JG, Gaudreault G, Honos GN, et al. Use of Valsalva maneuver to unmask left ventricular diastolic function abnormalities by Doppler echocardiography in patients with coronary artery disease or systemic hypertension. Am J Cardiol 1991;68: 515–9.
33. Marwick TH. Clinical applications of tissue Doppler imaging: a promise fulfilled. Heart 2003;89:1377.
34. Klein AL, Burstow DJ, Tajik AJ, et al. Effects of age on left ventricular dimensions and filling dynamics in 117 normal persons. Mayo Clin Proc 1994;69:212.
35. Nagueh SF, Kopellen HA, Quinones MA. Assessment of left ventricular filling pressures by Doppler in the presence of atrial fibrillation. Circulation 1996;94:2138–45.
36. Hurrell DG, Oh JK, Mahoney DW, et al. Short deceleration time of mitral inflow E velocity: prognostic implication with atrial fibrillation versus sinus rhythm. J Am Soc Echocardiogr 1998;11:450–7.
37. Ristow B, Ahmed S, Wang L, et al. Pulmonary regurgitation end-diastolic gradient is a Doppler marker of cardiac status: data from the Heart and Soul Study. J Am Soc Echocardiogr 2005;18:885–91.
38. Drazner MH, Hamilton MA, Fonarow G, et al. Relationship between right and left-sided filling pressures in 1000 patients with advanced heart failure. J Heart Lung Transplant 1999;18:1126.
39. Sohn DW, Chai IH, Lee DJ, et al. Assessment of mitral annulus velocity by Doppler tissue imaging in the evaluation of left ventricular diastolic function. J Am Coll Cardiol 1997;30:474–80.
40. Thomas JD, Greenberg NA, Vandervoort PM, et al. Digital analysis of transmitral color Doppler M-mode data: a potential new approach to the noninvasive assessment of diastolic function. Comput Cardiol 1992;1(1):631–4.
41. Moller JE, Sondergaard E, Seward JB, et al. Ratio of left ventricular peak E-wave velocity to flow propagation velocity assessed by color M-mode Doppler echocardiography in first myocardial infarction: prognostic and clinical implications. J Am Coll Cardiol 2000;35:363.
42. Bruch C, Gotzmann M, Sindermann J, et al. Prognostic value of a restrictive mitral filling pattern in patients with systolic heart failure and an implantable cardioverter-defibrillator. Am J Cardiol 2006;97: 676–80.
43. Liang HY, Cauduro SA, Pellikka PA, et al. Comparison of usefulness of echocardiographic Doppler variables to left ventricular end-diastolic pressure in predicting future heart failure events. Am J Cardiol 2006;97:866–71.
44. Klein AL, Hatle LK, Taliercio CP, et al. Prognostic significance of Doppler measures of diastolic function in cardiac amyloidosis: a Doppler echocardiography study. Circulation 1991;83:808–16.
45. Vanoverschelde JL, Raphael DA, Robert AR, et al. Left ventricular filling in dilated cardiomyopathy: relation to functional class and hemodynamics. J Am Coll Cardiol 1990;15:1288–95.
46. Pozzoli M, Traversi E, Cioffi G, et al. Loading manipulation improves the prognostic value of Doppler evaluation of mitral valve flow in patients with chronic heart failure. Circulation 1997;95:1222–30.
47. Temporelli PL, Corra U, Imparto A, et al. Reversible restrictive left ventricular diastolic filling with optimized oral therapy predicts a more favorable prognosis in patients with chronic heart failure. J Am Coll Cardiol 1998;31:1591–7.
48. Duncan AM, Lim E, Gibson DG, et al. Effect of dobutamine stress on left ventricular filling in ischemic dilated cardiomyopathy: pathophysiology and prognostic implications. J Am Coll Cardiol 2005;46:488–96.
49. Richardson P, McKenna W, Bristow M, et al. Report of the 1995 World Health Organization/International Society and Federation of Cardiology Task Force on the Definition and Classification of Cardiomyopathies. Circulation 1996;93:841–2.
50. Simonson JS, Schiller NB. Descent of the base of the left ventricle: an echocardiographic index of left ventricular function. J Am Soc Echocardiogr 1989; 2:25–35.
51. Vandenbossche JL, Massie BM, Schiller NB, et al. Relation of left ventricular shape to volume and mass in patients with minimally symptomatic chronic aortic regurgitation. Am Heart J 1988;116:1022–7.

52. Gorcsan J III, Denault A, Gasior TA, et al. Rapid estimation of left ventricular contractility from end-systolic relations by echocardiographic automated border detection and femoral arterial pressure. Anesthesiology 1994;81:553–62.
53. Yoerger DM, Marcus FL, Sherrill D, et al, Multidisciplinary Study of Right Ventricular Dysplasia Investigators. Echocardiographic findings in patients meeting task force criteria for arrhythmogenic right ventricular dysplasia: new insights from the multidisciplinary study of right ventricular dysplasia. J Am Coll Cardiol 2005;45:860–5.
54. Cerqueira MD, Weissman NJ, Dilsizian V, et al. Standardized myocardial segmentation and nomenclature for tomographic imaging of the heart. A statement for healthcare professionals from the Cardiac Imaging Committee of the Council on Clinical Cardiology of the American Heart Association. Circulation 2002;105:539–42.
55. Acquatella H, Schiller NB. Echocardiographic recognition of Chagas' disease and endomyocardial fibrosis. J Am Soc Echocardiogr 1988;1:60–8.
56. Bodiwala K, Miller AP, Nanda NC, et al. Live three-dimensional transthoracic echocardiographic assessment of ventricular noncompaction. Echocardiogr 2005;22:611–20.
57. Nanda NC, Gramiak R, Robinson TI, et al. Echocardiographic evaluation of pulmonary hypertension. Circulation 1974;50:575–81.
58. McConnell MV, Solomon SD, Rayan ME, et al. Regional right ventricular dysfunction detected by echocardiography in acute pulmonary embolism. Am J Cardiol 1996;78:469–73.
59. Kotler MN, Mintz GS, Parry WR, et al. Bedside diagnosis of organic murmurs in the elderly. Geriatrics 1981;36:107–25.
60. Baumgartner H, Hung J, Bernejo J, et al. Echocardiographic assessment of valve stenosis: EAE/ASE recommendations for clinical practice. J Am Soc Echocardiogr 2009;22:1–22.
61. Fan PH, Kapur KK, Nanda NC. Color-guided Doppler echocardiographic assessment in assessment of aortic valve stenosis. J Am Coll Cardiol 1998;12:441–9.
62. Naqvi TZ, Siegel RJ. Aortic stenosis: the role of transesophageal echocardiography. Echocardiogr 1999;16:677–88.
63. Bermejo J, Garcia-Fernandez MA, Antoranz JC, et al. Stress echocardiography in aortic stenosis: insights into valve mechanics and hemodynamics. Echocardiogr 1999;16:689–99.
64. Vengala S, Nanda NC, Dod H, et al. Usefulness of live three-dimensional transthoracic echocardiography in aortic valve stenosis evaluation. Am J Geriatr Cardiol 2004;13:279–84.
65. Zoghbi WA, Enriquez-Sarano M, Foster E, et al. Recommendations for evaluation of the severity of native valvular regurgitation with two-dimensional and Doppler echocardiography. J Am Soc Echocardiogr 2003;16:777–802.
66. Bargiggia GS, Tronconi L, Sahn DJ, et al. A new method for quantitation of mitral regurgitation based on color flow Doppler imaging of flow convergence proximal to regurgitant orifice. Circulation 1991;84:1481–9.
67. Khanna D, Vengala S, Miller AP, et al. Quantification of mitral regurgitation by live three-dimensional transthoracic echocardiographic measurements of vena contracta area. Echocardiography 2004;21:737–43.
68. Khanna D, Miller AP, Nanda NC, et al. Transthoracic and transesophageal echocardiographic assessment of mitral regurgitation severity: usefulness of qualitative and semi-quantitative techniques. Echocardiography 2005;22:748–69.
69. Ling LH, Enriquez-Sarano M, Seward JB, et al. Clinical outcome of mitral regurgitation due to flail leaflet. N Engl J Med 1996;335:1417–23.
70. Ghio S, Recusani F, Klersy C, et al. Prognostic usefulness of the tricuspid annular plane systolic excursion in patients with congestive heart failure secondary to idiopathic or ischemic dilated cardiomyopathy. Am J Cardiol 2000;85:837–42.
71. Rudski LG, Lai WW, Afilalo J, et al. Guidelines for the echocardiographic assessment of the right heart in adults: a report from the American Society of Echocardiography. J Am Soc Echocardiogr 2010;23:685–713.
72. Nath J, Vacek JL, Heidenreich PA. A dilated inferior vena cava is a marker of poor survival. Am Heart J 2006;151:730–5.
73. De Groote P, Millaire A, Foucher-Hossein C, et al. Right ventricular ejection fraction is an independent predictor of survival in patients with moderate heart failure. J Am Coll Cardiol 1998;32:948–54.
74. Hung J, Koelling T, Semigran MJ, et al. Usefulness of echocardiographic determined tricuspid regurgitation in predicting event-free survival in severe heart failure secondary to idiopathic-dilated cardiomyopathy or to ischemic cardiomyopathy. Am J Cardiol 1998;82:1301–3.
75. Bleeker GB, Schalij MJ, Molhoek SG, et al. Comparison of effectiveness of cardiac resynchronization therapy in patients <70 versus > or = 70 years of age. Am J Cardiol 2005;96:420–2.
76. Suffoletto MS, Dohi K, Cannesson M, et al. Novel speckle-tracking radial strain from routine black-and-white echocardiographic images to quantify dyssynchrony and predict response to cardiac resynchronization therapy. Circulation 2006;113:960–8.
77. Iriarte M, Murga N, Sagastagoitia D, et al. Congestive heart failure from left ventricular diastolic dysfunction in systemic hypertension. Am J Cardiol 1993;71:308–12.

78. Gola A, Pozzoli M, Capomolla S, et al. Comparison of Doppler echocardiography with thermodilution for assessing cardiac output in advanced congestive heart failure. Am J Cardiol 1996;78:708–12.
79. Tei C, Ling LH, Hodge DO, et al. New index of combined systolic and diastolic myocardial performance: a simple and reproducible measure of cardiac function: a study in normals and dilated cardiomyopathy. J Cardiol 1995;26:357–66.
80. Tei C, Dujardin KS, Hodge DO, et al. Doppler echocardiographic index for assessment of global right ventricular function. J Am Soc Echocardiogr 1996; 9:838–47.
81. Lee R, Hanekom L, Marwick TH, et al. Prediction of subclinical left ventricular dysfunction with strain rate imaging in patients with asymptomatic severe mitral regurgitation. Am J Cardiol 2004;94:1333–7.
82. Redfield MM, Jacobsen SJ, Burnett JC Jr, et al. Burden of systolic and diastolic ventricular dysfunction in the community: appreciating the scope of the heart failure epidemic. JAMA 2003;289:194–202.
83. Mosterd A, Hoes AW, de Bruyne MC, et al. Prevalence of heart failure and left ventricular dysfunction in the general population: the Rotterdam study. Eur Heart J 1999;20:447–55.
84. Davies M, Hobbs F, Davis R, et al. Prevalence of left-ventricular systolic dysfunction and heart failure in the Echocardiographic Heart of England Screening Study: a population-based study. Lancet 2001;358: 439–44.
85. McDonagh TA, Morrison CE, Lawrence A, et al. Symptomatic and asymptomatic left ventricular systolic dysfunction in an urban population. Lancet 1997;350:829–33.
86. Devereux RB, Roman MJ, Paranicas M, et al. A population-based assessment of left ventricular systolic dysfunction in middle-aged and older adults: the Strong Heart Study. Am Heart J 2001; 141:439–46.
87. Abhayaratna WP, Smith WT, Becker NG, et al. Prevalence of heart failure and systolic ventricular dysfunction in older Australians: the Canberra Heart Study. Med J Aust 2006;184:151–4.
88. Kannel WB. Epidemiology and prevention of cardiac failure: Framingham Study insights. Eur Heart J 1987;8(Suppl F):23–6.
89. Koilpillai C, Quinones MA, Greenberg B, et al. Relation of ventricular size and function to heart failure status and ventricular dysrhythmia in patients with severe left ventricular dysfunction. Am J Cardiol 1996;78:606–11.
90. Senni M, Rodeheffer RJ, Tribouilloy CM, et al. Use of echocardiography in the management of congestive heart failure in the community. J Am Coll Cardiol 1999;33:164–70.

Treatment of Heart Failure with Abnormal Left Ventricular Systolic Function in Older Adults

Wilbert S. Aronow, MD

KEYWORDS

- Heart failure • Myocardial infarction • Beta blockers • Angiotensin-converting enzyme inhibitors
- Nitrates • Aldosterone antagonists • Digoxin • Positive inotropic drugs

KEY POINTS

- Use diuretics and salt restriction in patients with heart failure (HF), abnormal left ventricular (LV) ejection fraction, and fluid retention.
- Use angiotensin-converting enzyme (ACE) inhibitors in patients with HF and abnormal LV ejection fraction.
- Use β-blockers (carvedilol, sustained-release metoprolol succinate, or bisoprolol) in patients with HF and abnormal LV ejection fraction.
- Use angiotensin II receptor blockers if intolerant to ACE inhibitors because of cough or angioneurotic edema in patients with HF and abnormal LV ejection fraction.
- Sacubitril/valsartan may be used instead of an ACE inhibitor or ARB in chronic symptomatic HF and abnormal LV ejection fraction class II or III.

The American College of Cardiology (ACC)/American Heart Association (AHA) guidelines for the evaluation and management of heart failure (HF) define 4 stages of HF.[1,2] Patients with stage A HF are at high risk of developing HF because of conditions strongly associated with the development of HF.[1,2] These patients have hypertension, coronary artery disease, diabetes mellitus, a history of cardiotoxic drug therapy, alcohol abuse, a history of rheumatic fever, or a family history of cardiomyopathy. These patients have no evidence of structural heart disease.

Patients with stage B HF have structural heart disease associated with the development of HF, but have never shown symptoms or signs of HF.[1,2] These patients have a prior myocardial infarction, left ventricular (LV) hypertrophy or fibrosis, LV dilatation or hypocontractility, or asymptomatic valvular heart disease.[1,2]

Patients with stage C HF have current or prior symptoms of HF associated with structural heart disease.[1,2] Patients with stage D HF have advanced structural heart disease and marked symptoms of HF at rest despite maximal medical therapy. These patients require specialized interventions.[1,2]

TREATMENT OF STAGE A HEART FAILURE

In patients with stage A HF, clinicians should treat hypertension[1–4] and lipid disorders[1,2,5–7]; encourage regular exercise; discourage smoking, alcohol consumption, and illicit drug use; control the ventricular

This is an updated version of an article that appeared in *Heart Failure Clinics*, Volume 3, Issue 4.
Disclosure Statement: The author has nothing to disclose.
Division of Cardiology, Department of Medicine, Westchester Medical Center, New York Medical College, Macy Pavilion, Room 141, Valhalla, NY 10595, USA
E-mail address: wsaronow@aol.com

Heart Failure Clin 13 (2017) 467–483
http://dx.doi.org/10.1016/j.hfc.2017.02.004
1551-7136/17/

rate in patients with supraventricular tachyarrhythmias; and use angiotensin-converting enzyme (ACE) inhibitors in patients with atherosclerotic vascular disease, diabetes mellitus, or hypertension.[1,2] Diabetics should be treated as if they had coronary artery disease.[8] Educational programs may be needed to increase the use of lipid-lowering drugs.[9,10]

TREATMENT OF STAGE B HEART FAILURE

The ACC/AHA guidelines recommend in patients with stage B HF treatment with all stage A measures, treatment with ACE inhibitors and β-blockers, and valve replacement or repair for patients with hemodynamically significant valvular stenosis or regurgitation.[1]

GENERAL MEASURE FOR TREATMENT OF STAGE C HEART FAILURE

Underlying and precipitating causes of HF should be identified and treated when possible. Hypertension should be treated with diuretics, ACE inhibitors, and β-blockers.[2,11] Myocardial ischemia should be treated with nitrates and β-blockers.[2,11]

Older persons who have HF without contraindications to coronary revascularization, and who have exercise-limiting angina pectoris, angina pectoris occurring frequently at rest, or recurrent episodes of acute pulmonary edema despite optimal medical therapy, should undergo coronary angiography. Coronary artery bypass graft surgery or percutaneous transluminal coronary angioplasty should be performed in selected patients with myocardial ischemia attributable to viable myocardium subserved by severely stenotic coronary arteries.

If indicated clinically, selected patients should undergo surgical correction of valvular lesions, surgical excision of a dyskinetic LV aneurysm, surgical correction of a systemic arteriovenous fistula, and surgical resection of the pericardium for constrictive pericarditis. Infective endocarditis should be treated with intravenous antibiotics and with surgical replacement of valvular lesions if indicated clinically. Anemia, infection, bronchospasm, hypoxia, tachyarrhythmias, bradyarrhythmias, obesity, hyperthyroidism, and hypothyroidism should be treated.

Oral warfarin should be given to patients with HF who have prior systemic or pulmonary embolism, atrial fibrillation, or cardiac thrombi detected by 2-dimensional echocardiography.[12] The dose of warfarin administered should achieve an International Normalized Ratio of 2.0 to 3.0. Newer oral anticoagulants such as dabigatran,[13] rivaroxaban,[14] apixaban,[15] or edoxaban[16] may be used instead of warfarin to prevent thromboembolic events in patients with cystic fibrosis who have nonvalvular atrial fibrillation.

A surgical procedure should be performed if anticoagulant therapy fails to prevent pulmonary embolism. Beriberi heart disease should be treated with thiamine. A transvenous pacemaker should be implanted into the right ventricle of a patient with HF and complete atrioventricular block or severe bradycardia.

Patients with HF should have their sodium intake reduced to 1.6 to 2.0 g of sodium daily (4–5 g of sodium chloride). Spices and herbs instead of sodium chloride should be used to flavor food. Normal fluid intake with sodium restriction is the general recommendation. Fluid intake should be restricted if dilutional hyponatremia develops and the serum sodium concentration falls below 130 mEq/L. Through patient education, patient compliance should be stressed, such as the need for salt restriction, fluid restriction, and daily weight checks.

Patients with HF should avoid exposure to heavy air pollution. Air conditioning is essential for patients with HF who are in hot, humid environments. Ethyl alcohol intake should be avoided. Medications that precipitate or exacerbate HF, such as nonsteroidal antiinflammatory and antiarrhythmic drugs, other than β-blockers, digoxin, amiodarone, and dofetilide, should be stopped (**Box 1**).[1] Regular physical activity, such as walking, should be encouraged in patients with mild-to-moderate HF to improve functional status and to decrease symptoms. Patients with HF who are dyspneic at rest at a low work level may benefit from a formal cardiac rehabilitation program (see **Box 1**).[1,2,17] A multidisciplinary approach to care is useful.[18] **Box 1** shows the class I recommendations for treating HF with a reduced LV ejection fraction.[2,19] **Box 2** shows the class IIa recommendations for treating HF with a reduced LV ejection fraction.[2,19]

DIURETICS

Diuretics are the first-line drugs in the treatment of older patients with HF and volume overload (see **Box 1**). Diuretics decrease venous return, reduce ventricular filling pressures, cause loss of fluid from the body, and decrease symptoms of pulmonary and systemic congestion and edema. Age-related decreases in renal function and in circulating plasma volume may reduce the efficacy of diuretics in elderly patients with HF.

A thiazide diuretic, such as hydrochlorothiazide, may be used to treat elderly patients with

Box 1
Class I recommendations for treating HF with abnormal LV systolic function

- Use all class I recommendations for treating stage A and B HF.
- Use diuretics and salt restriction in patients with fluid retention.
- Use ACE inhibitors.
- Use β-blockers (carvedilol, sustained-release metoprolol succinate, or bisoprolol).
- Use angiotensin II receptor blockers (candesartan or valsartan) if intolerant to ACE inhibitors because of cough or angioneurotic edema.
- Sacubitril/valsartan may be used instead of an ACE inhibitor or angiotensin II receptor blocker in patients with chronic symptomatic HF and abnormal LV ejection fraction class II or III to further reduce morbidity and mortality.
- Avoid or withdraw nonsteroidal antiinflammatory drugs, most antiarrhythmic drugs, and most calcium channel blockers.
- Recommend exercise training.
- Implant a cardioverter-defibrillator in patients with a history of cardiac arrest, ventricular fibrillation, or hemodynamically unstable ventricular tachycardia.
- Implant a cardioverter-defibrillator in selected patients with HF at least 40 days after acute MI with an LV ejection fraction of 35% or less or nonischemic cardiomyopathy and NYHA functional class II or III symptoms on chronic guided directed medical therapy with a reasonable expectation of meaningful survival for more than 1 year.
- Implant a cardioverter-defibrillator in patients with ischemic heart disease 40 or more days after an MI or nonischemic cardiomyopathy, a LV ejection fraction 30% or less, NYHA functional class I symptoms on optimal medical therapy, and an expectation of survival of 1 year or longer.
- Cardiac resynchronization therapy is indicated for patients with HF, a LV ejection fraction of 35% or less, NYHA functional class II, III, or ambulatory IV symptoms on guided, directed medical therapy, sinus rhythm, and left bundle branch block with a QRS duration of 150 ms or greater.
- Add an aldosterone antagonist (spironolactone or eplerenone) in selected patients with NYHA functional class II to IV HF who can be carefully monitored for renal function and potassium concentration (serum creatinine should be ≤2.5 mg/dL in men and ≤2.0 mg/dL in women; serum potassium should be <5.0 mEq/L).
- Add isosorbide dinitrate plus hydralazine in patients self-described as African Americans with NYHA functional class II to IV HF with abnormal LV ejection fraction who are being treated with diuretics, ACE inhibitors, and β-blockers

Abbreviations: ACE, angiotensin-converting enzyme; HF, heart failure; LV, left ventricular; MI, myocardial infarction; NYHA, New York Heart Association.

Adapted from Yancy CW, Jessup M, Bozkurt B, et al. 2013 ACCF/ AHA guideline for the management of heart failure: a report of the American College of Cardiology Foundation/American Heart Association Task Force on Practice Guidelines. J Am Coll Cardiol 2013;62:e147–239; and Yancy CW, Jessup M, Bozkurt B, et al. 2016 ACC/AHA/HFSA focused update on new pharmacologic therapy for heart failure: an update of the 2013 ACCF/AHA guideline for the management of heart failure: a report of the American College of Cardiology/American Heart Association Task Force on Clinical Practice Guidelines and the Heart Failure Society of America. J Am Coll Cardiol 2016;68(13):1476–88, with permission.

mild HF. However, a thiazide diuretic is ineffective if the glomerular filtration rate is less than 30 mL/min. Elderly patients with moderate or severe HF should be treated with a loop diuretic such as furosemide. These patients should not take nonsteroidal antiinflammatory drugs because these drugs may inhibit the induction of diuresis by furosemide. Elderly patients with severe HF or concomitant renal insufficiency may need the addition of metolazone to the loop diuretic. Severe volume overload should be treated with intravenous diuretics and hospitalization.

Older patients with HF treated with diuretics need close monitoring of their serum electrolytes. Hypokalemia and hypomagnesemia, both of which may precipitate ventricular arrhythmias and digitalis toxicity, may develop. Hyponatremia with activation of the renin–angiotensin–aldosterone system may occur.

Box 2
Class IIa recommendations for treating HF with abnormal left ventricular systolic function

- Angiotensin II receptor blockers may be used instead of ACE inhibitors if patients are already taking them for other indications.
- Hydralazine plus a nitrate may be used in patients with persistent symptoms who cannot be given an ACE inhibitor or angiotensin II receptor blocker because of drug intolerance, hypotension, or renal insufficiency
- Implant a cardioverter-defibrillator in patients with a LV ejection fraction of 30% to 35% of any origin with class II or III symptoms on optimal medical therapy with a life expectancy of greater than 1 year.
- Digoxin can be used in patients with persistent symptoms to reduce hospitalization for HF.
- CRT can be used in patients with HF, an LV ejection fraction of 35% or less, class III or ambulatory IV symptoms on guided directed medical therapy, sinus rhythm, and a non–LBBB pattern with a QRS duration of 150 ms or greater.
- CRT can be used in patients with HF, an LV ejection fraction of 35% or less, class II, III, or ambulatory IV symptoms on guided directed medical therapy, sinus rhythm, and an LBBB pattern with a QRS duration of 120 to 149 ms.
- CRT can be used in patients with HF, atrial fibrillation, an LV ejection fraction of 35% or less on guided directed medical therapy if a) the patient needs ventricular pacing or otherwise meets CRT criteria and b) atrioventricular nodal ablation or pharmacologic rate control will allow near 100% ventricular pacing with CRT.
- CRT can be used in patients with HF on guided directed medical therapy, an LVEF of 35% or less, and who are undergoing placement of a new or replacement device with anticipated need for more than 40% ventricular pacing.
- Ivabradine can be beneficial to reduce hospitalization for class II or III stable chronic HF and abnormal LV ejection fraction in patients on guided directed medical therapy receiving a β-blocker at the maximum tolerated dose, and who are in sinus rhythm with a heart rate of 70 beats per minute or greater at rest.

Abbreviations: ACE, angiotensin-converting enzyme; CRT, cardiac resynchronization therapy; HF, heart failure; LBBB, left bundle branch block.

Adapted from Yancy CW, Jessup M, Bozkurt B, et al. 2013 ACCF/ AHA guideline for the management of heart failure: a report of the American College of Cardiology Foundation/American Heart Association Task Force on Practice Guidelines. J Am Coll Cardiol 2013;62:e147–239; and Yancy CW, Jessup M, Bozkurt B, et al. 2016 ACC/AHA/HFSA focused update on new pharmacologic therapy for heart failure: an update of the 2013 ACCF/AHA guideline for the management of heart failure: a report of the American College of Cardiology/American Heart Association Task Force on Clinical Practice Guidelines and the Heart Failure Society of America. J Am Coll Cardiol 2016;68(13):1476–88, with permission.

Older patients with HF are especially sensitive to volume depletion. Dehydration and prerenal azotemia may occur if excessive doses of diuretics are given. Therefore, the minimum effective dose of diuretics should be used. The dose of diuretics should be reduced gradually and stopped if possible when fluid retention is not present in patients with HF. Patients on high doses of diuretics have an increased mortality.[20] The use of diuretics in older patients with HF is discussed elsewhere in this issue.

ANGIOTENSIN-CONVERTING ENZYME INHIBITORS

ACE inhibitors are balanced vasodilators that decrease both afterload and preload. ACE inhibitors reduce systemic vascular resistance, arterial pressure, LV and right ventricular end-diastolic pressures, cardiac work, and myocardial oxygen consumption, and they increase cardiac output. ACE inhibitors decrease circulating levels of angiotensin II, reduce sympathetic nervous system activity, stimulate prostaglandin synthesis, and decrease sodium and water retention by inhibiting angiotensin II stimulation of aldosterone release. ACE inhibitors are very effective in treating HF associated with an abnormal LV ejection fraction (**Table 1**). The ability of ACE inhibitors to block aldosterone production is only partial and limited to approximately the first 6 months of therapy, with loss of efficacy thereafter.

ACE inhibitors improve symptoms, quality of life, and exercise tolerance in patients with HF. ACE inhibitors also increase survival in patients with HF and abnormal LV ejection fraction (see

Table 1
Effect of ACE inhibitors on survival in patients with HF and abnormal left ventricular ejection fraction

Study	Results
Cooperative North Scandinavian Enalapril Survival Study[21]	Compared with placebo, enalapril significantly decreased mortality 40% at 6 mo, 31% at 1 y, and 27% at the end of the study.
Veterans Administration Cooperative Vasodilator–Heart Failure Trial II[22]	Compared with hydralazine plus isosorbide dinitrate, enalapril significantly decreased mortality 28% at 2 y.
Studies of Left Ventricular Dysfunction Treatment Trial[23]	At 41-mo follow-up, enalapril, compared with placebo, significantly decreased mortality by 16%, death owing to progressive HF by 22%, and mortality or hospitalization for worsening HF by 26%.
Acute Infarction Ramipril Efficacy Study[24]	At 15-mo follow-up of patients with myocardial infarction and HF, ramipril, compared with placebo, significantly decreased mortality by 36% in patients aged ≥65 y.
Overview of 32 randomized trials of ACE inhibitors on mortality and morbidity in patients with HF[25]	Compared with placebo, ACE inhibitors significantly decreased mortality by 23% and mortality or hospitalization for HF by 35%.

Abbreviations: ACE, angiotensin-converting enzyme; HF, heart failure

Table 1)[20–25] and should be used to treat patients with HF and abnormal LV ejection fraction with a class I indication (see **Box 1**).[2,19] ACE inhibitors also improve survival and reduce the incidence of HF and coronary events in patients with abnormal LV ejection fraction but without HF.[26–29] ACE inhibitors should be used to treat these patients with a class I indication.[2,19]

ACE inhibitors should be started in older patients with HF in low doses after correction of hyponatremia or volume depletion. Avoid overdiuresis before initiating treatment with ACE inhibitors because volume depletion may cause hypotension or renal insufficiency when ACE inhibitors are started or when the dose of these drugs is increased to full therapeutic levels. After the maintenance dose of ACE inhibitors is reached, it may be necessary to increase the dose of diuretics.

Patients with HF and an abnormal LV ejection fraction were randomized to lisinopril 2.5 to 5.0 mg/d versus 32.5 to 35 mg/d.[30] At the 39- to 58-month follow-up, compared with low-dose lisinopril, high-dose lisinopril caused an 8% insignificant reduction in mortality, a significant 12% reduction in mortality or all-cause hospitalization, and a significant 24% reduction in hospitalization for HF.[29] The discontinuation of study drug was similar for the 2 treatment groups. These data indicate that patients with HF should be treated with high doses of ACE inhibitors unless low doses are the only doses that can be tolerated.

In the Veterans Administration Cooperative Vasodilator–Heart Failure Trial II, enalapril, compared with isosorbide dinitrate plus hydralazine, significantly reduced 2-year mortality by 28% because of a greater response to enalapril in whites than in African Americans.[22] This finding led to the study of isosorbide dinitrate versus placebo in African Americans with HF.[31] A report from the Studies of Left Ventricular Dysfunction databases showed that whites but not African Americans randomized to enalapril had a significant reduction in the risk of hospitalization for HF.[32] However, a post hoc analysis of the 4054 African American and white participants in the Studies of Left Ventricular Dysfunction Prevention Trial was performed to investigate whether enalapril had similar efficacy in preventing symptomatic HF in African Americans versus whites.[33] Despite the increased absolute risk in African Americans compared with whites for the progression of asymptomatic LV dysfunction, enalapril was equally efficacious in reducing the risk of HF in African Americans versus whites.[33]

Older patients at risk for excessive hypotension should have their blood pressure monitored closely for the first 2 weeks of ACE inhibitor therapy and whenever the physician increases the dose of ACE inhibitor or diuretic. Renal function should be monitored in patients administered ACE inhibitors to detect increases in blood urea nitrogen and in serum creatinine, especially in elderly patients with renal artery stenosis. A doubling in serum creatinine should lead the physician to consider renal dysfunction caused by ACE inhibitors, a need to decrease the dose of diuretics, or exacerbation of HF. Potassium supplements and potassium-sparing diuretics should not be given to patients receiving ACE inhibitors because ACE inhibitor therapy may cause hyperkalemia by blocking aldosterone production.

Asymptomatic hypotension with a systolic blood pressure between 80 and 90 mm Hg and a serum creatinine of ≤2.5 mg/dL are side effects of ACE inhibitors that should not necessarily cause discontinuation of this drug, but should cause the physician to reduce the dose of diuretics if the jugular venous pressure is normal and to consider decreasing the dose of ACE inhibitor. Contraindications to the use of ACE inhibitors are symptomatic hypotension, progressive azotemia, angioneurotic edema, hyperkalemia, intolerable cough, and rash.

ACE inhibitors inhibit the metabolic degradation of bradykinin, which promotes vascular synthesis of vasodilating prostaglandins.[34] Aspirin is a cyclooxygenase inhibitor that dose-dependently inhibits synthesis of prostaglandins in vascular tissues.[35] Aspirin in doses of 100 mg/d or less provides the desired antiplatelet effect without inhibiting synthesis of prostaglandins.

There are conflicting data about the importance of the negative interaction of aspirin with ACE inhibitors in the treatment of patients with HF. Some hemodynamic studies support the importance of this negative interaction,[36,37] whereas other hemodynamic studies do not.[38,39] Retrospective analyses of clinical studies have also shown conflicting data, with some studies supporting[40,41] and other studies not supporting[42–44] a negative interaction between aspirin and ACE inhibitors. In a study of elderly patients with HF treated with ACE inhibitors, aspirin did not affect outcomes negatively.[44] Until data from controlled clinical trials are available, a prudent approach to this controversy might be to decrease the dose of aspirin to 80 to 100 mg/d or substitute clopidogrel as an antiplatelet drug in patients with HF treated with ACE inhibitors. The dose of ACE inhibitors could also be increased to overcome aspirin-related attenuation.

ANGIOTENSIN RECEPTOR BLOCKERS

Angiotensin II is a potent vasoconstrictor that may impair LV function and cause the progression of HF through increased impedance of LV emptying, adverse long-term structural effects on the heart and vasculature,[45] and activation of other neurohormonal agonists, including norepinephrine, aldosterone, and endothelin.[46]

The angiotensin II type 1 receptor blocker losartan significantly reduced the rate of first hospitalization for HF by 32%, compared with placebo, at the 3.4-year follow up of patients with type 2 diabetes mellitus and nephropathy.[47] Losartan also significantly reduced hospitalization for HF by 41% compared with atenolol at the 4.7-year follow-up of diabetics with hypertension and electrocardiographic LV hypertrophy.[48]

In the ELITE II trial (Losartan Heart Failure Survival Study), 3152 patients aged 60 years or greater with New York Heart Association (NYHA) functional class II through IV HF and an LV ejection fraction of 40% or less were randomized in a double-blind trial to receive losartan 50 mg/d or captopril 50 mg 3 times daily.[49] Median follow-up was 555 days. More patients discontinued captopril because of adverse effects (14.7%) than discontinued losartan (9.7%).[49]

Mortality was insignificantly 13% less in patients treated with captopril than in patients treated with losartan, significantly 77% less in patients treated with captopril plus β-blockers than in patients treated with losartan plus β-blockers, and insignificantly 5% less in patients treated with captopril without β-blockers than in patients treated with losartan without β-blockers.[49] Hospital admissions for any cause were insignificantly 4% higher in patients treated with losartan than in patients treated with captopril.[49]

The Valsartan Heart Failure Trial randomized 5010 patients with NYHA functional class II through IV HF and an abnormal LV ejection fraction to valsartan 160 mg/d or placebo.[50] Ninety-three percent of the patients were treated with ACE inhibitors, 85% with diuretics, 67% with digoxin, and 35% with β-blockers. At the 23-month follow-up, mortality was similar in the 2 treatment groups.[50] Mortality plus morbidity was significantly reduced 13% in patients treated with valsartan. Valsartan significantly decreased mortality in patients treated with neither an ACE inhibitor nor β-blocker.[50]

The Valsartan in Acute Myocardial Infarction trial randomized 14,703 patients after myocardial infarction complicated by LV systolic dysfunction, HF, or both to valsartan 160 mg twice daily, valsartan 80 mg twice daily plus captopril 50 mg 3 times daily, or captopril 50 mg 3 times daily.[51] At a median of 25 months of follow-up, all-cause mortality was similar in the 3 groups. Hypotension and renal dysfunction were more common in patients treated with valsartan, whereas cough, rash, and taste disturbance were more common in patients treated with captopril.[51] Combining valsartan with captopril increased the incidence of adverse effects without improving survival.[51]

In the Candesartan in Heart Failure: Assessment of Reduction in Mortality and Morbidity: Alternative Study, 2028 patients with HF, an abnormal LV ejection fraction, and intolerance to ACE inhibitors were randomized to candesartan 32 mg once daily or placebo.[52] At a median of 34 months of follow-up, candesartan significantly reduced the incidence of cardiovascular death or hospitalization for HF by 30%.[52]

In the Candesartan in Heart Failure: Assessment of Reduction in Mortality and Morbidity Added Study, 2548 patients with HF and an abnormal LV ejection fraction treated with ACE inhibitors were randomized to candesartan 32 mg/d or to placebo.[53] At a median of 41 months of follow-up, the addition of candesartan to an ACE inhibitor significantly reduced cardiovascular death or hospitalization for HF by 15%.[53]

On the basis of these data,[49–53] the author concurs with the ACC/AHA guidelines[2,19] that (1) an angiotensin receptor blocker (ARB) should be used for treating HF if the patient cannot tolerate an ACE inhibitor because of cough or angioneurotic edema with a class I indication (see **Boxes 1** and **2**); an ARB instead of an ACE inhibitor should be used if the patient is already on an ARB with a class IIa indication (see **Box 2**).[2,19]

β-BLOCKERS

Chronic administration of β-blockers after myocardial infarction decreases mortality, sudden cardiac death, and recurrent myocardial infarction, especially in elderly patients.[54–56] These benefits are more marked in patients with a history of HF.[56]

β-Blockers have been shown to reduce mortality in elderly patients with complex ventricular arrhythmias associated with prior myocardial infarction and an abnormal[57] or normal[58] LV ejection fraction. In patients with a prior myocardial infarction, abnormal LV ejection fraction, and complex ventricular arrhythmias, β-blockers caused a significant 32% decrease in occurrence of new or worsened HF.[57] The benefit of β-blockers in decreasing coronary events in elderly patients with a prior myocardial infarction is also especially increased in patients with diabetes mellitus,[59] peripheral arterial disease,[60] and abnormal LV ejection fraction.[29,61] β-Blockers significantly reduce mortality in elderly patients with HF and abnormal LV ejection fraction (**Table 2**).[62–66]

β-Blockers are effective in antagonizing neurohormonal systems that cause myocyte apoptosis, myocyte necrosis, myocyte hypertrophy, fetal gene program activation, extracellular matrix alterations, and β-receptor uncoupling.[67] β-Blockers may prevent or reverse increased systemic vascular resistance and increased afterload caused by excessive sympathetic nervous system activation. β-Blockers also reduce levels of atrial natriuretic peptide, brain natriuretic peptide, and tumor necrosis alpha levels.[68] β-Blockers are also effective in preventing cardiovascular events because of their antihypertensive, antiischemic, antiarrhythmic, and antiatherogenic effects.[69] The increase in ventricular rate that occurs after exercise can also be prevented with modest doses of β-blockers, especially in elderly patients.

β-Blockers reduce all-cause mortality, cardiovascular mortality, sudden death, and death from worsening HF in patients with HF.[62–66] β-Blockers significantly reduce mortality in African Americans[62,64,65] and in whites[62–66] with HF, in women and in men with HF,[62–66] in older and in younger patients with HF,[62–66] in diabetics and in nondiabetics with HF,[62–66] and in patients with severe HF and with mild or moderate HF.[62–64,66] β-Blockers should be used to treat patients with HF and abnormal LV ejection fraction with a class I indication (see **Table 2**)[2,19] unless there are contraindications to their use. Carvedilol and extended-release or controlled-release metoprolol are the only β-blockers that have been approved by the US Food and Drug Administration for the treatment of HF in the United States. Bisoprolol is also approved for the treatment of HF in Europe.

Patients with prior myocardial infarction and asymptomatic abnormal LV ejection fraction should be treated with ACE inhibitors plus β-blockers.[1,2,29,70,71] An observational prospective study was performed in 477 patients (196 men and 281 women; mean age, 79 years) with prior myocardial infarction and abnormal LV ejection fraction (mean LV ejection fraction, 31%).[29] At the 34-month follow-up, ACE inhibitors alone significantly reduced new coronary events by 17% and new HF by 32%, and β-blocker alone significantly reduced new coronary events by 25% and new HF by 41%, compared with no β-blocker or ACE inhibitor.[29] At the 41-month follow-up, ACE inhibitors plus β-blockers significantly reduced new coronary events by 37% and new HF by 61%, compared with no β-blocker or ACE inhibitor.[29] The significantly longer follow-up time in patients treated with ACE inhibitors plus β-blockers indicates that β-blockers plus ACE inhibitors delayed as well as decreased the occurrence of new coronary events and HF.[29]

Patients with HF should be treated with an ACE inhibitor or ARB and be in a relatively stable condition without the need of intravenous inotropic therapy and without signs of marked fluid retention before initiating β-blocker therapy.[72] β-Blockers should be initiated in a low dose, such as carvedilol 3.125 mg twice daily or extended-release or controlled-release metoprolol 12.5 mg/d if there is NYHA functional class III or IV HF, or 25 mg/d if there is NYHA functional class II HF. The dose of β-blockers should be doubled at 2- to 3-week

Table 2
Effect of β-blockers on mortality in patients with HF

Study	Results
Packer et al,[62] 1996 (n = 1094)	At 6- to 12-mo follow-up of patients with NYHA functional class II, III, or IV HF and abnormal LV ejection fraction, carvedilol, compared with placebo, significantly decreased mortality 65%.
The Cardiac Insufficiency Bisoprolol Study II (CIBIS II)[63] (n = 2647)	At 1.3-y follow-up of patients with NYHA functional class III or IV HF and abnormal LV ejection fraction, bisoprolol, compared with placebo, significantly decreased mortality 34%.
Metoprolol CR/XL Randomised Intervention Trial in Congestive Heart Failure (MERIT-HF)[64] (n = 3991)	At 1-y follow-up of patients with NYHA functional class II, III, or IV HF and abnormal LV ejection fraction, extended-release or controlled-release metoprolol (metoprolol CR/XL), compared with placebo, significantly decreased mortality 34%.
Carvedilol Prospective Randomized Cumulative Survival Trial (COPERNICUS)[65] (n = 2289)	At 10.4-mo follow-up of patients with severe HF and abnormal LV ejection fraction, carvedilol, compared with placebo, significantly reduced mortality 35%.
Randomized trial to determine the effect of nebivolol on mortality and cardiovascular hospital admission in elderly patients with HF (SENIORS)[66] (n = 1369)	At 32-mo follow-up of elderly patients with NYHA functional class II or III HF and LV ejection fraction of ≤35%, nebivolol, compared with placebo, significantly reduced mortality or cardiovascular hospital admission by 14%.

Abbreviations: HF, heart failure; LV, left ventricular; NYHA, New York Heart Association.

intervals with the maintenance dose of β-blockers reached over 3 months (carvedilol 25 mg twice daily or 50 mg twice daily if over 187 pounds or extended-release or controlled-release metoprolol 200 mg once daily). The patient may experience fatigue during the initiation or up-titration of the dose of β-blockers with this effect dissipating over time. The need to continue β-blockers in this patient must be stressed because of the importance of β-blockers in decreasing mortality.

During titration, the patient should be monitored for HF symptoms, fluid retention, hypotension, and bradycardia.[72] If there is worsening of symptoms, increase the dose of diuretics or ACE inhibitors. Temporarily reduce the dose of β-blockers if necessary. If there is hypotension, decrease the dose of vasodilators and temporarily decrease the dose of β-blockers if necessary. Reduce or discontinue drugs that may decrease the heart rate in the presence of bradycardia. Contraindications to the use of β-blockers in patients with HF are bronchial asthma, severe bronchial disease, symptomatic bradycardia, and symptomatic hypotension.[72]

ALDOSTERONE ANTAGONISTS

At the 2-year follow-up of 1663 patients (mean age, 65 years) with severe HF and an abnormal LV ejection fraction treated with diuretics, ACE inhibitors, 73% with digoxin, and 10% with β-blockers, spironolactone 25 mg/d significantly reduced mortality by 30% and hospitalization for worsening HF by 35%.[73] At the 16-month follow-up of 6632 patients (mean age, 64 years) with acute myocardial infarction complicated by HF and a low LV ejection fraction treated with diuretics, ACE inhibitors, and 75% with β-blockers, eplerenone 50 mg/d significantly reduced mortality by 15% and death from cardiovascular causes or hospitalization for cardiovascular events by 13%.[74] At the 21-month follow-up of 2737 patients with class II HF and abnormal LV ejection fraction, compared with placebo, eplerenone 50 mg/d decreased cardiovascular death or hospitalization for HF by 37%.[75]

The ACC/AHA guidelines recommend with a class I indication the addition of an aldosterone antagonist in selected patients with class II to IV HF and reduced LV ejection fraction who can be monitored carefully for preserved renal function and normal serum potassium concentration.[2,19] Patients should have a serum creatinine of 2.5 mg/dL or lower in men and 2.0 mg/dL or lower in women, and the serum potassium should be less than 5.0 mEq/L (see **Box 1**).[2,19]

ISOSORBIDE DINITRATE PLUS HYDRALAZINE

Oral nitrates reduce preload and pulmonary congestion in patients with HF. Hydralazine reduces afterload, improving perfusion at the same level of LV filling pressure. In the Veterans Administration Cooperative Vasodilator–Heart Failure Trial I, oral isosorbide dinitrate plus hydralazine, compared with placebo, significantly decreased mortality by 38% at 1 year, 25% at 2 years, and 23% at 3 years in men (mean age, 58 years) with abnormal LV ejection fraction.[76]

The African-American Heart Failure Trial randomized 1040 African Americans with class III through IV HF and an abnormal LV ejection fraction (only 23% with ischemic heart disease) treated with diuretics, ACE inhibitors, and β-blockers to isosorbide dinitrate plus hydralazine or to placebo.[30] At the 10-month follow-up, isosorbide dinitrate plus hydralazine significantly reduced mortality by 43% and rate of first hospitalization for HF by 33%.[31]

The ACC/AHA guidelines recommend using isosorbide dinitrate plus hydralazine in patients self-described as African Americans with NYHA functional class II through IV HF with an abnormal LV ejection fraction who are being treated with diuretics, ACE inhibitors, and β-blockers with a class I recommendation (see **Box 1**).[2,19]

The initial dose of oral isosorbide dinitrate in elderly patients with HF is 10 mg 3 times daily, with subsequent titration up to a maximum dose of 40 mg 3 times daily. Nitrates should be given no more than 3 times daily, with daily nitrate washout intervals of 12 hours to prevent nitrate tolerance from developing. The initial dose of oral hydralazine in older patients with HF is 10 to 25 mg 3 times daily, with subsequent titration up to a maximum dose of 100 mg 3 times daily.

DIGOXIN

At the 37-month follow-up of 6800 patients (mean age, 64 years) with HF and an LV ejection fraction of 45% or less in the DIG study (Digitalis Investigator Group), mortality was similar in patients treated with digoxin or placebo.[77,78] HF hospitalization was significantly reduced by 28% in patients with an abnormal LV ejection fraction.[77,78] Hospitalization for any cause was significantly reduced by 8% in patients with an abnormal LV ejection fraction.[78] Hospitalization for suspected digoxin toxicity in patients treated with digoxin was 0.67% in patients aged 50 to 59 years, 1.91% in patients aged 60 to 69 years, 2.47% in patients aged 70 to 79 years, and 4.42% in patients aged 80 years or greater.[78]

A post hoc subgroup analysis of data from women with an LV ejection fraction 45% or less in the DIG study showed by multivariate analysis that digoxin significantly increased the risk of death among women by 23% (absolute increase of 4.2%).[79] A post hoc subgroup analysis of data from men with an LV ejection fraction of 45% or less in the DIG study showed that digoxin significantly reduced mortality by 6% if the serum digoxin level was 0.5 to 0.8 ng/mL, insignificantly increased mortality by 3% if the serum digoxin level was 0.8 to 1.1 ng/mL, and significantly increased mortality by 12% if the serum digoxin level was 1.2 ng/mL or greater.[80]

Another post hoc subgroup analysis of data from all 1366 women with HF in the DIG study showed that digoxin significantly increased mortality for women by 80% if the serum digoxin level was 1.2 ng/mL or greater and insignificantly increased mortality by 5% if the serum digoxin level was 0.5 to 1.1 ng/mL.[81] If the serum digoxin level was 0.5 to 1.1 ng/mL and the LV ejection fraction was less than 35%, digoxin significantly reduced HF hospitalization by 37% in women.[81]

Digoxin reduces the rapid ventricular rate associated with supraventricular tachyarrhythmias and may be used along with β-blockers to treat elderly patients with HF and supraventricular tachyarrhythmias, such as atrial fibrillation. Digoxin may also be used to treat patients with persistent symptoms of HF and an abnormal LV ejection fraction despite treatment with diuretics, ACE inhibitors, and β-blockers to reduce HF hospitalization with a class IIa indication (see **Box 2**).[2,19] The maintenance dose of digoxin should be 0.125 mg/d in elderly patients with HF, and the serum digoxin level should be between 0.5 and 0.8 ng/mL.

Digoxin has a narrow therapeutic index, especially in elderly patients. An age-related reduction in renal function increases serum digoxin levels in older persons. The decrease in skeletal muscle mass in older patients reduces the volume of distribution of digoxin, increasing serum digoxin levels. Elderly patients are also more likely to be taking drugs that interact with digoxin by interfering with its bioavailability or excretion. For example, spironolactone, triamterene, amiodarone, quinidine, verapamil, propafenone, erythromycin, tetracycline, propantheline, and other drugs increase serum digoxin levels. Therefore, elderly patients receiving these drugs are at increased risk for developing digitalis toxicity. In addition, hypokalemia, hypomagnesemia, myocardial ischemia, hypoxia, acute and chronic lung disease, acidosis, hypercalcemia, and hypothyroidism may cause digitalis toxicity, despite normal serum digoxin levels.[82]

OTHER NEUROHORMONAL ANTAGONISTS

Other neurohormonal antagonists have not been shown to be effective in the treatment of HF.[83–87]

The OVERTURE (Omapatrilat vs Enalapril Randomized Trial of Utility in Reducing Events) trial was a phase III randomized double-blind trial that compared omapatrilat with enalapril in 5770 patients with class II through IV HF for a mean duration of 14.5 months.[83] Results from this trial showed that omapatrilat was neither superior nor inferior to enalapril in reducing the primary endpoint of combined all-cause mortality and HF hospitalizations requiring intravenous treatment.[83]

SACUBITRIL/VALSARTAN

The PARADIGM-HF (Prospective comparison of ARNI with ACEI to Determine Impact on Global Mortality and morbidity in Heart Failure) was a double-blind trial that randomized 8442 patients with class II through IV HF and an LV ejection fraction of EF of 40% or less (later amended to $\leq$ 35%) to receive twice daily dosing of either 200 mg of sacubitril (a neprilysin inhibitor)/valsartan or 10 mg of enalapril in addition to standard medical therapy for HF.[88] If participants tolerated both study drugs during 2 run-in periods, they were then randomized to double-blind treatment. The primary endpoint was a composite of death from cardiovascular causes or hospitalization for HF. At the 27-month follow-up, sacubitril/valsartan caused a significant 20% reduction in the primary endpoint.[88] Limitations to this study are discussed elsewhere.[89] The 2016 ACC/AHA/Heart Failure Society of America guidelines state with a class I recommendation that sacubitril/valsartan may be used instead of an ACE inhibitor or ARB in patients with chronic symptomatic HF and abnormal LV ejection fraction class II or III to further reduce morbidity and mortality[19] (see **Box 1**).

CALCIUM CHANNEL BLOCKERS

Calcium channel blockers, such as nifedipine, diltiazem, and verapamil, exacerbate HF in patients with HF and an abnormal LV ejection fraction.[90] Diltiazem significantly increased mortality in patients with pulmonary congestion and an abnormal LV ejection fraction after myocardial infarction.[91] The Multicenter Diltiazem Postinfarction Trial also showed in patients with an LV ejection fraction 40% or less that late HF at follow-up significantly increased in patients randomized to diltiazem (21%) compared with patients randomized to placebo (12%).[92]

The vasoselective calcium channel blockers amlodipine[93] and felodipine[94] did not significantly affect survival in patients with HF and an abnormal LV ejection fraction. In these studies, the incidence of pulmonary edema was significantly higher in patients treated with amlodipine (15%) than in patients treated with placebo (10%)[93] and the incidence of peripheral edema was significantly higher in patients treated with amlodipine[93] or felodipine[94] than in those treated with placebo. Based on the available data, calcium channel blockers should not be administered to patients with HF and an abnormal LV ejection fraction (see **Box 1**).[2,19]

IVABRADINE

Data were available for analysis of 6505 patients with HF and an LV ejection fraction of 35% or less in sinus rhythm with a heart rate of 70 beats per minute or more on background medical therapy including a β-blocker if tolerated who were randomized to ivabradine 7.5 mg twice daily or to placebo.[95] At the 22.9-month follow-up, the primary outcome of cardiovascular death or hospitalization for worsening HF was reduced 18% by ivabradine, driven mainly by hospitalization for worsening HF.[95] The 2016 ACC/AHA/Heart Failure Society of America guidelines state with a class IIa recommendation that ivabradine can be beneficial to reduce hospitalization for class II to III stable chronic HF and abnormal LV ejection fraction in patients on guided directed medical therapy receiving a β-blocker at the maximum tolerated dose, and who are in sinus rhythm with a heart rate of 70 beats per minute or greater at rest.[19]

SYNCHRONIZED PACING AND CARDIOVERTER-DEFIBRILLATORS

Implantable cardioverter-defibrillator therapy has a class I indication in selected patients with HF at least 40 days after acute myocardial infarction or nonischemic cardiomyopathy with an LV ejection fraction of 35% or less and NYHA functional class II or III symptoms on chronic guided directed medical therapy with a reasonable expectation of meaningful survival for more than 1 year.[2,19,96,97] Implantable cardioverter-defibrillator therapy also has a class I indication in selected patients with HF at least 40 days after acute myocardial infarction or nonischemic cardiomyopathy with an LV ejection fraction of 30% or less and NYHA functional class I symptoms on chronic guided directed medical therapy with a reasonable expectation of meaningful survival for more than 1 year.[2,19,98] Implantable cardioverter-defibrillator therapy is discussed elsewhere in this issue.

Cardiac resynchronization therapy (CRT) has a class I indication for patients with HF; an LV ejection fraction of 35% or less; class II, III, or ambulatory IV symptoms on guided directed medical therapy; sinus rhythm; and left bundle branch block with a QRS duration of 150 ms or greater.[2,19,99–104] CRT has a class IIa indication for patients with HF, an LV ejection fraction of 35% or less, class III or ambulatory IV symptoms on guided directed medical therapy, sinus rhythm, and a non–left bundle branch block pattern with a QRS duration of 150 ms or greater.[2,19,99,103] CRT has a class IIa indication for patients with HF; an LV ejection fraction of 35% or less; class II, III, or ambulatory IV symptoms on guided directed medical therapy; sinus rhythm; and a left bundle branch block pattern with a QRS duration of 120 to 149 ms.[2,19,100,103–105] CRT has a class IIa indication in patients with HF, atrial fibrillation, an LV ejection fraction of 35% or less on guided directed medical therapy if (a) the patient needs ventricular pacing or otherwise meets CRT criteria and (b) atrioventricular nodal ablation or pharmacologic rate control will allow near 100% ventricular pacing with CRT.[2,19,106] CRT also has a class IIa indication in patients with HF on guided directed medical therapy, an LV ejection fraction of 35% or less, and who are undergoing placement of a new or replacement device with anticipated need for more than 40% ventricular pacing[2,19,107] (see **Boxes 1** and **2**).[2,19] CRT therapy is discussed elsewhere in this issue.

INOTROPIC THERAPY

Inotropic therapy significantly increases mortality in patients with HF and abnormal LV ejection fraction.[108–116] The use of inotropic therapy in the treatment of elderly patients with acute decompensated HF is discussed elsewhere in this issue.

NESIRITIDE

Intravenous nesiritide (human B-type natriuretic peptide) causes hemodynamic and symptomatic improvement in hospitalized patients with decompensated HF through balanced vasodilatory effects, neurohormonal suppression, and enhanced natriuresis and diuresis.[117] Nesiritide improved hemodynamic function and some self-reported symptoms more effectively than intravenous nitroglycerin or placebo in a randomized, double-blind trial of 489 patients with dyspnea at rest from decompensated HF in the VMAC study (Vasodilation in the Management of Acute HF).[117]

However, in the VMAC study, intravenous nesiritide, compared with intravenous nitroglycerin, insignificantly increased hospital stay and 30-day and 6-month mortality.[117,118] This trial was also not powered for mortality. A review of US Food and Drug Administration files available via the website also showed that nesiritide (1) significantly increases the risk of worsening renal function in patients with acute decompensated HF[119] and (2) that nesiritide insignificantly increased mortality 1.8 times in patients with acute decompensated HF with an abnormal LV ejection fraction.[120] In a study of 7141 patients (median age, 67 years) with acute decompensated HF randomized to intravenous nesiritide or to placebo, compared with placebo, nesiritide caused no significant effect on dyspnea at 6 or 24 hours, caused no significant effect on rehospitalization for HF or death within 30 days, and caused a significant increase in hypotension (26.6% for nesiritide vs 15.3% for placebo).[121] These data do not support the use of nesiritide in patients with acute decompensated HF.

SURGICAL THERAPY

Surgical ventricular reconstruction (SVR) was used to reduce LV volume in patients with HF and abnormal LV ejection fraction caused by ischemic heart disease.[122] The STICH trial (Surgical Treatment for Ischemic Heart Failure) randomized 1000 patients with an LV ejection fraction of 35% or less, coronary artery disease amenable to coronary artery bypass grafting (CABG), and dominant anterior LV dysfunction amenable to SVR to CABG alone or to CABG plus SVR.[123] At the 48-month median follow-up, adding SVR to CABG reduced LV end-systolic volume by 19% as compared with 6% by CABG alone. Cardiac symptoms and exercise tolerance improved to a similar degree in the 2 study groups. The primary outcome of all-cause mortality or hospitalization for cardiac causes was similar in both groups.[123]

The STICH trial also randomized 1212 patients with an LV ejection fraction of 35% or less and coronary artery disease amenable to CABG to medical therapy alone or to medical therapy plus CABG.[124] At a median of 56 months of follow-up, the primary outcome of all-cause mortality was not different between the groups (41% for medical therapy alone vs 36% for medical therapy plus CABG).[124] Of the 1212 patients randomized in the STICH trial to medical therapy alone or to medical therapy plus CABG, 601 underwent assessment of myocardial viability.[125] The presence of viable myocardium was associated with a greater likelihood of survival, but this association was not significant after adjustment for other baseline variables.[125] At a median of 9.8 years of follow-up in the STICH trial, all-cause mortality was significantly reduced 16% by medical therapy plus CABG from 66.1% for medical therapy alone to 58.9% for medical therapy plus CABG.[126] All-cause mortality or hospitalization for cardiovascular causes was significantly reduced by 28% with medical therapy plus CABG from 87.0% for medical therapy alone to 76.6% for medical therapy plus CABG.[126] Surgical therapy in the treatment of HF is discussed elsewhere in this issue.

END-STAGE HEART FAILURE

An implantable LV assist device (LVAD) has benefited patients with end-stage HF as a bridge to cardiac transplantation. However, cardiac transplantation is not a viable option for the vast majority of patients with end-stage HF. One hundred twenty-nine transplant-ineligible patients (mean age, 67 years) with end-stage HF were randomized to medical therapy or to an LVAD.[127] The 2-year survival was 23% in the LVAD-treated group versus 8% in the medical therapy group.[127] Patients with advanced HF ineligible for cardiac transplantation were randomized to implantation of a continuous flow device (134 patients) or the pulsatile flow device (66 patients).[128] Actuarial 2-year survival rates were higher in patients with continuous flow devices (58%) than in patients with pulsatile flow devices (24%).[128] These data suggest using an LVAD as an alternative therapy in selected patients who are not candidates for cardiac transplantation. LVADs in the treatment of HF is discussed elsewhere in this issue.

Other therapies for older patients with end-stage HF include continuous intravenous inotropic infusions for palliation and hospice care.[2,19] End-of-life care in the treatment of HF is discussed elsewhere in this issue.

REFERENCES

1. Hunt SA, Abraham WT, Chin MH, et al. ACC/AHA 2005 guideline update for the diagnosis and management of chronic heart failure in the adult: summary article. Circulation 2005;112:1825–52.
2. Yancy CW, Jessup M, Bozkurt B, et al. 2013 ACCF/AHA guideline for the management of heart failure: a report of the American College of Cardiology Foundation/American Heart Association Task Force on Practice Guidelines. J Am Coll Cardiol 2013;62:e147–239.
3. Aronow WS. What is the appropriate treatment of hypertension in elders? J Gerontol A Biol Sci Med Sci 2002;57A:M483–6.
4. Aronow WS, Fleg JL, Pepine CJ, et al. ACCF/AHA 2011 expert consensus document on hypertension in the elderly: a report of the American College of Cardiology Foundation Task Force on Clinical Expert Consensus Documents Developed in collaboration with the American Academy of Neurology, American Geriatrics Society, American Society for Preventive Cardiology, American Society of Hypertension, American Society of Nephrology, Association of Black Cardiologists, and European Society of Hypertension. J Am Coll Cardiol 2011;57:2037–114.
5. Aronow WS. Treatment of older persons with hypercholesterolemia with and without cardiovascular disease. J Gerontol A Biol Sci Med Sci 2001;56A:M138–45.
6. Aronow WS, Ahn C. Frequency of congestive heart failure in older persons with prior myocardial infarction and serum low-density lipoprotein cholesterol ≥125 mg/dL treated with statins versus no lipid-lowering drug. Am J Cardiol 2002;90:147–9.
7. Stone NJ, Robinson J, Lichtenstein AH, et al. 2013 ACC/AHA guideline on the treatment of blood cholesterol to reduce atherosclerotic cardiovascular risk in adults: a report of the American College of Cardiology/American Heart Association Task Force on Practice Guidelines. J Am Coll Cardiol 2014;63:2889–934.
8. Aronow WS, Ahn C. Elderly diabetics with peripheral arterial disease and no coronary artery disease have a higher incidence of new coronary events than elderly nondiabetics with peripheral arterial disease and prior myocardial infarction treated with statins and with no lipid-lowering drug. J Gerontol A Biol Sci Med Sci 2003;58A:M573–5.
9. Sanal S, Aronow WS. Effect of an educational program on the prevalence of use of antiplatelet drugs, beta blockers, angiotensin-converting enzyme inhibitors, lipid-lowering drugs, and calcium channel blockers prescribed during hospitalization and at hospital discharge in patients with coronary artery disease. J Gerontol A Biol Sci Med Sci 2003;58A:M1046–8.
10. Ghosh S, Aronow WS. Utilization of lipid-lowering drugs in elderly persons with increased serum low-density lipoprotein cholesterol associated with coronary artery disease, symptomatic peripheral arterial disease, prior stroke, or diabetes mellitus before and after an educational program on dyslipidemia treatment. J Gerontol A Biol Sci Med Sci 2003;58A:M432–5.
11. Rosendorff C, Lackland DT, Allison M, et al. AHA/ACC/ASH scientific statement. Treatment of hypertension in patients with coronary artery disease: a scientific statement from the American Heart Association, American College of Cardiology, and American Society of Hypertension. J Am Coll Cardiol 2015;65:1998–2038.
12. Aronow WS. Management of atrial fibrillation in the elderly. Minerva Med 2009;100:3–24.
13. Connolly SJ, Ezekowitz MD, Yusuf S, et al. Dabigatran versus warfarin in patients with atrial fibrillation. N Engl J Med 2009;361:1139–51.

14. Patel MR, Mahaffey KW, Garg J, et al. Rivaroxaban versus warfarin in nonvalvular atrial fibrillation. N Engl J Med 2011;365:883–91.
15. Granger CB, Alexander JH, McMurray JJ, et al. Apixaban versus warfarin in patients with atrial fibrillation. N Engl J Med 2011;365:981–92.
16. Giugliano RP, Ruff CT, Braunwald E, et al. Edoxaban versus warfarin in patients with atrial fibrillation. N Engl J Med 2013;369:2093–104.
17. Aronow WS. Exercise therapy for older persons with cardiovascular disease. Am J Geriatr Cardiol 2001;10:245–52.
18. Rich MW, Beckham V, Wittenberg C, et al. A multidisciplinary intervention to prevent the readmission of elderly patients with congestive heart failure. N Engl J Med 1995;333:1190–5.
19. Yancy CW, Jessup M, Bozkurt B, et al. 2016 ACC/AHA/HFSA focused update on new pharmacologic therapy for heart failure: an update of the 2013 ACCF/AHA guideline for the management of heart failure: a report of the American College of Cardiology/American Heart Association Task Force on Clinical Practice Guidelines and the Heart Failure Society of America. J Am Coll Cardiol 2016;68:1488.
20. Neuberg GW, Miller AB, O'Connor CM, et al. Diuretic resistance predicts mortality in patients with advanced heart failure. Am Heart J 2002; 144:31–8.
21. Effect of enalapril on mortality in severe congestive heart failure: results of the Cooperative North Scandinavian Enalapril Survival Study (CONSENSUS). The CONSENSUS Trial Study Group. N Engl J Med 1987;316:1429–35.
22. Cohn J, Johnson G, Ziesche S, et al. A comparison of enalapril with hydralazine-isosorbide dinitrate in the treatment of chronic congestive heart failure. N Engl J Med 1991;325:303–10.
23. Effect of enalapril on survival in patients with reduced left ventricular ejection fractions and congestive heart failure. The SOLVD Investigators. N Engl J Med 1991;325:293–302.
24. Effect of ramipril on mortality and morbidity of survivors of acute myocardial infarction with clinical evidence of heart failure. The Acute Infarction Ramipril Efficacy (AIRE) Study Investigators. Lancet 1993;342:821–8.
25. Garg R, Yusuf S. Overview of randomized trials of angiotensin-converting enzyme inhibitors on mortality and morbidity in patients with heart failure. JAMA 1995;273:1450–6.
26. Pfeffer MA, Braunwald E, Moye LA, et al. Effect of captopril on mortality and morbidity in patients with left ventricular dysfunction after myocardial infarction. Results of the Survival and Ventricular Enlargement Trial. N Engl J Med 1992;327:669–77.
27. Effect of enalapril on mortality and the development of heart failure in asymptomatic patients with reduced left ventricular ejection fractions. The SOLVD Investigators. N Engl J Med 1992; 327:685–91.
28. Kober L, Torp-Pedersen C, Carlsen JE, et al. A clinical trial of the angiotensin-converting-enzyme inhibitor trandolapril in patients with left ventricular dysfunction after myocardial infarction. N Engl J Med 1995;333:1670–6.
29. Aronow WS, Ahn C, Kronzon I. Effect of beta blockers alone, of angiotensin-converting enzyme inhibitors alone, and of beta blockers plus angiotensin-converting enzyme inhibitors on new coronary events and on congestive heart failure in older persons with healed myocardial infarcts and asymptomatic left ventricular systolic dysfunction. Am J Cardiol 2001;88:1298–300.
30. Packer M, Poole-Wilson PA, Armstrong PW, et al. Comparative effects of low and high doses of the angiotensin-converting enzyme inhibitor, lisinopril, on morbidity and mortality in chronic heart failure. Circulation 1999;100:2312–8.
31. Taylor AL, Ziesche S, Yancy C, et al. Combination of isosorbide dinitrate and hydralazine in blacks with heart failure. N Engl J Med 2004;351:2049–57.
32. Exner DV, Dries DL, Domanski MJ, et al. Lesser response to angiotensin-converting enzyme inhibitor therapy in black as compared with white patients with left ventricular dysfunction. N Engl J Med 2001;344:1351–7.
33. Dries DL, Strong MH, Cooper RS, et al. Efficacy of angiotensin-converting enzyme inhibition in reducing progression from asymptomatic left ventricular dysfunction to symptomatic heart failure in black and white patients. J Am Coll Cardiol 2002; 40:311–7.
34. Vanhoutte PM, Auch-Schwelk W, Biondi ML, et al. Why are converting enzyme inhibitors vasodilators? Br J Clin Pharmacol 1989;28:95S–104S.
35. Weksler BB, Pett SB, Alonso D, et al. Differential inhibition by aspirin of vascular and platelet prostaglandin synthesis in atherosclerotic patients. N Engl J Med 1983;308:800–5.
36. Hall D, Zeitler H, Rudolph W. Counteraction of the vasodilator effects of enalapril by aspirin in severe heart failure. J Am Coll Cardiol 1994;20:1549–55.
37. Boger RH, Bodeboger SM, Kramme P, et al. Effect of captopril on prostacyclin and nitric oxide formation in healthy human subjects: interaction with low dose acetylsalicylic acid. Br J Clin Pharmacol 1996;42:721–7.
38. Evans MA, Burnett JC Jr, Redfield MM. Effect of low dose aspirin on cardiorenal function and acute hemodynamic response to enalaprilat in a canine model of severe heart failure. J Am Coll Cardiol 1995;25:1445–50.
39. Katz SD, Radin M, Graves T, et al. Effect of aspirin and ifetroban on skeletal muscle blood flow in

patients with congestive heart failure treated with enalapril. J Am Coll Cardiol 1999;34:170–6.
40. Nguyen KN, Aursnes I, Kjekshus J. Interaction between enalapril and aspirin on mortality after acute myocardial infarction: subgroup analysis of the Cooperative New Scandinavian Enalapril Survival Study II (CONSENSUS II). Am J Cardiol 1997;79: 115–9.
41. Al-Khadra AS, Salem DN, Rand WM, et al. Antiplatelet agents and survival: a cohort analysis from the Studies of Left Ventricular Dysfunction (SOLVD) trial. J Am Coll Cardiol 1998;31:419–25.
42. Leor J, Reicher-Reiss H, Goldbourt U, et al. Aspirin and mortality in patients treated with angiotensin-converting enzyme inhibitors. A cohort study of 11,575 patients with coronary artery disease. J Am Coll Cardiol 1999;33:1920–5.
43. Flather MD, Yusuf S, Kober L, et al. Long-term ACE-inhibitor therapy in patients with heart failure or left-ventricular dysfunction: a systematic overview of data from individual patients. Lancet 2000;355:1575–81.
44. Lapane KL, Hume AL, Barbour MM, et al. Does aspirin attenuate the effect of angiotensin-converting enzyme inhibitors on health outcomes of very old patients with heart failure? J Am Geriatr Soc 2002;50:1198–204.
45. Dzau VJ. Tissue renin-angiotensin system in myocardial hypertrophy and failure. Arch Intern Med 1993;153:937–42.
46. Jilma B, Krejcy K, Dirnberger E, et al. Effects of angiotensin-II infusion at pressor and subpressor doses on endothelin-1 plasma levels in healthy men. Life Sci 1997;60:1859–66.
47. Brenner BM, Cooper ME, de Zeeuw D, et al. Effects of losartan on renal and cardiovascular outcomes in patients with type 2 diabetes and nephropathy. N Engl J Med 2001;345:861–9.
48. Lindholm LH, Ibsen H, Dahlof B, et al. Cardiovascular morbidity and mortality in patients with diabetes in the Losartan Intervention for Endpoint reduction in hypertension study (LIFE): a randomised trial against atenolol. Lancet 2002;359: 1004–10.
49. Pitt B, Poole-Wilson PA, Segal R, et al. Effect of losartan compared with captopril on mortality in patients with symptomatic heart failure: randomised trial: the Losartan Heart Failure Survival Study ELITE II. Lancet 2000;355:1582–7.
50. Cohn JN, Tognoni G. A randomized trial of the angiotensin-receptor blocker valsartan in chronic heart failure. N Engl J Med 2001;345:1667–75.
51. Pfeffer MA, McMurray JJ, Velazquez EJ, et al. Valsartan, captopril, or both in myocardial infarction complicated by heart failure, left ventricular dysfunction, or both. N Engl J Mod 2003;349: 1893–906.
52. Granger CB, McMurray JJ, Yusuf S, et al. Effects of candesartan in patients with chronic heart failure and reduced left-ventricular systolic function intolerant to angiotensin-converting-enzyme inhibitors: the CHARM-Alternative trial. Lancet 2003;362: 772–6.
53. McMurray JJ, Ostergren J, Swedberg K, et al. Effects of candesartan in patients with chronic heart failure and reduced left-ventricular systolic function taking angiotensin-converting-enzyme inhibitors: the CHARM-Added trial. Lancet 2003;362: 767–71.
54. Beta-Blocker Heart Attack Trial Research Group. A randomized trial of propranolol in patients with acute myocardial infarction. JAMA 1982;247: 1707–14.
55. Pedersen TR. Six-year follow-up of the Norwegian Multicentre Study on Timolol after acute myocardial infarction. N Engl J Med 1985;313:1055–8.
56. Chadda K, Goldstein S, Byington R, et al. Effect of propranolol after acute myocardial infarction in patients with congestive heart failure. Circulation 1986;73:503–10.
57. Kennedy HL, Brooks MM, Barker AH, et al. Beta blocker therapy in the Cardiac Arrhythmia Suppression Trial. Am J Cardiol 1994;74:674–80.
58. Aronow WS, Ahn C, Mercando AD, et al. Effect of propranolol versus no antiarrhythmic drug on sudden cardiac death, total cardiac death, and total death in patients R62 years of age with heart disease, complex ventricular arrhythmias, and left ventricular ejection fraction R40%. Am J Cardiol 1994;74:267–70.
59. Aronow WS, Ahn C. Effect of beta blockers on incidence of new coronary events in older persons with prior myocardial infarction and diabetes mellitus. Am J Cardiol 2001;87:780–1.
60. Aronow WS, Ahn C. Effect of beta blockers on incidence of new coronary events in older persons with prior myocardial infarction and symptomatic peripheral arterial disease. Am J Cardiol 2001;87: 1284–6.
61. Furberg CD, Hawkins CM, Lichstein E. Effect of propranolol in postinfarction patients with mechanical or electrical complications. Circulation 1984; 69:761–5.
62. Packer M, Bristow MR, Cohn JN, et al. The effect of carvedilol on morbidity and mortality in patients with chronic heart failure. N Engl J Med 1996; 334:1349–55.
63. CIBIS-II Investigators and Committees. The Cardiac Insufficiency Bisoprolol Study II (CIBIS-II): a randomised trial. Lancet 1999;353:9–13.
64. MERIT-HF Study Group. Effect of metoprolol CR/XL in chronic heart failure: Metoprolol CR/XL Randomised Intervention Trial in Congestive Heart Failure (MERIT-HF). Lancet 1999;353:2001–7.

65. Packer M, Coats AJS, Fowler MB, et al. Effect of carvedilol on survival in chronic heart failure. N Engl J Med 2001;344:651–8.
66. Flather MD, Shibata MC, Coats AJ, et al. Randomized trial to determine the effect of nebivolol on mortality and cardiovascular hospital admission in elderly patients with heart failure (SENIORS). Eur Heart J 2005;26:215–25.
67. Mann DL, Deswal A, Bozkurt B, et al. New therapeutics for chronic heart failure. Annu Rev Med 2002;53:59–74.
68. Ohtsuka T, Hamada M, Hiasa G, et al. Effect of beta-blockers on circulating levels of inflammatory and anti-inflammatory cytokines in patients with dilated cardiomyopathy. J Am Coll Cardiol 2001; 37:412–7.
69. Wiklund O, Hulthe J, Wikstrand J, et al. Effect of controlled release/extended release metoprolol on carotid intima-media thickness in patients with hypercholesterolemia: a 3-year randomized study. Stroke 2002;33:572–7.
70. Moye L, Pfeffer M. Additional beneficial effects of beta-blockers to angiotensin-converting enzyme inhibitors in the Survival and Ventricular Enlargement (SAVE) Study. J Am Coll Cardiol 1997;29: 229–36.
71. Exner DV, Dries DL, Waclawiw MA, et al. Beta adrenergic blocking agent use and mortality in patients with asymptomatic and symptomatic left ventricular systolic dysfunction: a post hoc analysis of the Studies of Left Ventricular Dysfunction. J Am Coll Cardiol 1999;33:916–23.
72. Task Force for the Diagnosis and Treatment of Chronic Heart Failure. Guidelines for the diagnosis and treatment of chronic heart failure. Eur Heart J 2001;22:1527–60.
73. Pitt B, Zannad F, Remme WJ, et al. The effect of spironolactone on morbidity and mortality in patients with severe heart failure. N Engl J Med 1999;341:709–17.
74. Pitt B, Remme W, Zannad F, et al. Eplerenone, a selective aldosterone blocker, in patients with left ventricular dysfunction after myocardial infarction. N Engl J Med 2003;348:1309–21.
75. Zannad F, McMurray JJ, Krun H, et al. Eplerenone in patients with systolic heart failure and mild symptoms. N Engl J Med 2011;364:11–21.
76. Cohn JN, Archibald DG, Ziesche S, et al. Effect of vasodilator therapy on mortality in chronic congestive heart failure: results of a Veterans Administration Cooperative Study. N Engl J Med 1986;314: 1547–52.
77. The Digitalis Investigation Group. The effect of digoxin on mortality and morbidity in patients with heart failure. N Engl J Med 1997;336:525–33.
78. Rich MW, McSherry F, Williford WO, et al. Effect of age on mortality, hospitalizations and response to digoxin in patients with heart failure: the DIG Study. J Am Coll Cardiol 2001;38:806–13.
79. Rathore SS, Wang Y, Krumholz HM. Sex-based differences in the effect of digoxin for the treatment of heart failure. N Engl J Med 2002;347: 1403–11.
80. Rathore SS, Curtis JP, Wang Y, et al. Association of serum digoxin concentration and outcomes in patients with heart failure. JAMA 2003;289:871–8.
81. Ahmed A, Aban IB, Weaver MT, et al. Serum digoxin concentration and outcomes in women with heart failure: a bi-directional effect and a possible effect modification by ejection fraction. Eur J Heart Fail 2006;8(4):409–19.
82. Aronow WS. Digoxin or angiotensin converting enzyme inhibitors for congestive heart failure in geriatric patients. Which is the preferred treatment? Drugs Aging 1991;1:98–103.
83. Packer M, Califf RM, Konstam MA, et al. Comparison of omapatrilat and enalapril in patients with chronic heart failure. The Omapatrilat Versus Enalapril Randomized Trial of Utility in Reducing Events (OVERTURE). Circulation 2002;106: 920–6.
84. Abraham WT, Ascheim D, Demarco T, et al. Effects of enrasentan, a nonselective endothelin receptor antagonist in class II to III heart failure: results of the Enrasentan Cooperative Randomized (ENCOR) Evaluation. J Am Coll Cardiol 2001;38:612.
85. McMurray J, Pfeffer MA. New therapeutic options in congestive heart failure: part II. Circulation 2002;105:2223–8.
86. Gheorghiade M, Gattis WA, O'Connor CM, et al. Effects of tolvaptan, a vasopressin antagonist, in patients hospitalized with worsening heart failure: a randomized controlled trial. JAMA 2004;291: 1963–71.
87. Francis GS, Tang WH. Vasopressin receptor antagonists. Will the "vaptans" fulfill their promise? JAMA 2004;291:2017–8.
88. McMurray JJ, Packer M, Desai AS, et al. Angiotensin-neprilysin inhibition versus enalapril in heart failure. N Engl J Med 2014;371:993–1004.
89. Yandrapalli S, Aronow WS, Mondal P, et al. Limitations of sacubitril/valsartan in the management of heart failure. Am J Ther 2017;24:e234–9.
90. Elkayam U, Amin J, Mehra A, et al. A prospective, randomized, double-blind, crossover study to compare the efficacy and safety of chronic nifedipine therapy with that of isosorbide dinitrate and their combination in the treatment of chronic congestive heart failure. Circulation 1990;82: 1954–61.
91. The Multicenter Diltiazem Postinfarction Trial Research Group. The effect of diltiazem on mortality and reinfarction after myocardial infarction. N Engl J Med 1988;319:385–92.

92. Goldstein RE, Boccuzzi SJ, Cruess D, et al. Diltiazem increases late-onset congestive heart failure in postinfarction patients with early reduction in ejection fraction. Circulation 1991;83:52–60.
93. Packer M, O'Connor CM, Ghali JK, et al. Effect of amlodipine on morbidity and mortality in severe chronic heart failure. N Engl J Med 1996;335: 1107–14.
94. Cohn JN, Ziesche S, Smith R, et al. Effect of the calcium antagonist felodipine as supplementary vasodilator therapy in patients with chronic heart failure treated with enalapril. V-HeFT III. Vasodilator-Heart Failure Trial (V-HeFT) Study Group. Circulation 1997;96:856–63.
95. Swedberg K, Komajda M, Bohm M, et al. Ivabradine and outcomes in chronic heart failure (SHIFT): a randomised placebo-controlled study. Lancet 2010;376:875–85.
96. Bardy GH, Lee KL, Mark DB, et al. Amiodarone or an implantable cardioverter-defibrillator for congestive heart failure. N Engl J Med 2005;352: 225–37.
97. Moss AJ, Zareba W, Hall WJ, et al. Prophylactic implantation of a defibrillator in patients with myocardial infarction and reduced ejection fraction. N Engl J Med 2002;346:877–83.
98. Moss AJ, Hall WJ, Cannom DS, et al. Improved survival with an implanted defibrillator in patients with coronary disease at high risk for ventricular arrhythmia. N Engl J Med 1996;335:1933–40.
99. Aronow WS. CRT plus ICD in congestive heart failure. Use of cardiac resynchronization therapy and an implantable cardioverter-defibrillator in heart failure patients with abnormal left ventricular dysfunction. Geriatrics 2005;60(2):24–8.
100. Cleland JGF, Daubert J-C, Erdmann E, et al. The effect of cardiac resynchronization on morbidity and mortality in heart failure. N Engl J Med 2005;352: 1539–49.
101. Young JB, Abraham WT, Smith AL, et al. Combined cardiac resynchronization and implantable cardioversion defibrillation in advanced chronic heart failure. The MIRACLE ICD trial. JAMA 2003;289: 2685–94.
102. Bristow MR, Saxon LA, Boehmer J, et al. Cardiac resynchronization therapy with or without an implantable defibrillator in advanced chronic heart failure. N Engl J Med 2004;350:2140–50.
103. Moss AJ, Hall WJ, Cannom DS, et al. Cardiac- resynchronization therapy for the prevention of heart-failure events. N Engl J Med 2009;361: 1329–38.
104. Tang AS, Wells GA, Talajic M, et al. Cardiac-resynchronization therapy for mild-to-moderate heart failure. N Engl J Med 2010;363:2385–95.
105. Lindo C, Abraham WT, Gold MR, et al. Randomized trial of cardiac resynchronization in mildly symptomatic heart failure patients and in asymptomatic patients with left ventricular dysfunction and previous heart failure symptoms. J Am Coll Cardiol 2008;52:1834–43.
106. Brignole M, Botto G, Mont L, et al. Cardiac resynchronization in patients undergoing atrioventricular junction ablation for permanent atrial fibrillation: a randomized trial. Eur Heart J 2011; 32:2420–9.
107. Vatankulu MA, Goktekin O, Kaya MG, et al. Effect of long-term resynchronization therapy on left ventricular remodeling in pacemaker patients upgraded to biventricular devices. Am J Cardiol 2009;103:1280–4.
108. Packer M, Carver JR, Rodeheffer RJ, et al. Effect of oral milrinone on mortality in severe chronic heart failure. N Engl J Med 1991;325:1468–75.
109. Packer M, Rouleau J, Swedberg K, et al. Effect of flosequinan on survival in chronic heart failure: preliminary results of the PROFILE study [abstract]. Circulation 1993;88(Suppl I):I-301.
110. Uretsky BF, Jessup F, Konstan MA, et al. Multicenter trial of oral enoximone in patients with moderate to moderately severe congestive heart failure. Circulation 1990;82:774–80.
111. Cohn JN, Goldstein SO, Greenberg BH, et al. A dose-dependent increase in mortality with vesnarinone among patients with severe heart failure. N Engl J Med 1998;339:1810–6.
112. Pimobendan in Congestive Heart Failure (PICO) Investigators. Effect of pimobendan on exercise capacity in patients with heart failure: main results from the Pimobendan in Congestive Heart Failure (PICO) Trial. Heart 1996;76:223–31.
113. Xamoterol in Severe Heart Failure Study Group. Xamoterol in severe heart failure. Lancet 1990; 336:1–6.
114. Hampton JR, Van Veldhusisen DJ, Kleber FX, et al. Randomized study of effect of ibopamine on survival in patients with advanced heart failure. Lancet 1997;349:971–7.
115. O'Connor CM, Gattis WA, Uretsky BF, et al. Continuous intravenous dobutamine is associated with an increased risk of death in patients with advanced heart failure: insights from the Flolan International Randomized Survival Trial (FIRST). Am Heart J 2000;138:78–86.
116. Tariq S, Aronow WS. Use of inotropic agents in treatment of systolic heart failure. Int J Mol Sci 2015;16:29060–8.
117. Publication Committee for the VMAC Investigators. Intravenous nesiritide vs nitroglycerin for treatment of decompensated congestive heart failure. A randomized controlled trial. JAMA 2002;287:1531–40.
118. Teerlink JR, Massie BM. Nesiritide and worsening of renal function. The emperor's new clothes? Circulation 2005;111:1459–61.

119. Sackner-Bernstein JD, Skopicki HA, Aaronson KD. Risk of worsening renal function with nesiritide in patients with acutely decompensated heart failure. Circulation 2005;111:1487–91.
120. Sackner-Bernstein JD, Kowalski M, Fox M, et al. Short-term risk of death after treatment with nesiritide for decompensated heart failure. A pooled analysis of randomized controlled trials. JAMA 2005;293:1900–5.
121. O'Connor CM, Starling RC, Hernandez PW, et al. Effect of nesiritide in patients with acute decompensated heart failure. N Engl J Med 2011;365: 32–43.
122. Athanasuleas CL, Stanley AW Jr, Buckberg GD, et al. Surgical anterior ventricular endocardial restoration (SAVER) in the dilated remodeled ventricle after anterior myocardial infarction. J Am Coll Cardiol 2001;37:1210–3.
123. Jones RH, Velazquez EJ, Michler RE, et al. Coronary bypass surgery with or without surgical ventricular reconstruction. N Engl J Med 2009; 360:1705–17.
124. Velazquez EJ, Lee KL, Deja MA, et al. Coronary-artery bypass surgery in patients with left ventricular dysfunction. N Engl J Med 2011;364:1607–16.
125. Bonow RO, Maurer G, Lee KL, et al. Myocardial viability and survival in ischemic left ventricular dysfunction. N Engl J Med 2011;364:1617–25.
126. Velazquez EJ, Lee KL, Jones RH, et al. Coronary-artery bypass surgery in patients with ischemic cardiomyopathy. dysfunction. N Engl J Med 2016; 374:1511–20.
127. Rose EA, Gelijns AC, Moskowitz AJ, et al. Long-term use of a left ventricular assist device for endstage heart failure. N Engl J Med 2001;345: 1435–43.
128. Slaughter MS, Rogers JG, Milano CA, et al. Advanced heart failure treated with continuous-flow left ventricular assist device. N Engl J Med 2009;361:2241–51.

Heart Failure with Preserved Ejection Fraction in Older Adults

Bharathi Upadhya, MD, Dalane W. Kitzman, MD*

KEYWORDS

• Heart failure • Preserved ejection fraction • Elderly • Aging • Comorbidities

KEY POINTS

- Heart failure with preserved ejection fraction (HFpEF) is a diverse syndrome, strongly influenced by aging, with likely systemic, multifactorial causes that affect all organ systems.
- The overwhelming majority of HFpEF patients have multiple comorbidities that also drive phenotypic heterogeneity and multifactorial pathophysiology.
- So far, only exercise training and weight loss appear to improve exercise intolerance and quality of life.
- New drugs that target underlying inflammation, oxidative stress, and aging-related dysfunction may prove to be particularly effective for HFpEF.

INTRODUCTION

Clinical Significance

There has been growing recognition over the past 2 decades that a substantial proportion of heart failure (HF) patients, particularly the elderly, have preserved systolic left ventricular (LV) function. An epidemiologic study from Olmstead County, Minnesota found that the prevalence of HF with preserved ejection fraction (HFpEF) relative to HF with reduced ejection fraction (HFrEF) is increasing at a rate of 1% per year.[1] Among elderly women living in the community, HFpEF comprises nearly 90% of incident HF cases.[2] The annual incidence of HF in both men and women doubles with every decade after age 65, and the prevalence increases from less than 0.5% in the age group of 20 to 39 years to more than 10% in those 80 years and older.[3] By 2020, the prevalence of HFpEF is projected to exceed 8% of persons older than 65 years of age, and because of the current pandemic of obesity, the prevalence of HFpEF in persons younger than 65 years of age is expected to increase exponentially.[4]

The health and economic impact of HFpEF is at least as great as that of HFrEF, with similar severity of acute hospitalization rates, and substantial mortality.[1,5] Get With The Guidelines–HF, a very large, nationwide study of HF hospitalization in the United States (N >110,000), showed that the

This is an updated version of an article that appeared in *Heart Failure Clinics*, Volume 3, Issue 4.
Supported in part by NIH grants R01AG18915 and P30AG12232, and by the Kermit Glenn Phillips II Endowed Chair in Cardiovascular Medicine.
Potential Financial Conflicts of Interest: Dr D.W. Kitzman declares the following relationships: Consultant for Abbvie, Bayer, Merck, Medtronic, GSK, Relypsa, Regeneron, Merck, Corvia Medical, and Actavis; research grant funding from Novartis; and stock ownership in Gilead Sciences and Relypsa. Dr B. Upadhya has received research funding from Novarits and Corvia.
Cardiovascular Medicine Section, Department of Internal Medicine, Wake Forest School of Medicine, Winston-Salem, NC 27101, USA
* Corresponding author. Wake Forest School of Medicine, Medical Center Boulevard, Winston-Salem, NC 27157-1045.
E-mail address: dkitzman@wakehealth.edu

Heart Failure Clin 13 (2017) 485–502
http://dx.doi.org/10.1016/j.hfc.2017.02.005
1551-7136/17/

proportion of patients hospitalized with HFpEF increased from 33% in 2005 to 39% in 2010.[6] Outcomes following hospitalization for decompensated HFpEF are poor with about one-third of patients rehospitalized or dead within 90 days of discharge.[7] Noncardiovascular hospital readmissions and mortality are more frequent in HFpEF than in HFrEF, and the number of comorbidities correlate with increased all-cause hospitalization and mortality.[7]

Diagnostic Dilemma of Heart Failure with Preserved Ejection Fraction in Older Adults

Diagnosing HF in older adults poses specific challenges; false-positive clinical diagnoses are not uncommon.[6] The most common symptoms of HFpEF are exertional dyspnea. However, symptoms of reduced exercise tolerance are common in the elderly and have been shown to reflect normal physiologic changes related to aging or could be related to noncardiac causes. Furthermore, the diagnosis of HF in the elderly may be difficult due to the presence of multiple comorbidities, some of which can mimic HF signs and further confound the diagnosis of HF. In addition, there is no universally agreed on definition to define HFpEF. The American College of Cardiology/American Heart Association (AHA) consensus states that the diagnosis of HFpEF is based on typical symptoms and signs of HF in a patient with a normal range LV ejection fraction (EF), and no significant valvular abnormalities by echocardiography and no other obvious precipitating factors for HF or other disorders that could account for the HF symptoms.[8] By contrast, the European Society of Cardiology (ESC) requires diastolic dysfunction for the diagnosis of HFpEF, along with symptoms and signs of HF and normal or mildly abnormal LV function.[9]

Why Is Heart Failure with Preserved Ejection Fraction Increasing in Prevalence as the Population Ages?

Aging associated with heart failure with preserved ejection fraction epidemic

There are several normal age-related changes in cardiovascular (CV) structure and function that are likely relevant to the development of HFpEF. These changes include increased arterial stiffening, increased myocardial stiffness, decreased diastolic myocardial relaxation, increased LV mass, decreased peak contractility, reduced myocardial and vascular responsiveness to β-adrenergic stimulation, decreased coronary flow reserve, and decreased mitochondrial response to increased demand for adenosine triphosphate production.[10] As observed by Borlaug and colleagues,[11] LV stiffness increases with normal aging, despite excellent control of blood pressure (BP) and reductions in LV mass. Although aging may have no effects on resting heart rate (HR), contractility, or cardiac output (CO) at rest, it blunts the capacity to enhance HR, systolic function, and CO in response to β-adrenoceptor stimulation and exercise. Aging is also associated with impaired endothelium-dependent vasodilatation.[12,13] These normal age-related changes result in decreased CV reserve, which contributes, along with reduced skeletal muscle mass and function, an approximately 1% per year decline in maximal exercise oxygen consumption (peak V_{O_2}).[14] In addition, insults from acute myocardial ischemia/infarction, poorly controlled hypertension, atrial fibrillation (AF), iatrogenic volume overload, and pneumonia that would be tolerated in younger patients can cause acute HF in older persons.[10]

Why Is Heart Failure with Preserved Ejection Fraction so Common Among Elderly Women?

Among healthy normal subjects, older women tend to have higher LVEF, independent of their smaller chamber size, compared with men.[15,16] In addition, the LV in female mammals has a distinctly different response to pressure load, such as is typical of systemic hypertension. In hypertensives in the Framingham study, the predominant pattern of hypertrophic remodeling in women was concentric, whereas in men it was eccentric, and this has been reported also in several other studies.[17] Douglas and colleagues[18] showed the female rats developed concentric hypertrophy in response to increased afterload, and thereby maintained near-normal wall stress, and normal (or even a trend toward supranormal) contractility. In contrast, the male LV is less able to tolerate a pressure load, and in the presence of chronic systolic hypertension becomes dilated with thin walls and a depressed EF. However, the long-term cost of this female pattern of LV adaptation to a pressure load is impaired LV diastolic function. In addition, women have also been shown to have different CV physiologic responses to exercise than men, particularly in HR and stroke volume, independent of age and body size.[14,19,20]

Aging-related body changes/skeletal muscle changes

Aging is associated with a decline in a variety of neural, hormonal, and environmental trophic signals to muscle that can result in loss of muscle mass and mass-specific strength and[21–23] changes in body composition, including decreases in lean body mass and muscle strength, and increases in adiposity.[24] In addition, aging is associated with a systemic proinflammatory state and increased levels of cytokines[25,26] that may lead to a functional decline in multiple organs even in absence of a specific disease.[27]

Haykowsky and colleagues[28] found that percent body fat and percent leg fat were significantly increased, whereas percent body lean and leg lean mass were significantly reduced, in older HFpEF patients compared with healthy controls. When peak V_{O_2} was indexed to total lean body mass or leg lean mass, it remained significantly reduced, and there was a downward shift in the relationship of leg lean mass to peak V_{O_2} in HFpEF versus healthy, age-matched controls (**Fig. 1**).[28] These data suggest that poor "quality" of skeletal muscle may contribute to the reduced peak V_{O_2} found in older HFpEF patients.

Haykowsky and colleagues[29] subsequently extended these results by showing that there is abnormal fat infiltration into the thigh skeletal muscle, and this is associated with reduced peak exercise V_{O_2} in HFpEF (**Fig. 2**). Kitzman and colleagues[30] also showed that compared with healthy control subjects, older HFpEF patients had a shift in skeletal muscle fiber type distribution with a reduced percentage of slow twitch type I fibers and reduced type I to type II fiber ratio as well as reduced capillary-to-fiber ratio. Furthermore, both the capillary-to-fiber ratio and percentage of type I fibers were significant, independent predictors of peak V_{O_2} (**Fig. 3**).[30] A reduction in the percentage of type I fibers could be associated with reduced oxidative capacity and mitochondrial density and thereby contribute to the reduced peak V_{O_2} in HFpEF. The same investigators subsequently reported that skeletal muscle oxidative capacity, mitochondrial content, and mitochondrial fusion are abnormal in older patients with HFpEF.[31] The findings of abnormal mitochondrial function were also demonstrated by others in an animal model of HFpEF.[32] In addition to this, it is known that aging results in alterations in skeletal muscle, including a reduction in the relative number of type II fibers,[33] and in capillary density,[34] and that these are associated with a decline in physical performance. The loss of skeletal muscle and age-related alterations in skeletal muscle function are major factors in the age-associated decline in peak V_{O_2}.[35–37] These, along with sedentary behavior as HFpEF symptoms worsen, further exacerbate exercise intolerance.[38] Taken together, these findings may help explain why older HFpEF patients have such severely reduced exercise capacity, and why this has usually not improved with medications aimed solely at cardiac function in trials.[39,40]

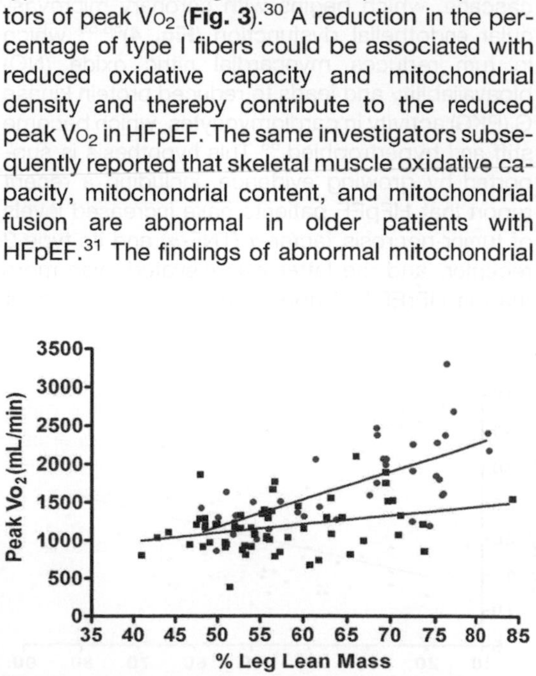

Fig. 1. Relationship between peak V_{O_2} (mL/min) and percent leg lean mass in HFpEF and healthy controls (HC) HFpEF (*filled squares*) and HC (*filled circles*).

Marked increase in prevalence of cardiac and noncardiac comorbidities with aging and heart failure with preserved ejection fraction

Cardiac comorbidities: coronary artery disease and atrial fibrillation Although several epidemiologic and observational studies have found that coronary artery disease (CAD) is less common in HFpEF compared with HFrEF,[6,41] the pooled data across studies suggest that the prevalence of CAD in HFpEF is approximately 40% to 50%.[42] Large retrospective studies showed CAD is common in patients with HFpEF and is associated with increased risk of CV death, especially sudden death.[43,44] An autopsy study recently showed epicardial CAD was frequent and extensive in HFpEF.[45] In addition, with increasing life expectancy, decreased mortality, and increased salvage of the myocardium with revascularization in the setting of acute coronary syndromes, patients with CAD are more likely aged and more likely to have a preserved EF. Moreover, myocardial ischemia acutely causes both systolic and diastolic dysfunction and may contribute to abnormal CV reserve with stress.[46] Thus, it is not surprising that CAD has been associated with increased risk of developing HFpEF.

HFpEF and AF are inextricably linked, both to each other and to adverse CV outcomes.[47,48] AF prevalence has been increasing due to an aging general population and increased longevity. AF in HFpEF is associated with impaired LV systolic, diastolic function and functional reserve, larger left atrium (LA) with poor LA function, more severe neurohumoral activation, and impaired exercise tolerance.[49,50]

Noncardiac comorbidities and the epidemic of obesity Noncardiac comorbidities are highly prevalent in HFpEF, and most older HFpEF patients

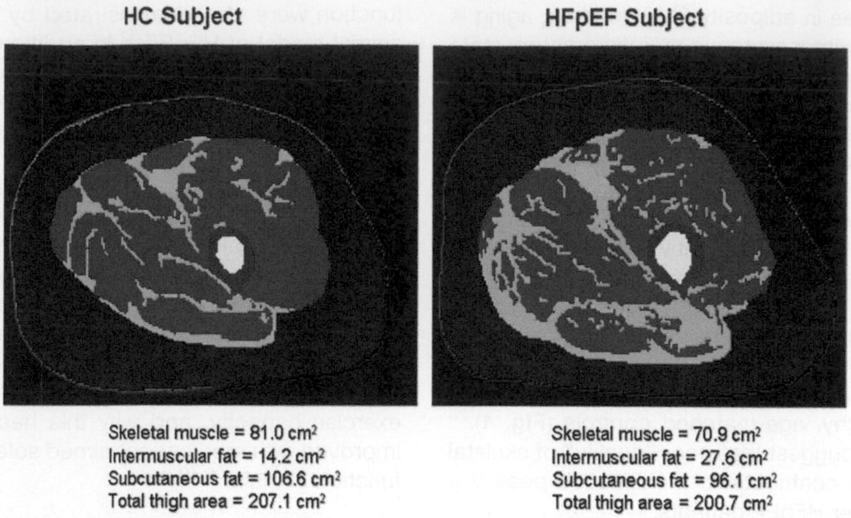

Fig. 2. MRI axial image of the midthigh in a patient with HFpEF and HC. (*red*) Skeletal muscle; (*blue*) subcutaneous fat; (*purple*) femoral cortex; (*yellow*) femoral medulla. Intermuscular fat (IMF; *green*) is substantially increased in the patient with HFpEF compared with the HC despite similar subcutaneous fat.

have multiple and often severe noncardiac comorbidities.[51] The most important noncardiac comorbidities for HFpEF are obesity, hypertension, diabetes, chronic obstructive pulmonary disease (COPD), anemia, and chronic kidney disease. Approximately 85% of elderly HFpEF patients are overweight or obese, and the HFpEF epidemic has largely paralleled the obesity epidemic.[52] Adiposity-induced inflammation has wide-ranging adverse effects, including endothelial dysfunction, capillary rarefaction, and mitochondrial dysfunction in both the cardiac and the systemic vascular beds.[53] A recent study demonstrated that body mass index was a key contributor to symptoms of breathlessness in patients with HFpEF.[54] Nearly two-thirds of HFpEF patients have COPD.[55] Moreover, patients with preserved EF do not have the alternative diagnosis of low EF; they are more likely to receive a COPD diagnosis as an explanation for dyspnea.[56] In addition, even in the absence of formal COPD diagnosis, patients with HFpEF have multiple pulmonary abnormalities and may contribute to their poor outcomes.[57]

Aging and the aforementioned comorbidities may initiate and/or aggravate chronic systemic inflammation that may affect myocardial remodeling and dysfunction in HFpEF through a signaling cascade, which begins with coronary microvascular endothelial dysfunction (**Fig. 4**)[58,59] which in turn reduces myocardial nitric oxide (NO) bioavailability and leads to reduced protein kinase G (PKG) activity in cardiomyocytes, which become stiff and hypertrophied.[58] This hypothesis is supported by growing evidence, including a recent report that HFpEF patients have increased levels of tumor necrosis factor-α (TNF-α) and its type 2 receptor, and the latter was elevated even more than in HFrEF.[60] Support for a systemic trigger

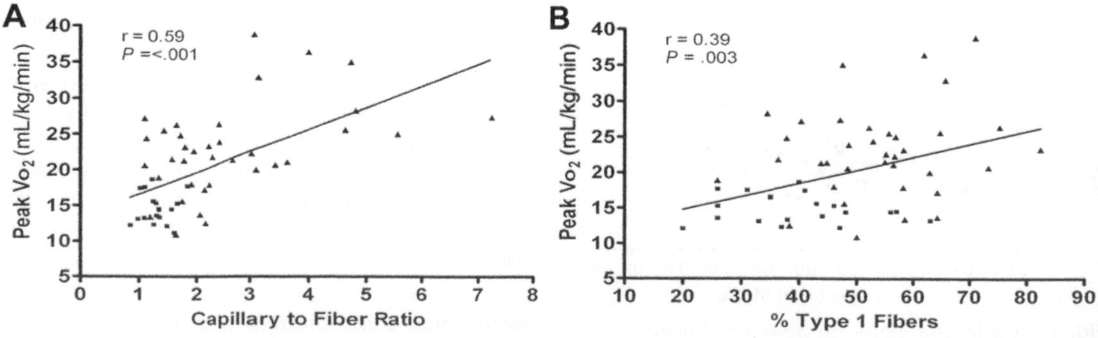

Fig. 3. Relationship of capillary-to-fiber ratio (*A*) and percentage of type I muscle fibers (*B*) with peak O_2 uptake (Vo_2) in older patients with HFpEF (■) and age-matched healthy control subjects (▲).

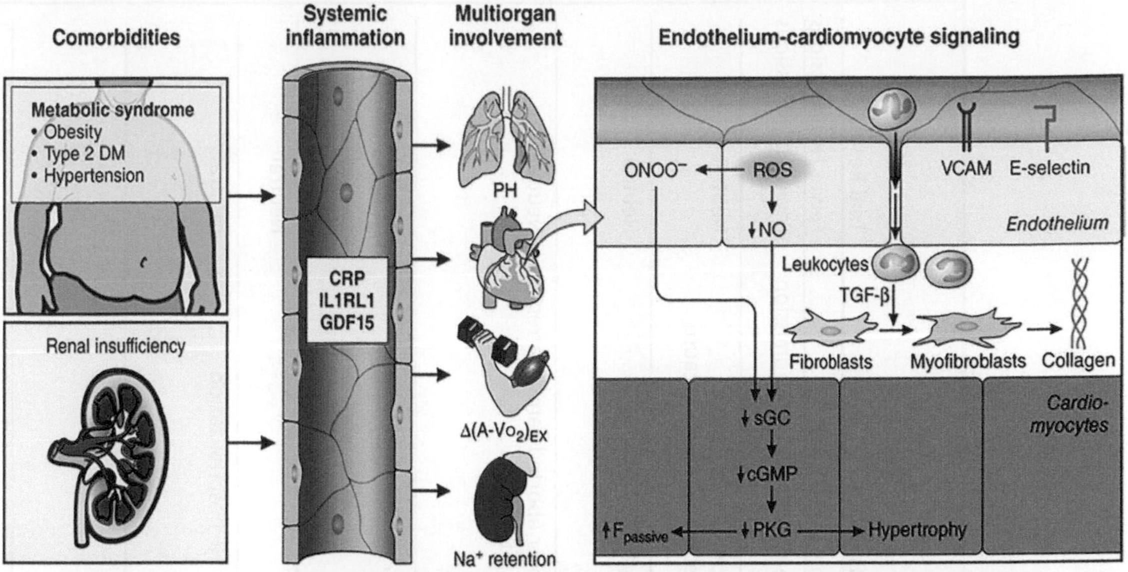

Fig. 4. Systemic and myocardial signaling in HFpEF. Comorbidities induce systemic inflammation, evident from elevated plasma levels of inflammatory biomarkers such as soluble interleukin 1 receptor-like 1 (IL1RL1), C-reactive protein (CRP), and growth differentiation factor 15 (GDF15). Chronic inflammation affects the lungs, myocardium, skeletal muscle, and kidneys leading to diverse HFpEF phenotypes with variable involvement of pulmonary hypertension (PH), myocardial remodeling, deficient skeletal muscle oxygen extraction (ΔA-Vo_2) during exercise (Ex), and renal Na+ retention. Myocardial remodeling and dysfunction begins with coronary endothelial microvascular inflammation manifest from endothelial expression of adhesion molecules such as vascular cell adhesion molecule (VCAM) and E-selectin. Expression of adhesion molecules attracts infiltrating leukocytes secreting transforming growth factor-β (TGF-β), which converts fibroblasts to myofibroblasts with enhanced interstitial collagen deposition. Endothelial inflammation also results in the presence of reactive oxygen species (ROS), reduced NO bioavailability, and production of peroxynitrite ($ONOO^-$). This reduces soluble guanylate cyclase (sGC) activity, cGMP content, and the favorable effects of PKG on cardiomyocyte stiffness and hypertrophy. DM, diabetes mellitus.

for HFpEF came from parabiosis experiments in which hearts of young animals acquired HFpEF-like features when exposed to blood from old animals and vice versa.[61]

Key Knowledge Gaps

1. What are the mechanisms whereby aging, noncardiac comorbidities impact physical function outcomes in HFpEF?
2. How can we develop and test novel exercise and physical function interventions that directly address the adverse impact of multiple comorbidities in older patients with HFpEF?

Pharmacologic Interventions

Summary of traditional clinical trials

Targeting the renin-angiotensin-aldosterone system (RAAS) pathway has long been considered a logical intervention for HFpEF, based on animal models as well as human hypertensives without HF and its link to LV hypertrophy, interstitial fibrosis, and fluid imbalance.[62–65] Angiotensin II promotes LV hypertrophy and fibrosis, both of which are contributors to HFpEF, as well as vasoconstriction and vascular remodeling.[66] Aldosterone can promote interstitial collagen deposition and fibrosis, leading to ventricular stiffness, and its inhibition might be expected to reduce the ventricular-vascular stiffening and diastolic dysfunction. **Table 1** summarizes the important randomized trials. Of the 3 large randomized trials of angiotensin-converting enzyme inhibitors (ACEI)/angiotensin receptor blockers (ARB) performed to date in HFpEF, only the CHARM-Preserved study found nominal benefit for reducing HF hospitalizations over 3 years of follow-up. However, most importantly, none of the trials showed benefit for their preplanned primary endpoints.[67–69] Similarly, Kitzman and colleagues[39] studied a 12-month, randomized controlled trial of the ACEI enalapril in elderly patients with established HFpEF and showed no improvement in exercise capacity or quality of life.

Table 1
Summary of few important randomized trials

First Author/Trial (Ref.)	Intervention	HFpEF Patient Type	Primary Endpoint	Trial Result
CHARM-Preserved[67]	Candesartan	≥18 y/NYHA class II-IV HF	CV death or HF admission	Fewer HF admissions
The PEP-CHF[68]	Perindopril	≥70 y/diagnosis of HF and treated with diuretics and an Echo-DD	All-cause mortality and HF admission	Fewer HF admissions
I-PRESERVE[69]	Irbesartan	≥60 y/hospitalized for HF during the previous 6 mo and have current NYHA class II-IV symptoms	Death from any cause or hospitalization for a CV cause	Neutral
Kitzman et al[39]	Enalapril	Elderly (70 ± 1 y), predominant woman (80%) with compensated HF	Peak Vo_2 and 6 MWD	Neutral
TOPCAT[70]	Spironolactone	≥50 y, Symptomatic HF. Patients had a history of HF hospitalization within previous 12 mo and elevated BNP within 60 d before randomization	CV death or aborted cardiac arrest, HF hospitalization	Neutral
Aldo-DHF[40]	Spironolactone	≥50 y ambulatory patients/NYHA class II-III symptoms, grade 1 DD and normal or near-normal BNP levels	Peak Vo_2, change in E/e′	Neutral
RAAM-PEF[71]	Eplerenone	Elderly, symptomatic NYHA class II/III, increased BNP within 60 d	6 MWD	Neutral
J-DHF[74]	Carvedilol (low-dose)	≥20 y/ambulatory patients with NYHA class II-III symptoms, grade I DD, and normal or near-normal BNP levels	Death or HF hospitalization	Neutral
ELANDD[75]	Nebivolol	≥40 y/ambulatory patients with NYHA class II-III symptoms, grade I DD, and normal or near-normal BNP levels	6 MWD	Neutral

NEAT-HFPEF trial[100]	Isosorbide mononitrate	≥50 y/ambulatory HF patients, prior hospitalization for HF within 12 mo or increased invasively measured LV filling pressure or elevated BNP or echo-DD	Daily activity level, 6 MWD	Neutral
RELAX[99,100]	Sildenafil	≥18 y/elevated BNP or elevated invasively measured LV filling pressure and reduced exercise capacity	Peak V_{O_2}	Neutral
DILATE-1[114]	Riociguat	≥18 y/stable symptomatic HF, mean PAP ≥25 mm of Hg and PCWP >15 mm of Hg	Change in mean PAP	Neutral
Zile et al[119]	Sitaxsentan	NYHA class II-III HF, Echo-DD	Change in treadmill exercise time	Positive
PARAMOUNT[78]	LCZ696(ARNI)	≥40 y/NYHA class II-III HF, NT-pro BNP >400 pg/nL and be on a diuretic therapy	Change in NT-proBNP	Positive
Kosmala et al[112]	Ivabradine	≥50 y/ambulatory patients with NYHA class II-III symptoms, grade I DD, and normal or near-normal BNP levels	Peak V_{O_2}, Peak E/e′	Positive
Kitzman et al[131]	ET	≥60 y/ambulatory HF patients with NYHA class II-III symptoms	Peak V_{O_2}	Positive
Kitzman et al[134]	Caloric restriction and ET	≥60 y/ambulatory HF patients with NYHA class II-III symptoms	Peak V_{O_2} and quality of life	Positive
CHAMPION[127]	CardioMEMS sensor	≥18 y, NYHA class III HF, hospitalization for HF in last 12 mo	HF hospitalization	Positive

Abbreviations: ARNI, angiotensin receptor-neprilysin inhibitor; DD, diastolic dysfunction; E, mitral early diastolic velocity; e′, mitral annular velocity; NYHA, New York Heart Association; PAP, pulmonary artery pressure; PCWP, pulmonary capillary wedge pressure.

Aldosterone antagonists have also been examined in HFpEF. The Aldo-DHF trial showed improvement in some measures of diastolic dysfunction; the RAAM-PEF trial showed reductions in circulating markers of collagen turnover and modest improvements in diastolic function, and the larger TOPCAT trial showed a modest decline in hospitalizations but not mortality.[40,70,71] However, a post hoc regional analysis of TOPCAT indicated that the cohort from the Americas most closely matched characteristics observed in other randomized trials and also appeared most responsive to spironolactone.[72]

Slowing the HR should result in an increase in the diastolic filling period in an abnormally stiff LV, thus potentially allowing greater filling of LV. As shown in **Table 1**, beta-blocker data on HFpEF to date have not been promising.[73–76] In the Digitalis Interaction Group, there were no significant reductions in the amount of hospitalizations or mortality secondary to HF with digoxin, although trends toward decreased hospitalization and improved exercise tolerance were noted.[77] Ivabridine, a novel agent for reducing HR, is discussed later.

Why have clinical pharmacologic intervention trials fail to meet their primary endpoints?

Relative lack of success of prior trials has led to a reevaluation of paradigms regarding HFpEF physiology. To date, trials have largely targeted solely targets previously thought to be specific to and universally present in HFpEF, such as LVH, diastolic dysfunction, and other features. However, more recent data have challenged these assumptions. For instance, in the recently reported PARAMOUNT trial of well-characterized HFpEF patients, only 8% of patients had LVH at baseline, and 50% had significant/severe diastolic function at rest.[78] With treatment, even though there was a positive signal on B-type natriuretic peptide (BNP), there was no difference in LV mass. Similarly, Maurer and colleagues[79] found no significantly increased LV mass in older HFpEF patients compared with controls with hypertension but not HF.[80] The magnitude of increase in fibrosis in HFpEF patients also appears to be modest at most.[81] Absence of increased LV mass indicates LV hypertrophy may not be unique to, or required for, diagnosis of HFpEF. This might explain the agents that had a proven ability to ameliorate LV hypertrophy, fibrosis, and other cardiac abnormalities typically found in HFpEF have failed to produce a positive effect.

Studies of patients with all the clinical hallmarks of HF and an EF greater than 50% showed that many patients appear to have modest diastolic dysfunction under resting conditions.[78,82] Furthermore, similar changes can be seen in elderly patients with hypertensive heart disease with no clinical HF, and diastolic dysfunction in HFpEF patients may not be greater than age-matched sedentary controls and has not prevented a successful target for intervention.[83–87] Most HFpEF trials measured diastolic or other CV measures at rest and not during exercise. Importantly, most measures used to assess diastolic function (echocardiographic or radionuclide techniques or invasive measurements) do not assess the key passive component of diastole. Furthermore, using direct invasive measurements, Kawaguchi and colleagues[88] showed that during exercise, patients with HFpEF were able to increase preload volume with very little if any effect on the ventricular end-diastolic pressure-volume relation, despite a substantial prolongation of time constant of relaxation. Although other studies have had varying results in this respect, these data suggest that diastolic function abnormalities may not be the sole contributor to symptoms in HFpEF.[85]

Across reports from a variety of sources, lower HR at peak exercise (chronotropic incompetence [CI]) has been the most consistently reported cardiac abnormality during exercise in HFpEF.[46,89–91] In some studies, CI appears to be the primary mechanism accounting for reduced CO during exercise in HFpEF and the primary or sole cardiac contributor to exercise intolerance.[92] In addition, there is a high prevalence of CI in HFpEF, and limitations in chronotropic reserve might be a key factor to reduce CO and exercise capacity.[46,93] Beta-blockers may result in pharmacologically induced CI and obscure identification of an underlying intrinsic abnormality in neural balance.[94] In addition, unfavorable effect of beta-blockers on COPD and diabetes could complicate the overall effect of these drugs in HFpEF patients with such conditions.[95,96]

The neutral outcomes were often attributed to patient recruitment with inclusion of many HFrEF or noncardiac patients or nonadherence to diagnostic guidelines that might have led to excessive enrollment of HF patients with eccentric LV remodeling and CAD rather than concentric remodeling and hypertension.[58] For example, in the TOPCAT trial, neutral outcome in the overall population has been attributed to aberrant patient enrollment in Russia/Republic of Georgia rather than to inefficacy of spironolactone.[72]

Perhaps most importantly, HFpEF is strongly influenced by aging, a progressive process affecting all organ systems, including the heart and arterial system, those most implicated in

HFpEF. In addition, recent data, discussed above, indicate that HFpEF may be best understood as a systemic disorder, triggered by one or more circulating factors, involving virtually all organ systems, in addition to the heart, and also involves important contributions from peripheral abnormalities of vascular and skeletal muscle function that have not been addressed in trials to date. Finally, multiple comorbidities, including noncardiovascular comorbidities, may play a much greater role in the development of symptoms and treatment response than previously recognized. If so, they may not be addressed by agents and strategies that are primarily targeted at cardiac function. These concepts have led to the proposal of key phenotypes in HFpEF, with each phenotype having distant pathophysiologic and treatment implications.[97] However, past and current HFpEF studies make no or little effort to enroll specific etiologic/pathophysiologic subtypes.

Novel pharmacotherapies in heart failure with preserved ejection fraction

Sildenafil Sildenafil is an inhibitor of phosphodiesterase 5 that increases cyclic guanosine monophosphate (cGMP) levels by blocking catabolism, thus augmenting PKG activity in multiple organs relevant to HF. Increased availability of cGMP could provide benefits for both vascular and myocardial remodeling, including attenuating hypertrophy, fibrosis, and impaired cardiac relaxation.[98] In the RELAX trial, sildenafil did not improve 6-minute walk distance (MWD) or quality of life.[99]

Nitrates In the NEAT-HFpEF trial, the isosorbide mononitrate, an organic nitrate, did not improve in 6 MWD, quality-of-life scores, or NT-pro BNP levels compared with placebo.[100] Recently, 2 randomized studies showed that intravenous or inhaled sodium nitrite, which unlike inorganic nitrate is a direct NO donor, improved CO reserve, LV stroke work, biventricular filling pressures, and pulmonary artery pressures at rest and during exercise in HFpEF.[101,102] These trials led to the launch of 2 clinical trials sponsored by the National Heart, Lung, and Blood Institute (NCT02742129 and NCT02713126). A recent study with a relatively small patient sample showed that 1 week of daily dosing with beet root juice (supplying 6.1 mmol inorganic nitrate) significantly improved submaximal aerobic endurance and BP in elderly 20 HFpEF patients.[103]

Neprilysin inhibitors Neprilysin is a zinc-dependent metalloprotease that degrades biologically active natriuretic peptides and does not affect the biologically inactive NT-pro BNP.[78] LCZ696 is a new combination drug of the angiotensin II type 1 receptor blocker valsartan and the neprilysin inhibitor prodrug AHU377. This dual combination exerts a powerful vasodilatory and natriuresis effect by blocking angiotensin II activity on the one hand, although augmenting plasma levels of natriuretic peptides, such as BNP, on the other. In the PARAMOUNT study (see **Table 1**), the group randomized to receive LCZ696 had significantly lower NT-pro BNP levels, and at 36 weeks, decreased LA size and showed a trend toward improved functional class.[78] This agent also appears to reduce TNF-α levels, and this finding correlates with improvements in cardiac features of HFpEF.[104] The promising findings of this phase 2 study led to an ongoing large, multicenter trial, PARAGON, which is comparing LCZ696 to valsartan in patients with HFpEF with the primary composite outcome of CV death or first hospitalization for HF (ClinicalTrials.gov; NCT01920711).

Statins By blocking the activity of several guanosine triphosphate binding proteins and inhibiting some of the inflammatory processes, statins can suppress LV hypertrophy and decrease collagen synthesis in experimental models.[105,106] Even though observational data in HFpEF patients suggest a mortality benefit with use of HMG-Coa reductase inhibitors, definitive trials have not been performed in HFpEF patients.[107,108] A recent meta-analyses suggested a potential mortality benefit with statin.[109] Likewise, in a recent prospective study of HFpEF patients, statin use was associated with a higher rate of 1-year survival compared with those who were not treated.[110]

Ivabradine Ivabradine is a selective sinus node If sodium channel inhibitor that reduces HR without affecting contractility or lusitropy. The role of ivabradine in HFpEF has not been well established. In a diabetic mouse model of HFpEF, ivabradine reduced aortic stiffness and fibrosis and improved LV contractility and diastolic function.[111] In a 7-day study, ivabradine increased peak V_{O_2} and reduced exercise E/e′ ratio in 61 patients with HFpEF.[112] However, in contrast, a short-term, placebo-controlled, randomized, crossover study found that 2 weeks of HR reduction with ivabradine in patients with HFpEF almost uniformly exacerbated already abnormal exercise physiology.[113]

Riociguat Riociguat is a soluble guanylate cyclase stimulator that targets the NO-soluble guanylate cyclase–cGMP signaling pathway. The DILATE-1 study showed that riociguat did not impact the primary end point of peak change in mean pulmonary artery pressure in patients with HFpEF and pulmonary hypertension.[114] Other studies using these agents for other endpoints are planned or underway.

Ranolazine Ranolazine blocks inward sodium current, promotes Ca^{2+} extrusion through the Na^{+}/Ca^{2+} exchanger, and thereby improves diastolic tension and relaxation. The RALI-DHF study showed improvement in some measures of hemodynamics but no improvement in relaxation parameters.[115,116] Reduction of filling pressures did occur with ranolazine, but it also appeared to decrease CO.[116]

Alagebrium (ALT-711) Advanced glycation end products (AGEs) are formed when glucose interacts nonenzymatically with proteins. AGEs can cause increased stiffness of the extracellular matrix directly by cross-linking collagen or elastin and indirectly by stimulating the production of collagen and depleting NO, thereby increasing oxidative stress.[117] A small open-label study found that administration of alagebrium chloride was associated with slightly reduced LV mass and improved diastolic filling; however, there were no changes in EF, BP, peak V_{O_2}, and aortic dispensability (the latter 2 were the primary outcomes).[118]

Sitaxsentan The effects of treatment with a selective endothelin type A (ET_A) receptor antagonist on characteristics commonly found in patients with HFpEF, such as pulmonary hypertension, diastolic dysfunction, and LV hypertrophy, suggest the potential for its therapeutic application in HFpEF patients. In a moderate-sized trial of HFpEF patients, with 6-months treatment with sitaxsentan, a selective ET_A receptor antagonist appeared to provide a modest increase in treadmill exercise time but did not improve any secondary endpoints, such as LV mass or diastolic function.[119]

New drugs in development or testing

Anakinra Interleukin-1 (IL-1 [alpha]) and IL-1 (beta) are potent proinflammatory cytokines implicated in adverse ventricular-vascular remodeling.[120] IL-1 blockade with anakinra for 14 days significantly reduced the systemic inflammatory response and improved aerobic exercise capacity in patients with HFpEF and elevated plasma CRP levels.[121]

Inhibitors of sodium-glucose cotransporters type 2 The inhibitors of sodium-glucose cotransporters type 2 (SGLT2) empagliflozin was shown to reduce HF admissions in patients with type 2 diabetes and high CV risk, with a consistent benefit in patients with and without baseline HF.[122] The ongoing CANDLE trial in patients with type 2 diabetes mellitus and chronic HF (both HFpEF and HFrEF) has the potential to evaluate the clinical safety and efficacy on HF of another SGLT2 inhibitor canagliflozin in comparison with glimepiride.[123]

Nifedipine and isosorbide dinitrate/hydralazine Two classic medications, nifedipine and isosorbide dinitrate/hydralazine (HISDN), are currently being tested for their potential benefit to HFpEF patients (NCT01157481 and NCT01516346, respectively). Preclinical data showed HISDN improved diastolic function, exercise capacity, and reduced soluble vascular cell adhesion molecule 1 levels in mice, but there were no reductions in LV hypertrophy, cardiac fibrosis, or pulmonary congestion.[124] Recently, exciting studies have revealed that microRNAs (miRNA)-34a might have an important role in cardiac aging via effects on apoptosis, DNA damage, and telomere shortening.[125] The strategy of replacement of miRNAs of interest or of blockade of potentially harmful miRNAs is currently being tested in preclinical studies.[125] Endothelial NO synthase activators were studied in the Dahl salt–sensitive rat model of HFpEF. Diastolic dysfunction was reduced, as were both cardiac hypertrophy and fibrosis.[126]

Device Therapy

The CardioMEMS device is a wireless, implanted pulmonary artery pressure monitor implanted in the distal pulmonary artery during a right heart catheterization procedure. Patients transmit hemodynamic data daily using a wireless radiofrequency transmitter. The CHAMPION trial, a single-blind clinical trial of the CardioMEMS device in patients with HF of any cause, showed a significant reduction in HF hospitalizations.[127] In HFpEF, the CardioMEMS device reduced decompensation leading to hospitalization compared with standard HF management strategies.[128]

Given that increases in LA pressure and pulmonary venous congestion are shown to herald HF decompensation events in patients with HFpEF, creating a controlled left-to-right interatrial shunt to allow LA decompression could be a rational nonpharmacologic strategy for alleviating symptoms in patients with HFpEF. Hemodynamic modeling based on clinical measurements suggested that an appropriately sized iatrogenic atrial septal defect could attenuate exercise-induced increases in LA pressure in patients with HFpEF.[129] Subsequently, an open-label study demonstrated reductions in LA pressure during exercise with improvements in functional capacity and quality of life 6 months after implantation of this device.[130] A prospective, multicenter, randomized, and single-blinded trial is underway to confirm this finding (NCT02600234).

What Treatments Have Worked so Far?

Exercise training

Exercise intolerance is the primary manifestation of chronic HFpEF and is a strong determinant of prognosis and of reduced quality of life. Exercise training (ET) has been shown to improve exercise intolerance in HFrEF. Kitzman and colleagues[131] performed the first randomized, single-blinded trial comparing the effects of 16 weeks of endurance ET versus attention control in older patients with HFpEF. They found increased peak Vo_2, ventilatory anaerobic threshold, 6 MWD, and physical quality-of-life scores with exercise therapy. These results were confirmed in a subsequent multicenter, randomized trial of 3 months of combined ET and strength training in HFpEF patients.[132] In a second, separate, randomized, attention-controlled, single-blind trial of 4 months upper and lower extremity endurance ET, Kitzman and colleagues[133] found a significant increase in peak Vo_2 without altering carotid arterial stiffness or brachial artery flow mediated dilation. Edelmann and colleagues[132] confirmed in a multicenter trial that ET improves exercise capacity and symptoms. Recently, Kitzman and colleagues[134] further extended these results in obese older patients with HFpEF by revealing a combination of diet with endurance ET training was additive and produced a relatively large increase in peak Vo_2. In a recent pilot study, 4 weeks of high-intensity interval training significantly improved peak Vo_2 and LV diastolic dysfunction in HFpEF patients.[135] Taken together, ET is an effective nonpharmacologic therapy in clinically stable patients with HFpEF to improve exercise tolerance. Despite the increasing evidence for the benefits of ET in HFpEF and calls for additional exercise-oriented research, the Center for Medicare and Medicaid Services excluded HFpEF patients from reimbursement for cardiac rehabilitation in their 2014 funding decision.[136,137]

How Does Exercise Training Improve Exercise Intolerance in Heart Failure with Preserved Ejection Fraction Patients?

Aerobic ET may improve exercise capacity either by increasing exercise CO (via increased HR or stroke volume) or by increasing arteriovenous oxygen difference (A-Vo_2 diff) by improvement in peripheral vascular function leading to increase diffusive oxygen transport or by increased oxygen utilization by the skeletal muscle. Haykowsky and colleagues[92] showed that an ET-induced increase in A-Vo_2 diff was the primary contributor to improved peak Vo_2.[92] Similarly, Hundley and colleagues[138] reported that resting and flow-mediated increases in leg blood flow in elderly HFpEF patients may not be significantly impaired; thus, it is possible that in this elderly population with HFpEF muscle adaptation plays a more important role compared with vascular changes. Indeed, Bhella and colleagues[139] showed impaired skeletal muscle oxidative metabolism in elderly patients with HFpEF at baseline that can be favorably shifted by ET to a more efficient muscle O_2 utilization. In addition, Fujimoto and colleagues[140] found no ET-related beneficial effect on LV diastolic function in HFpEF elderly patients, even after 1 year of exercise.

Although the above studies support mechanisms for the beneficial effects of ET that are independent of LV systolic or diastolic function, some studies have attributed ET-related improvements to exercise-induced favorable changes in LV function and CO, atrial reverse remodeling, and improved LV diastolic function.[132,135,141]

Key Knowledge Gaps

1. What will be the optimal ET to improve CV and skeletal muscle function, and physical functional performance in elderly HFpEF patients?
2. Can we develop the most cost-effective models of ET for these patients?
3. Can we start ET early, even shortly after a hospitalization for acute decompensated HF in elderly patients?

Dietary Caloric Restriction

Up to 80% of older patients with HFpEF are overweight or obese, and excess adipose tissue adversely affects cardiac, arterial, and skeletal muscle function. Recently, Kitzman and colleagues[134] showed, among obese older patients with clinically stable HFpEF, that caloric restriction significantly improved exercise capacity and quality of life, and the effect was additive to ET (**Fig. 5**). They demonstrated that caloric restriction was feasible and appeared safe in older, obese HFpEF patients. Caloric restriction improved quality of life much more than ET. The improvements from caloric restriction appeared to be mediated by reduced total body and skeletal muscle adipose and reduced inflammation.

Current guidelines in heart failure with preserved ejection fraction: what is the evidence?

Current guidelines for the management of HFpEF recommend management of volume status with appropriate diuretic dosing, control of BP, management of comorbidities, and dietary

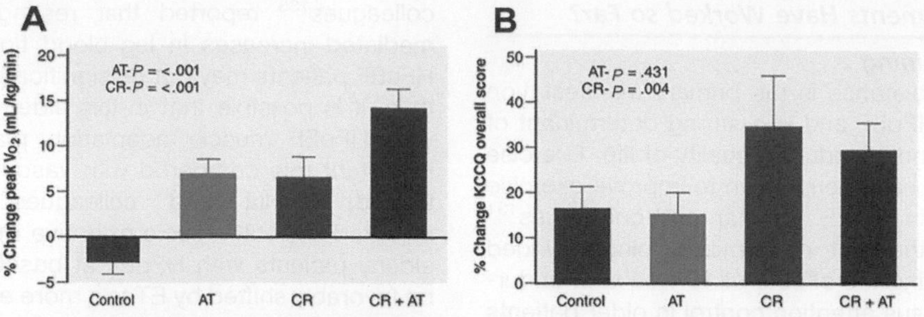

Fig. 5. Effects of a 20-week caloric restriction diet on exercise capacity and quality of life in HFpEF. The graph displays percent changes ± standard errors at the 20-week follow-up relative to baseline by randomized group for peak Vo_2 ($mL \cdot kg^{-1} \cdot min^{-1}$; *A*), and Kansas City Cardiomyopathy Questionnaire (KCCQ) overall score (Quality of Life Score; *B*). *P* values represent effects for aerobic exercise training (AT) and caloric restriction diet (CR).

education.[142] The 2013 American College of Cardiology Foundation (ACCF)/AHA HF guidelines indicate that systolic and diastolic hypertension should be controlled in accordance with published clinical practice guidelines to prevent morbidity, and diuretics should be used to relieve symptoms due to volume overload (class I with level of evidence B).[142] ACCF/AHA guidelines support the use of beta-blockers, ACEI, and ARB for hypertension (IIa recommendation, level of evidence C) and recommend ARBs be considered to decrease hospitalizations (IIb recommendation, level of evidence B).[142] Beta-blockers are recommended for HFpEF patients with a history of myocardial infarction, hypertension, or AF. The ESC guidelines have similar recommendations.[143] To avoid the activation of the RAAS and renal insufficiency or electrolyte disturbances, lowest dose of diuretics should be used to maintain euvolemia. Nonsteroidal anti-inflammatory medications, frequently used in older patients, can cause relative diuretic resistance and should be discontinued if possible.

Screening for ischemic heart disease with a noninvasive stress test or coronary angiography should be considered, especially in patients with chest pain and/or "flash pulmonary edema" to exclude severe CAD.[144] When found, manifest ischemia should be treated, including invasively if indicated (class IIa with level of evidence C). Control of hypertension may be the single most important treatment strategy for HFpEF (class I).[145] Recently, the SPRINT trial demonstrated that intensive BP reduction reduced the risk of acute decompensated HF.[146] The ACCF/AHA guideline recommends management of AF for symptom control for HFpEF (class IIa with level of evidence C). Even though ESC guidelines support restoring sinus rhythm by cardioversion along with anticoagulation, strong evidence is still deficient.[143] The HR control and permanent anticoagulation become mandatory in HFpEF.

Management goals in elders with HFpEF include relief of symptoms, improvement in functional capacity and quality of life, prevention of acute exacerbations and related hospital admissions, and prolongation of survival. A systematic approach should comprise several elements: diagnosis and staging of disease, search for reversible cause, judicious use of medications, patient education, enhancement of self-management skills, coordination of care across disciplines, and effective follow-up. Elders with HF often have severe deconditioning and severe exercise intolerance, and they should be encouraged to undertake regular moderate physical activity. It is likely optimal for this to be under medical supervision, at least initially, but reimbursement barriers can make this a challenge.

Recently, Shah and colleagues[97] proposed a detailed, phenotype-specific roadmap for treatment of HFpEF patients. However, although informative and synthesizing the most current understanding of HFpEF, this strategy has not been prospectively evaluated.

SUMMARY

Multiple lines of evidence suggest that HFpEF may be a systemic disorder with several phenotypes, influenced by aging and affecting all organ systems, including the CV system principally. Moreover, the overwhelming majority of HFpEF patients have multiple comorbidities that also drive phenotypic heterogeneity and multifactorial pathophysiology. Furthermore, noncardiovascular hospital readmissions and mortality are more frequent in HFpEF than in HFrEF. So far, only ET and calorie restriction seem to improve exercise intolerance and quality of life. Given such a multifactorial, complex milieu, it is not surprising that drugs and interventions aimed primarily at a central hemodynamics repeatedly failed to strongly impact overall outcomes in HFpEF. New drugs that target underlying inflammation, oxidative stress, and aging-related dysfunction may prove to be effective for improving outcomes in HFpEF, a rapidly growing disorder among older persons.

REFERENCES

1. Owan TE, Hodge DO, Herges RM, et al. Trends in prevalence and outcome of heart failure with preserved ejection fraction. N Engl J Med 2006;355:251–9.
2. Gottdiener JS, Arnold AM, Aurigemma GP, et al. Predictors of congestive heart failure in the elderly: the Cardiovascular Health Study. J Am Coll Cardiol 2000;35:1628–37.
3. Roger V, Go A, Lloyd-Jones D, et al. Heart disease and stroke statistics - 2011 update - a report from the American Heart Association Statistics committee and stroke statistics subcommittee. Circulation 2011;123:e18–209.
4. van der Velden J, van der Wall EE, Paulus WJ. Heart failure with preserved ejection fraction: current status and challenges for the future. Neth Heart J 2016;24:225–6.
5. Dunlay SM, Redfield MM, Weston SA, et al. Hospitalizations after heart failure diagnosis: a community perspective. J Am Coll Cardiol 2009;54:1695–702.
6. Steinberg BA, Zhao X, Heidenreich PA, et al. Trends in patients hospitalized with heart failure and preserved left ventricular ejection fraction: prevalence, therapies, and outcomes. Circulation 2012;126:65–75.
7. Fonarow GC, Stough WG, Abraham WT, et al. Characteristics, treatments, and outcomes of patients with preserved systolic function hospitalized for heart failure: a report from the OPTIMIZE-HF Registry. J Am Coll Cardiol 2007;50:768–77.
8. Hunt SA, Abraham WT, Chin MH, et al. 2009 focused update incorporated into the ACC/AHA 2005 guidelines for the diagnosis and management of heart failure in adults: a report of the American College of Cardiology Foundation/American Heart Association Task Force on Practice Guidelines developed in collaboration with the International Society for Heart and Lung Transplantation. J Am Coll Cardiol 2009;53:e1–90.
9. McMurray JJ, Adamopoulos S, Anker SD, et al. ESC guidelines for the diagnosis and treatment of acute and chronic heart failure 2012: the task force for the diagnosis and treatment of acute and chronic heart failure 2012 of the European Society of Cardiology. Developed in collaboration with the Heart Failure Association (HFA) of the ESC. Eur Heart J 2012;14:803–69.
10. Rich MW, Kitzman DW. Heart failure in octogenarians: a fundamentally different disease. Am J Geriatr Cardiol 2000;9:97–104.
11. Borlaug B, Redfield M, Melenovsky V, et al. Longitudinal changes in left ventricular stiffness: a community-based study. Circ Heart Fail 2013;6:944–52.
12. DeSouza CA, Shapiro LF, Clevenger CM, et al. Regular aerobic exercise prevents and restores age-related declines in endothelium-dependent vasodilation in healthy men. Circulation 2000;102:1351–7.
13. Gerhard M, Roddy MA, Creager SJ, et al. Aging progressively impairs endothelium-dependent vasodilation in forearm resistance vessels of humans. Hypertension 1996;27:849–53.
14. Ogawa T, Spina RJ, Martin WH, et al. Effect of aging, sex, and physical training on cardiovascular responses to exercise. Circulation 1992;86:494–503.
15. Gerdts E, Zabalgoitia M, Bjornstad H, et al. Gender differences in systolic left ventricular function in hypertensive patients with electrocardiographic left ventricular hypertrophy (the LIFE study). Am J Cardiol 2001;87:980–3.
16. Kane GC, Hauser MF, Behrenbeck TR, et al. Impact of gender on rest Tc-99m sestamibi-gated left ventricular ejection fraction. Am J Cardiol 2002;89:1238–41.
17. Bella JN, Wachtell K, Palmieri V, et al. Relation of left ventricular geometry and function to systemic hemodynamics in hypertension: the LIFE Study. Losartan intervention for endpoint reduction in hypertension study. J Hypertens 2001;19:127–34.
18. Douglas PS, Katz SE, Weinberg EO, et al. Hypertrophic remodeling: gender differences in the early response to left ventricular pressure overload. J Am Coll Cardiol 1998;32:1118–25.
19. Spina RJ, Ogawa T, Miller TR, et al. Effect of exercise training on left ventricular performance in older women free of cardiopulmonary disease. Am J Cardiol 1993;71:99–194.
20. Sullivan M, Cobb F, Higginbotham M. Stroke volume increases by similar mechanisms during upright exercise in normal men and women. Am J Cardiol 1991;67:1405–12.
21. Marcell TJ. Sarcopenia: causes, consequences, and preventions. J Gerontol A Biol Sci Med Sci 2003;58:M911–6.
22. Morley JE, Baumgartner RN, Roubenoff R, et al. Sarcopenia. J Lab Clin Med 2001;137:231–43.
23. Roubenoff R. Sarcopenia: effects on body composition and function. J Gerontol A Biol Sci Med Sci 2003;58:1012–7.
24. Forbes GB, Halloran E. The adult decline in lean body mass. Hum Biol 1976;48:161–73.
25. Collier P, Watson C, Voon V, et al. Can emerging biomarkers of myocardial remodelling identify asymptomatic hypertensive patients at risk for diastolic dysfunction and diastolic heart failure? Eur J Heart Fail 2011;13:1087–95.

26. Kalogeropoulos A, Georgiopoulou V, Psaty B, et al. Inflammatory markers and incident heart failure risk in older adults: the Health ABC (health, aging, and body composition) study. J Am Coll Cardiol 2010; 55:2129–37.
27. Franceschi C, Bonafe M, Valensin S, et al. Inflamm-aging: an evolutionary perspective on immunosenescence. Ann N Y Acad Sci 2000;908:244–54.
28. Haykowsky MJ, Brubaker PH, Morgan TM, et al. Impaired aerobic capacity and physical functional performance in older heart failure patients with preserved ejection fraction: role of lean body mass. J Gerontol A Biol Sci Med Sci 2013;68: 968–75.
29. Haykowsky M, Kouba EJ, Brubaker PH, et al. Skeletal muscle composition and its relation to exercise intolerance in older patients with heart failure and preserved ejection fraction. Am J Cardiol 2014; 113:1211–6.
30. Kitzman DW, Nicklas B, Kraus WE, et al. Skeletal muscle abnormalities and exercise intolerance in older patients with heart failure and preserved ejection fraction. Am J Physiol Heart Circ Physiol 2014;306:H1364–70.
31. Molina AJ, Bharadwaj MS, Van Horn C, et al. Skeletal muscle mitochondrial content, oxidative capacity, and Mfn2 expression are reduced in older patients with heart failure and preserved ejection fraction and are related to exercise intolerance. JACC Heart Fail 2016;4:636–45.
32. Bowen TS, Rolim NP, Fischer T, et al. Heart failure with preserved ejection fraction induces molecular, mitochondrial, histological, and functional alterations in rat respiratory and limb skeletal muscle. Eur J Heart Fail 2015;17:263–72.
33. Larsson L, Sjodin B, Karlsson J. Histochemical and biochemical changes in human skeletal muscle with age in sedentary males, age 22-65 years. Acta Physiol Scand 1978;103:31–9.
34. Coggan AR, Spina RJ, King DS. Histochemical and enzymatic comparison of the gastrocnemius muscle of young and elderly men and women. J Gerontol 1992;47:B71–6.
35. Franssen F, Wouters E, Schols A. The contribution of starvation, deconditioning and ageing to the observed alterations in peripheral skeletal muscle in chronic organ diseases. Clin Nutr 2002;21: 1–14.
36. Coats A, Clark A, Piepoli M, et al. Symptoms and quality of life in heart failure: the muscle hypothesis. Br Heart J 1994;72:S39.
37. Middlekauff HR. Making the case for skeletal myopathy as the major limitation of exercise capacity in heart failure. Circ Heart Fail 2010;3:537–46.
38. Fried LP, Hadley EC, Walston JD, et al. From bedside to bench: research agenda for frailty. Sci Aging Knowledge Environ 2005;2005:e24.
39. Kitzman DW, Hundley WG, Brubaker P, et al. A randomized, controlled, double-blinded trial of enalapril in older patients with heart failure and preserved ejection fraction; effects on exercise tolerance, and arterial distensibility. Circ Heart Fail 2010;3:477–85.
40. Edelmann F, Aldo-DHF Investigators. Effect of spironolactone on diastolic function and exercise capacity in patients with heart failure with preserved ejection fraction: The Aldo-DHF randomized controlled trial. JAMA 2013;309:781–91.
41. Yancy C, Lopatin M, Stevenson L, et al, ADHERE Scientific Advisory Committee and Investigators. Clinical presentation, management, and in-hospital outcomes of patients admitted with acute decompensated heart failure with preserved systolic function: a report from the Acute Decompensated Heart Failure National Registry (ADHERE) Database. J Am Coll Cardiol 2006;47:76–84.
42. Shah SJ. Evolving approaches to the management of heart failure with preserved ejection fraction in patients with coronary artery disease. Curr Treat Options Cardiovasc Med 2010;12:58–75.
43. Hwang SJ, Melenovsky V, Borlaug BA. Implications of coronary artery disease in heart failure with preserved ejection fraction. J Am Coll Cardiol 2014;63: 2817–27.
44. Rusinaru D, Houpe D, Szymanski C, et al. Coronary artery disease and 10-year outcome after hospital admission for heart failure with preserved and with reduced ejection fraction. Eur J Heart Fail 2014;16:967–76.
45. Mohammed SF, Hussain S, Mirzoyev SA, et al. Coronary microvascular rarefaction and myocardial fibrosis in heart failure with preserved ejection fraction. Circulation 2015;131:550–9.
46. Borlaug BA, Olson TP, Lam CSP, et al. Global cardiovascular reserve dysfunction in heart failure with preserved ejection fraction. J Am Coll Cardiol 2010;56:845–54.
47. Vermond RA, Geelhoed B, Verweij N, et al. Incidence of atrial fibrillation and relationship with cardiovascular events, heart failure, and mortality: a community-based study from the Netherlands. J Am Coll Cardiol 2015;66:1000–7.
48. Chamberlain AM, Redfield MM, Alonso A, et al. Atrial fibrillation and mortality in heart failure: a community study. Circ Heart Fail 2011;4:740–6.
49. Zakeri R, Borlaug BA, McNulty SE, et al. Impact of atrial fibrillation on exercise capacity in heart failure with preserved ejection fraction: a RELAX trial ancillary study. Circ Heart Fail 2014;7:123–30.
50. Lam CS, Rienstra M, Tay WT, et al. Atrial fibrillation in heart failure with preserved ejection fraction: association with exercise capacity, left ventricular filling pressures, natriuretic peptides, and left atrial volume. JACC Heart Fail 2017;5(2):92–8.

51. Ather S, Chan W, Bozkurt B, et al. Impact of noncardiac comorbidities on morbidity and mortality in a predominantly male population with heart failure and preserved versus reduced ejection fraction. J Am Coll Cardiol 2012;59:998–1005.
52. Ndumele CE, Coresh J, Lazo M, et al. Obesity, subclinical myocardial injury, and incident heart failure. JACC Heart Fail 2014;2:600–7.
53. Kitzman DW, Shah SJ. The HFpEF obesity phenotype: the elephant in the room. J Am Coll Cardiol 2016;68:200–3.
54. Dalos D, Mascherbauer J, Zotter-Tufaro C, et al. NYHA functional class is associated with diastolic pulmonary pressure and predicts outcome in patients with heart failure and preserved ejection fraction. J Am Coll Cardiol 2016;68:189–99.
55. Kitzman DW, Gardin JM, Gottdiener JS, et al. Importance of heart failure with preserved systolic function in patients > or = 65 years of age. CHS Research Group. Cardiovascular health study. Am J Cardiol 2001;87:413–9.
56. Caruana L, Petrie MC, Davie AP, et al. Do patients with suspected heart failure and preserved left ventricular systolic function suffer from "diastolic heart failure" or from misdiagnosis? A prospective descriptive study. BMJ 2000;321:215–8.
57. Kitzman DW, Guazzi M. Impaired alveolar capillary membrane diffusion: a recently recognized contributor to exertional dyspnea in heart failure with preserved ejection fraction. JACC Heart Fail 2016;4:499–501.
58. Paulus W, Tschope C. A novel paradigm for heart failure with preserved ejection fraction: comorbidities drive myocardial dysfunction and remodeling through coronary microvascular endothelial inflammation. J Am Coll Cardiol 2013;62:263–71.
59. Franssen C, Chen S, Unger A, et al. Myocardial microvascular inflammatory endothelial activation in heart failure with preserved ejection fraction. JACC Heart Fail 2015;4:312–24.
60. Putko BN, Wang Z, Lo J, et al. Circulating levels of tumor necrosis factor-alpha receptor 2 are increased in heart failure with preserved ejection fraction relative to heart failure with reduced ejection fraction: evidence for a divergence in pathophysiology. PLoS ONE 2014;9:e99495.
61. Loffredo FS, Steinhauser ML, Jay SM, et al. Growth differentiation factor 11 is a circulating factor that reverses age-related cardiac hypertrophy. Cell 2013;153:828–39.
62. Groban L, Pailes NA, Bennett C, et al. Growth hormone replacement attenuates diastolic dysfunction and cardiac angiotensin ii expression in senescent rats. J Gerontol A Biol Sci Med Sci 2006;61:28–35.
63. Groban L, Yamaleyeva LM, Westwood BM, et al. Progressive diastolic dysfunction in the female mRen(2). Lewis rat: influence of salt and ovarian hormones. J Gerontol A Biol Sci Med Sci 2008; 63:3–11.
64. Lasocki S, Iglarz M, Seince PF, et al. Involvement of renin-angiotensin system in pressure-flow relationship: role of angiotensin-converting enzyme gene polymorphism. Anesthesiology 2002;96:271–5.
65. Little WC, Wesley-Farrington DJ, Hoyle J, et al. Effect of candesartan and verapamil on exercise tolerance in diastolic dysfunction. J Cardiovasc Pharmacol 2004;43:288–93.
66. Wright JW, Mizutani S, Harding JW. Pathways involved in the transition from hypertension to hypertrophy to heart failure. Treatment strategies. Heart Fail Rev 2008;13:367–75.
67. Yusuf S, Pfeffer MA, Swedberg K, et al. Effects of candesartan in patients with chronic heart failure and preserved left-ventricular ejection fraction: the CHARM-Preserved Trial. Lancet 2003;362:777–81.
68. Cleland JGF, Tendera M, Adamus J, et al. The perindopril in elderly people with chronic heart failure (PEP-CHF) study. Eur Heart J 2006;27: 2338–45.
69. Massie BM, Carson PE, McMurray JJ, et al. Irbesartan in patients with heart failure and preserved ejection fraction. N Engl J Med 2008;359:2456–67.
70. Pitt B, Pfeffer M, Assmann S, et al. Spironolactone for heart failure with preserved ejection fraction. N Engl J Med 2014;370:1383–92.
71. Deswal A, Richardson P, Bozkurt B, et al. Results of the randomized aldosterone antagonism in heart failure with preserved ejection fraction trial (RAAM-PEF). J Card Fail 2011;17:634–42.
72. Pfeffer MA, Claggett B, Assmann SF, et al. Regional variation in patients and outcomes in the treatment of preserved cardiac function heart failure with an Aldosterone Antagonist (TOPCAT) Trial. Circulation 2015;131:34–42.
73. Aronow WS, Ahn C, Kronzon I. Effect of propranolol versus no propranolol on total mortality plus nonfatal myocardial infarction in older patients with prior myocardial infarction, congestive heart failure, and left ventricular ejection fraction > or = 40% treated with diuretics plus angiotensin-converting enzyme inhibitors. Am J Cardiol 1997; 80:207–9.
74. Yamamoto K, Origasa H, Hori M, J-DHF Investigators. Effects of carvedilol on heart failure with preserved ejection fraction: the Japanese Diastolic Heart Failure Study (J-DHF). Eur J Heart Fail 2013;15:110–8.
75. Conraads V, Metra M, Kamp O, et al. Effects of the long-term administration of nebivolol on the clinical symptoms, exercise capacity, and left ventricular function of patients with diastolic dysfunction: results of the ELANDD study. Eur J Heart Fail 2012; 14:219–25.

76. Hernandez AF, Hammill BG, O'Connor CM, et al. Clinical effectiveness of beta-blockers in heart failure: findings from the OPTIMIZE-HF (organized program to initiate lifesaving treatment in hospitalized patients with heart failure) registry. J Am Coll Cardiol 2009;53:184–92.
77. Ahmed A, Pitt B, Rahimtoola SH, et al. Effects of digoxin at low serum concentrations on mortality and hospitalization in heart failure: A propensity-matched study of the DIG trial. Int J Cardiol 2008; 123:138–46.
78. Solomon S, Zile M, Pieske B, et al. The angiotensin receptor neprilysin inhibitor LCZ696 in heart failure with preserved ejection fraction: a phase 2 double-blind randomised controlled trial. Lancet 2012;380: 1387–95.
79. Maurer MS, Burkhoff D, Fried LP, et al. Ventricular structure and function in hypertensive participants with heart failure and a normal ejection fraction: the Cardiovascular Health Study. J Am Coll Cardiol 2007;49:972–81.
80. Solomon SD, Verma A, Desai A, et al. Effect of intensive versus standard blood pressure lowering on diastolic function in patients with uncontrolled hypertension and diastolic dysfunction. Hypertension 2010;55:241–8.
81. Su MY, Lin LY, Tseng YH, et al. CMR-verified diffuse myocardial fibrosis is associated with diastolic dysfunction in HFpEF. JACC Cardiovasc Imaging 2014;7:991–7.
82. Kitzman D, Upadhya B. Heart failure with preserved ejection fraction: a heterogenous disorder with multifactorial pathophysiology. J Am Coll Cardiol 2014;63:457–9.
83. Zile MR, Gaasch WH, Carroll JD, et al. Heart failure with a normal ejection fraction: is measurement of diastolic function necessary to make the diagnosis of diastolic heart failure? Circulation 2001; 104:779–82.
84. Zile MR, Brutsaert DL. New concepts in diastolic dysfunction and diastolic heart failure: part I: diagnosis, prognosis, and measurements of diastolic function. Circulation 2002;105:1387–93.
85. Burkhoff D, Maurer MS, Packer M. Heart failure with a normal ejection fraction: is it really a disorder of diastolic function? Circulation 2003;107:656–8.
86. Melenovsky V, Borlaug BA, Rosen B, et al. Cardiovascular features of heart failure with preserved ejection fraction versus nonfailing hypertensive left ventricular hypertrophy in the urban Baltimore community: the role of atrial remodeling/dysfunction. J Am Coll Cardiol 2007;49:198–207.
87. Maurer MS, Hummel SL. Heart failure with a preserved ejection fraction: what is in a name? J Am Coll Cardiol 2011;58:275–7.
88. Kawaguchi M, Hay I, Fetics B, et al. Combined ventricular systolic and arterial stiffening in patients with heart failure and preserved ejection fraction. Circulation 2003;107:714–20.
89. Brubaker PH, Joo KC, Stewart KP, et al. Chronotropic incompetence and its contribution to exercise intolerance in older heart failure patients. J Cardiopulm Rehabil 2006;26:86–9.
90. Borlaug BA, Melenovsky V, Russell SD, et al. Impaired chronotropic and vasodilator reserves limit exercise capacity in patients with heart failure and a preserved ejection fraction. Circulation 2006; 114:2138–47.
91. Pham PP, Balaji S, Shen I, et al. Impact of conventional versus biventricular pacing on hemodynamics and tissue Doppler imaging indexes of resynchronization postoperatively in children with congenital heart disease. J Am Coll Cardiol 2005; 46:2284–9.
92. Haykowsky MJ, Brubaker PH, Stewart KP, et al. Effect of endurance training on the determinants of peak exercise oxygen consumption in elderly patients with stable compensated heart failure and preserved ejection fraction. J Am Coll Cardiol 2012;60:120–8.
93. Phan TT, Abozguia K, Nallur Shivu G, et al. Heart failure with preserved ejection fraction is characterized by dynamic impairment of active relaxation and contraction of the left ventricle on exercise and associated with myocardial energy deficiency. J Am Coll Cardiol 2009;54:402–9.
94. Witte KK, Cleland J, Clark AL. Chronic heart failure, chronotropic incompetence, and the effects of beta blockers. Heart 2006;92:481–6.
95. Hawkins NM, Petrie MC, MacDonald MR, et al. Heart failure and chronic obstructive pulmonary disease: the quandary of beta-blockers and beta-agonists. J Am Coll Cardiol 2011;57:2127–38.
96. Bangalore S, Parkar S, Grossman E, et al. A meta-analysis of 94,492 patients with hypertension treated with beta blockers to determine the risk of new-onset diabetes mellitus. Am J Cardiol 2007; 100:1254–62.
97. Shah SJ, Kitzman DW, Borlaug BA, et al. Phenotype-specific treatment of heart failure with preserved ejection fraction: a multiorgan roadmap. Circulation 2016;134:73–90.
98. Kanwar M, Agarwal R, Barnes M, et al. Role of phosphodiesterase-5 inhibitors in heart failure: emerging data and concepts. Curr Heart Fail Rep 2013;10:26–35.
99. Redfield M, Chen H, Borlaug B, et al. Effect of phosphodiesterase-5 inhibition on exercise capacity and clinical status in heart failure with preserved ejection fraction: a randomized clinical trial. JAMA 2013;309:1268–77.
100. Redfield M, Anstrom K, Levine J, et al. Isosorbide mononitrate in heart failure with preserved ejection fraction. N Engl J Med 2015;373(24):2314–24.

101. Borlaug BA, Melenovsky V, Koepp KE. Inhaled sodium nitrite improves rest and exercise hemodynamics in heart failure with preserved ejection fraction. Circ Res 2016;119:880–6.
102. Thomas GR, DiFabio JM, Gori T, et al. Once daily therapy with isosorbide-5-mononitrate causes endothelial dysfunction in humans: evidence of a free-radical-mediated mechanism. J Am Coll Cardiol 2007;49:1289–95.
103. Eggebeen J, Kim-Shapiro DB, Haykowsky MJ, et al. One week of daily dosing with beetroot juice improves submaximal endurance and blood pressure in older patients with heart failure and preserved ejection fraction. JACC Heart Fail 2015;4:428–37.
104. Jhund PS, Claggett BL, Voors AA, et al. Elevation in high-sensitivity troponin T in heart failure and preserved ejection fraction and influence of treatment with the angiotensin receptor neprilysin inhibitor LCZ696. Circ Heart Fail 2014;7:953–9.
105. Hattori T, Shimokawa H, Higashi M, et al. Long-term inhibition of Rho-kinase suppresses left ventricular remodeling after myocardial infarction in mice. Circulation 2004;109:2234–9.
106. Martin J, Denver R, Bailey M, et al. In vitro inhibitory effects of atorvastatin on cardiac fibroblasts: implications for ventricular remodelling. Clin Exp Pharmacol Physiol 2005;32:697–701.
107. Fukuta H, Little W. Observational studies of statins in heart failure with preserved systolic function. Heart Fail Clin 2008;4:209–16.
108. Fukuta H, Sane DC, Brucks S, et al. Statin therapy may be associated with lower mortality in patients with diastolic heart failure: a preliminary report. Circulation 2005;112:357–63.
109. Fukuta H, Goto T, Wakami K, et al. The effect of statins on mortality in heart failure with preserved ejection fraction: a meta-analysis of propensity score analyses. Int J Cardiol 2016;214:301–6.
110. Alehagen U, Benson L, Edner M, et al. Association between use of statins and outcomes in heart failure with reduced ejection fraction: prospective propensity score matched cohort study of 21 864 patients in the Swedish Heart Failure Registry. Circ Heart Fail 2015;8:252–60.
111. Reil JC, Hohl M, Reil GH, et al. Heart rate reduction by If-inhibition improves vascular stiffness and left ventricular systolic and diastolic function in a mouse model of heart failure with preserved ejection fraction. Eur Heart J 2013;34:2839–49.
112. Kosmala W, Holland DJ, Rojek A, et al. Effect of if-channel inhibition on hemodynamic status and exercise tolerance in heart failure with preserved ejection fraction: a randomized trial. J Am Coll Cardiol 2013;62:1330–8.
113. Pal N, Sivaswamy N, Mahmod M, et al. Effect of selective heart rate slowing in heart failure with preserved ejection fraction. Circulation 2015;132:1719–25.
114. Bonderman D, Pretsch I, Steringer-Mascherbauer R, et al. Acute hemodynamic effects of riociguat in patients with pulmonary hypertension associated with diastolic heart failure (dilate-1): a randomized, double-blind, placebo-controlled, single-dose study. Chest J 2014;146:1274–85.
115. Jacobshagen C, Belardinelli L, Hasenfuss G, et al. Ranolazine for the treatment of heart failure with preserved ejection fraction: background, aims, and design of the RALI-DHF Study. Clin Cardiol 2011;34:426–32.
116. Maier LS, Layug B, Karwatowska-Prokopczuk E, et al. RAnoLazIne for the treatment of diastolic heart failure in patients with preserved ejection fraction: the RALI-DHF proof-of-concept study. JACC Heart Fail 2013;1:115–22.
117. Borbely A, Papp Z, Edes I, et al. Molecular determinants of heart failure with normal left ventricular ejection fraction. Pharmacol Rep 2009;61:139–45.
118. Little WC, Zile MR, Kitzman DW, et al. The effect of alagebrium chloride (ALT-711), a novel glucose cross-link breaker, in the treatment of elderly patients with diastolic heart failure. J Card Fail 2005;11:191–5.
119. Zile MR, Bourge RC, Redfield MM, et al. Randomized, double-blind, placebo-controlled study of sitaxsentan to improve impaired exercise tolerance in patients with heart failure and a preserved ejection fraction. JACC Heart Fail 2014;2:123–30.
120. Bujak M, Frangogiannis NG. The role of IL-1 in the pathogenesis of heart disease. Arch Immunol Ther Exp (Warsz) 2009;57:165–76.
121. Van Tassell BW, Arena R, Biondi-Zoccai G, et al. Effects of interleukin-1 blockade with anakinra on aerobic exercise capacity in patients with heart failure and preserved ejection fraction (from the D-HART pilot study). Am J Cardiol 2014;113:321–7.
122. Fitchett D, Zinman B, Wanner C, et al. Heart failure outcomes with empagliflozin in patients with type 2 diabetes at high cardiovascular risk: results of the EMPA-REG OUTCOME(R) trial. Eur Heart J 2016;37:1526–34.
123. Tanaka A, Inoue T, Kitakaze M, et al. Rationale and design of a randomized trial to test the safety and non-inferiority of canagliflozin in patients with diabetes with chronic heart failure: the CANDLE trial. Cardiovasc Diabetol 2016;15:57.
124. Wilson RM, De Silva DS, Sato K, et al. Effects of fixed-dose isosorbide dinitrate/hydralazine on diastolic function and exercise capacity in hypertension-induced diastolic heart failure. Hypertension 2009;54:583–90.
125. Boon RA, Iekushi K, Lechner S, et al. MicroRNA-34a regulates cardiac ageing and function. Nature 2013;495:107–10.

126. Westermann D, Riad A, Richter U, et al. Enhancement of the endothelial NO synthase attenuates experimental diastolic heart failure. Basic Res Cardiol 2009;104:499–509.
127. Abraham WT, Adamson PB, Bourge RC, et al. Wireless pulmonary artery haemodynamic monitoring in chronic heart failure: a randomised controlled trial. Lancet 2011;377:658–66.
128. Adamson PB, Abraham WT, Bourge RC, et al. Wireless pulmonary artery pressure monitoring guides management to reduce decompensation in heart failure with preserved ejection fraction. Circ Heart Fail 2014;7:935–44.
129. Kaye D, Shah SJ, Borlaug BA, et al. Effects of an interatrial shunt on rest and exercise hemodynamics: results of a computer simulation in heart failure. J Card Fail 2014;20:212–21.
130. Hasenfuss G, Hayward C, Burkhoff D, et al. A transcatheter intracardiac shunt device for heart failure with preserved ejection fraction (REDUCE LAP-HF): a multicentre, open-label, single-arm, phase 1 trial. Lancet 2016;387:1298–304.
131. Kitzman D, Brubaker P, Morgan T, et al. Exercise training in older patients with heart failure and preserved ejection fraction. Circ Heart Fail 2010;3:659–67.
132. Edelmann F, Gelbrich G, Dungen H, et al. Exercise training improves exercise capacity and diastolic function in patients with heart failure with preserved ejection fraction: results of the Ex-DHF (exercise training in diastolic heart failure) pilot study. J Am Coll Cardiol 2011;58:1780–91.
133. Kitzman DW, Brubaker PH, Herrington DM, et al. Effect of endurance exercise training on endothelial function and arterial stiffness in older patients with heart failure and preserved ejection fraction: a randomized, controlled, single-blind trial. J Am Coll Cardiol 2013;62:584–92.
134. Kitzman DW, Brubaker P, Morgan T, et al. Effect of caloric restriction or aerobic exercise training on peak oxygen consumption and quality of life in obese older patients with heart failure with preserved ejection fraction: a randomised clinical trial. JAMA 2016;315:36–46.
135. Angadi SS, Mookadam F, Lee CD, et al. High-intensity interval training vs. moderate-intensity continuous exercise training in heart failure with preserved ejection fraction: a pilot study. J Appl Physiol 2014;95:15–27.
136. Suchy C, Massen L, Rognmo O, et al. Optimising exercise training in prevention and treatment of diastolic heart failure (OptimEx-CLIN): rationale and design of a prospective, randomised, controlled trial. Eur J Prev Cardiol 2014;21:18–25.
137. Koifman E, Grossman E, Elis A, et al. Multidisciplinary rehabilitation program in recently hospitalized patients with heart failure and preserved ejection fraction: rationale and design of a randomized controlled trial. Am Heart J 2014;168:830–7.
138. Hundley WG, Bayram E, Hamilton CA, et al. Leg flow-mediated arterial dilation in elderly patients with heart failure and normal left ventricular ejection fraction. Am J Physiol Heart Circ Physiol 2007;292:H1427–34.
139. Bhella PS, Prasad A, Heinicke K, et al. Abnormal haemodynamic response to exercise in heart failure with preserved ejection fraction. Eur J Heart Fail 2011;13:1296–304.
140. Fujimoto N, Prasad A, Hastings JL, et al. Cardiovascular effects of 1 year of progressive endurance exercise training in patients with heart failure with preserved ejection fraction. Am Heart J 2012;164:869–77.
141. Hambrecht R, Gielen S, Linke A, et al. Effects of exercise training on left ventricular function and peripheral resistance in patients with chronic heart failure. JAMA 2000;283:3095–101.
142. Yancy CW, Jessup M, Bozkurt B, et al. 2013 ACCF/AHA guideline for the management of heart-failure: a report of the American College of Cardiology Foundation/American Heart Association Task Force on Practice Guidelines. J Am Coll Cardiol 2013;62:e147–239.
143. Ponikowski P, Voors AA, Anker SD, et al. 2016 ESC Guidelines for the diagnosis and treatment of acute and chronic heart failure: the Task Force for the diagnosis and treatment of acute and chronic heart failure of the European Society of Cardiology (ESC). Developed with the special contribution of the Heart Failure Association (HFA) of the ESC. Eur J Heart Fail 2016;18:891–975.
144. Mendes LA, Davidoff R, Cupples LA, et al. Congestive heart failure in patients with coronary artery disease: the gender paradox. Am Heart J 1997;134:207–12.
145. Moser M, Hebert PR. Prevention of disease progression, left ventricular hypertrophy and congestive heart failure in hypertension treatment trials. J Am Coll Cardiol 1996;27:1214–8.
146. Wright JT Jr, Williamson JD, Whelton PK, et al. A randomized trial of intensive versus standard blood-pressure control. N Engl J Med 2015;373:2103–16.

Use of Diuretics in the Treatment of Heart Failure in Older Adults

Domenic A. Sica, MD[a], Todd W.B. Gehr, MD[b], William H. Frishman, MD[c,*]

KEYWORDS

• Heart failure • Diuretics • Fluid congestion • Elderly patients

KEY POINTS

- Diuretic therapy remains a cornerstone of heart failure (HF) therapy.
- In the treatment of volume-overloaded patients, diuretics clearly improve symptoms and quality of life.
- Despite the acceptance of diuretic therapy for the treatment of symptoms, considerable debate has ensued for many decades about the impact of this class of agent on mortality, cardiac function, and disease progression.
- Accordingly, diuretics should be used judiciously in patients with HF, at the minimum effective dose, with careful monitoring of electrolyte balance, and continued only if there is a demonstrable ongoing clinical need.
- Aldosterone receptor antagonists (ARAs) should be distinguished from both loop and thiazide-type diuretics in that outcomes data support their routine use in advanced systolic HF and in patients after myocardial infarction with clinical HF symptoms and a left ventricular ejection fraction less than 40%.
- ARAs also can be considered for use in patients with diastolic HF and a normal ejection fraction.

Most therapies used in the contemporary management of heart failure (HF) have been rigorously evaluated in large-scale clinical trials to assess their beneficial effects on quality of life and prognosis. Such therapies include angiotensin-converting enzyme (ACE) inhibitors, angiotensin-receptor blockers, β-adrenergic-blockers, and aldosterone receptor antagonists (ARAs). Diuretics are the most commonly prescribed class of drugs in patients with HF and in the short term they remain the most effective treatment for relief from fluid congestion. Diuretic therapy in the patient with HF often is as much an art as a science. Moreover, as a class of drugs, diuretics are fairly heterogeneous in their effects. Diuretic therapy in HF always should be accompanied by dietary sodium restriction. Important considerations in defining diuretic effect include issues of dose amount, frequency of dosing, concomitant medications, blood pressure, and, most importantly, the degree to which cardiac function is compromised. Diuretic combinations are often quite effective in the more advanced stages of HF. Diuretic-related electrolyte side effects are common and require ongoing vigilance both to detect their occurrence as well as to track their correction.

Diuretics are tools of considerable therapeutic importance. First, they effectively reduce blood pressure, while at the same time decreasing the morbidity and mortality associated with

This is an updated version of an article that appeared in *Heart Failure Clinics*, Volume 3, Issue 4.
[a] Clinical Pharmacology and Hypertension, Box 980160, MCV Station, Medical College of Virginia of Virginia Commonwealth University, 1101 East Marshall Street, Richmond, VA 23298, USA; [b] Division of Nephrology, Box 980160, MCV Station, Medical College of Virginia of Virginia Commonwealth University, Richmond, VA 23298, USA; [c] Department of Medicine, Westchester Medical Center, New York Medical College, Valhalla, NY 10595, USA
* Corresponding author.
E-mail address: William_Frishman@nymc.edu

Heart Failure Clin 13 (2017) 503–512
http://dx.doi.org/10.1016/j.hfc.2017.02.006
1551-7136/17/

hypertension. The Joint National Committee on Prevention, Detection, Evaluation, and Treatment of Hypertension continues to recommend diuretics as first-line therapy for the treatment of hypertension.[1] In addition, they remain an important component of HF therapy, in that they improve the symptoms of congestion, which typify the more advanced stages of HF.[2–6] This article reviews the mode of action of the various diuretic classes and the physiologic adaptations that follow and sets up the basis for their use in the treatment of volume-retaining states, particularly as applies to the elderly. In addition, the article reviews the common side effects related to diuretics.

OVERVIEW

Guideline-promulgating committees have positioned diuretics as necessary adjuncts in the medical therapy for HF when symptoms of volume overload exist.[2–6] Diuretics are typically used first for the acute relief of congestion and thereafter for achieving and maintaining a target or "dry" weight. Diuretic doses are typically higher in the case of congestion relief and can generally be scaled back in the chronic treatment phase of HF. Diuretic therapy typically results in rapid improvement of dyspnea and increased exercise tolerance.[7] No controlled randomized trials have assessed the effect on symptoms or survival of thiazide and loop diuretics, and they should always be administered in combination with ACE inhibitors and β-blockers if tolerated.

The relation of systolic to diastolic HF is clearly shifted toward diastolic HF in elderly patients, especially in women.[8] Mortality increases with systolic dysfunction in elderly patients compared with younger patients with HF.[9] Mortality is less with diastolic dysfunction, but still higher compared with elderly individuals without HF.[10] In addition, morbidity is increased both with diastolic and systolic HF in elderly patients. Drug therapy for systolic HF in elderly patients is similar to younger patients, although guideline recommendations for drug therapy are based in most cases on studies conducted in younger patients with systolic HF. However, when administering drug therapy for systolic HF in the elderly, clinicians should be mindful of the physiologic decrease in renal function with age and the more frequent renal impairment that occurs in elderly patients receiving diuretics for HF management.[11] In addition, loop diuretic treatment of any patient with HF always should be at the lowest effective dose. This is particularly so in the elderly patient with HF because the hypercalciuria, produced in a dose-dependent manner by loop diuretics,[12] increases the bone-fracture rate, a clinical finding also observed with thiazide-type diuretics.[13]

TREATMENT ALGORITHM FOR DIURETIC USE IN HEART FAILURE

A diuretic treatment algorithm for the treatment of HF can become extremely complicated. No one such algorithm can ever meet the treatment needs of all patients, particularly elderly patients. In cases involving the elderly, negative effects of excessive diuresis on blood pressure and renal function often have an impact on decisions related to diuretic dose and frequency. **Table 1** offers some guidance on the order of medication choice and the basis for such choices. Loop diuretics offer short-term benefits in HF because of symptomatic relief. However, in the long term, they have the potential to adversely influence outcome due to electrolyte changes or excessive neurohumoral activation.[14–16] Consequently, in the long term, diuretic withdrawal or dosage reduction is desirable.[17] Diuretic withdrawal (or interruption) is facilitated by adherence to a low-sodium (low-Na^+) diet. Such withdrawal is typically better tolerated in patients requiring lower diuretic doses, a patient subset characterized by having both smaller ventricles and a higher left ventricular ejection fraction.[17]

INDIVIDUAL CLASSES OF DIURETICS

Interclass and intraclass differences exist for all diuretic classes. The diuretic classes of note include carbonic anhydrase inhibitors, loop and distal tubular diuretics, and potassium (K^+)-sparing agents.[16]

Carbonic Anhydrase Inhibitors

Acetazolamide is the only carbonic anhydrase inhibitor with relevant diuretic effects. Acetazolamide is readily absorbed and undergoes renal elimination predominantly by tubular secretion. Its administration is ordinarily accompanied by a brisk alkaline diuresis. Although carbonic anhydrase inhibitors are proximal tubular diuretics (where the bulk of Na^+ reabsorption occurs), their net diuretic effect is modest, because Na^+ reabsorption in more distal nephron segments offsets proximal Na^+ losses. Acetazolamide use is constrained by both its transient action as well as the development of metabolic acidosis with its prolonged administration. Alternatively, acetazolamide (250–500 mg daily) can correct the metabolic or contraction alkalosis that on occasion occurs with aggressive thiazide or loop diuretic therapy.[18]

Table 1
Diuretic treatment in heart failure

Treatment Situation	Comments
Initial treatment given with a loop or a thiazide diuretic in conjunction with an angiotensin-converting enzyme (ACE) inhibitor.	Severity of volume overload and level of heart failure dictate initial choice and whether drug is given orally or intravenously.
Higher total doses given as needed.	Higher total doses can be given by increasing the individual dose amount, by giving the diuretic more frequently, or both. If diuretic doses need to be titrated upward, excessive dietary sodium intake needs to be considered as a factor contributing to the change in dose.
Single diuretic therapy fails to produce the desired response.	Factors that may reduce diuretic response, such as insufficient blood pressure, poor diuretic absorption, suboptimal neurohumoral blockade, or use of nonsteroidal anti-inflammatory drugs, should be considered before moving to combination therapy.
Single diuretic therapy fails to produce the desired response and combination therapy is started.	Metolazone can be added to a loop diuretic but is poorly absorbed. Poor absorption needs to be considered in determining the timing of its dosing. Metolazone has a very long half-life and may not need to be given on a daily basis.
Potassium-sparing diuretics are started at varying times in the overall treatment.	These drugs are used to facilitate treatment of diuretic-related hypokalemia or hypomagnesemia. Serum potassium needs to be regularly measured until it is stable.
Once a dry weight is established and maintained, some consideration can be given to reducing the amount of diuretic being given.	Optimizing neurohumoral blockade with ACE inhibition and β-blockade will often allow lowering or sometimes discontinuation of diuretics.

Loop Diuretics

Loop diuretics act predominantly at the apical membrane in the thick ascending limb of the loop of Henle, where they compete with chloride (Cl^-) for binding to the $Na^+/K^+/2Cl^-$ cotransporter, thereby inhibiting both Na^+ and Cl^- reabsorption.[19] Loop diuretics also affect Na^+ reabsorption within other nephron segments. However, these effects are qualitatively minor compared with their action at the thick ascending limb. Other clinically important effects of loop diuretics include a decrease in both free water excretion during water loading and free water absorption during dehydration, an approximately 30% increase in fractional calcium (Ca^{++}) excretion, a significant increase in magnesium (Mg^{++}) excretion, and a decrease in uric acid excretion.

The available loop diuretics include bumetanide, ethacrynic acid, furosemide, and torsemide. These compounds are typically highly protein-bound. To gain access to the tubular lumen (site of action), they must undergo secretion. The same applies to thiazide-type diuretics. Tubular secretion is by way of probenecid-sensitive organic anion transporters localized in the proximal tubule. The pharmacologic characteristics of all loop diuretics are similar. Therefore, a lack of response to adequate doses of one loop diuretic reasons against the administration of another loop diuretic. Instead, combinations of diuretics with different sites of action should be given if aggressive diuresis is truly needed.

The rate of diuretic excretion approximates drug delivery to the medullary thick ascending limb and corresponds to the observed natriuretic response.[20,21] The relationship between the urinary loop diuretic excretion rate and the natriuretic effect is described by a sigmoidal curve and can be distorted (downward and rightward shifted) by a variety of circumstances, ranging from volume depletion (''braking phenomenon'') and the use of nonsteroidal anti-inflammatory drugs (NSAIDs), to HF or nephrotic syndrome (disease-state alterations).[22]

Furosemide is the most widely used diuretic in this class. However, its use in elderly individuals (and probably in all subjects) is confused by extremely erratic absorption with a bioavailability range of 12% to 112%.[23] The coefficient of variation for absorption varies from 25% to 43% for different furosemide products. Thus, exchanging one furosemide formulation for another will not standardize patient absorption (and thus response) to oral furosemide.[23] Bumetanide and especially torsemide are more predictably absorbed than furosemide. The consistency of absorption of torsemide and its longer duration of action are pharmacologic features to consider when loop diuretic therapy is called for in the elderly patient with HF.[24]

Thiazide Diuretics

The main site of action for thiazide-type diuretics is the early distal convoluted tubule where the coupled reabsorption of Na^+ and Cl^- is inhibited. Besides effects on Na^+ excretion, thiazide diuretics also impair urinary diluting capacity (while preserving urinary concentrating mechanisms and thus the greater likelihood of their causing diuretic-related hyponatremia), reduce Ca^{++} and uric acid excretion, and increase Mg^{++} excretion. The latter is especially the case with long-acting thiazide-type diuretics, such as chlorthalidone.[25]

Hydrochlorothiazide is the most widely used thiazide-type diuretic in the United States, and is given mainly for its blood-pressure–reducing properties. Hydrochlorothiazide is little used in HF because of its variable absorption, short duration of action, and limited potency. However, metolazone, chlorthalidone, and other thiazide-type diuretics with much longer durations of action can be safely and effectively used in the earlier stages of HF.[26–29] In addition, chlorthalidone therapy has been shown to be superior to calcium channel blockers and, at least in the short term, ACE inhibitors, in preventing HF in hypertensive individuals.[30]

Metolazone is a quinazoline diuretic with a chief site of action in the distal tubule and a minor inhibitory effect on proximal Na^+ reabsorption through a carbonic-anhydrase–independent mechanism. Metolazone is lipid soluble and has a wide volume of distribution, which plays a role in its extended duration of action in the setting of either renal insufficiency or diuretic-resistant situations when being given together with a loop diuretic.[22,26] Oral metolazone is absorbed slowly and fairly unpredictably, which can confuse the diagnosis of "diuretic resistance" in a volume-overloaded patient with HF. Diuretic resistance, the failure to respond to a diuretic regimen, is usually taken to signify a worsening of the primary volume-retaining state, but with metolazone, it can be a consequence of failure to absorb sufficient amounts of drug in a timely manner to effect a diuresis.[22,26]

Distal Potassium-Sparing Diuretics

There are 2 classes of K^+-sparing diuretics: competitive antagonists of aldosterone, such as spironolactone and eplerenone, and compounds, such as amiloride and triamterene, that act independent of aldosterone. The large majority of the treatment experience with K^+-sparing diuretics in HF is with the ARA spironolactone and eplerenone. Spironolactone is a highly protein-bound and well-absorbed, lipid-soluble compound with a 20-hour half-life. The onset of action for spironolactone is characteristically slow, with a peak diuretic response at times 48 hours or more after the first dose. Two metabolites of spironolactone that are responsible for much of its antimineralocorticoid activity are 7α-thiomethyl-spirolactone and canrenone.[31] Eplerenone, a highly selective ARA compound (reduced affinity for androgen and progesterone receptors), is associated with fewer endocrine side effects than occur with spironolactone.[32] ARAs are used in the patient with HF, elderly or otherwise, for 3 primary reasons: for their diuretic effect, to reduce K^+ or Mg^{++} losses produced by non–K^+-sparing diuretics, and to improve the morbidity and mortality of HF. First, drugs in this class work by way of inhibiting active Na^+ absorption in the late distal tubule and the collecting duct. Typically, eplerenone has a mild diuretic effect, which may relate to its having a short half-life and no active metabolites.[33] Conversely, spironolactone can generate a more significant diuretic response in HF, particularly when used in combination with a loop diuretic and an ACE inhibitor.[34] Spironolactone can remain active as a diuretic in states of reduced renal function because it gains access to its tubular site of action independent of the glomerular filtration rate.

Spironolactone and eplerenone both have a propensity to cause hyperkalemia, which limits use in many elderly patients with HF or chronic kidney disease.[32,35,36] Conversely, these compounds are effective in attenuating diuretic-related K^+ or Mg^{++} losses.[37] Spironolactone and eplerenone both have also been shown to improve the morbidity and mortality associated with various forms of HF.[38–40] In this regard, the Randomized Aldactone Evaluation Study showed that, when added to standard treatment (including an ACE inhibitor), a 25-mg dose of the ARA spironolactone reduced the risk of death by 30% over an average follow-up period of 2 years among carefully selected patients with current or recent HF of New York Heart Association functional class IV.[39] Also, in the Eplerenone Post-Acute Myocardial Infarction HF Efficacy and Survival Study, the addition of 50 mg eplerenone to standard medical therapy significantly improved mortality and morbidity within 30 days of randomization in patients with left ventricular systolic dysfunction and clinical evidence of HF following acute myocardial infarction.[38,40] These positive survival benefits with ARA therapy in HF are independent of patient age and have been suggested (but not proved) to relate to any of a number of processes, including positive vascular, immunologic, cellular, and electrolyte changes that follow from ARA therapy.[41–44]

In addition to showing a mortality benefit when used in patients post myocardial infarction with clinical symptoms of HF and a diminished left ventricular ejection fraction, ARA therapy with spironolactone also seems to favorably affect mortality in patients with heart failure and a normal ejection fraction.[45]

SPECIAL CONSIDERATIONS WITH DIURETIC THERAPY

A range of common variables, which are, in general, age-independent, can unfavorably influence the response to diuretic therapy. Such variables include body position, dietary Na^+ intake, blood pressure, the pattern of diuretic absorption, the use of NSAIDs, and the braking phenomenon. These are important factors to identify, because otherwise patients are incorrectly viewed as being diuretic resistant, which is a much worse prognostic category.[46]

Bed rest is a useful ancillary treatment measure when patients are being actively diuresed.[47] This may be particularly so in the elderly patient, in whom excessive orthostatic changes in blood pressure and posturally induced neurohumoral activation may serve to attenuate the response to a diuretic. Noncompliance with prescribed Na^+ and fluid intake is a major cause of apparent diuretic resistance and an important precipitant of HF exacerbations.[48] An excessive Na^+ intake as a cause of apparent diuretic resistance can be established by the measurement of 24-hour Na^+ excretion in the steady state. In volume-expanded subjects receiving diuretic therapy, dietary noncompliance can be presumed when daily Na^+ excretion is high (>100 mmol/d) without concurrent weight loss.

For a diuretic to work effectively, blood pressure must be sufficient to allow for drug delivery into the intratubular space and filtrate to be produced. What constitutes an effective blood pressure for diuretic action is highly variable in HF but, in general, is a systolic value higher than 100 to 110 mm Hg.[49] Atheromatous disease is commonly seen in many elderly patients. This disease, if present in the renal vascular bed, often dictates that even higher systemic blood pressure values be maintained for diuretic action. Also, conventional doses of an ACE inhibitor, such as captopril, can inhibit the natriuretic and diuretic responses to furosemide if systemic blood pressure is excessively reduced or glomerular hemodynamics are adversely affected.[50] On a practical note, separating the administration of each drug by several hours can minimize this interaction between an ACE inhibitor and a loop diuretic.

For the best natriuretic response to a loop diuretic, urinary drug delivery must be timed precisely and take into account many potential variables that influence the rate of delivery. Absorption and subsequent urinary delivery of orally administered loop diuretics must occur at a rate sufficient to exceed a response threshold. Disease states, such as HF, which slow diuretic absorption and thereby the rate of urinary delivery, can influence the response to a diuretic solely by slow absorption.[51] This is even more apparent when diuretic absorption is inherently erratic, as is the case with furosemide, and low doses of drug are used (eg, furosemide 40–80 mg).[23] Such difficulties can be minimized by choosing a diuretic, such as torsemide, with an absorptive profile that is rapid and complete and thus more compatible with the pharmacologic needs of HF.[52] The use of NSAIDs is a major cause of apparent diuretic resistance. These drugs interfere with prostaglandin synthesis by inhibiting cyclooxygenase and thereby antagonize the natriuretic response to loop diuretics. Consumption of NSAIDs is associated with an increased risk of hospital admission because of HF in patients with preexisting HF.[53]

Pharmacodynamic alterations presenting as "apparent" resistance to the effects of a diuretic frequently surface with repetitive administration of diuretics. This tolerance evolves sequentially, and commences abruptly at the time of the first dose of a diuretic. This braking phenomenon or "postdiuretic sodium retention" ultimately determines the influence of a diuretic on net Na^+ balance.[54] The braking phenomenon involves a complex series of counterbalancing changes that ultimately serve to stimulate Na^+ and water absorption at tubular sites, which are proximal and distal to the site of action of the particular diuretic in question.[22] The braking phenomenon can be attenuated by the more frequent administration of a diuretic or, on occasion, by the judicious use of multiple-site diuretic combinations, such as hydrochlorothiazide and furosemide, or metolazone and furosemide.[26] Diuretics active at the distal tubule, such as the thiazide diuretics, not only block this increase in Na^+ reabsorption, but may also prevent the development of cellular hypertrophy at this location.[55] These structural adaptations in the nephron may contribute to postdiuretic Na^+ retention and to diuretic tolerance in humans. The adaptations also may cause persistent Na^+ retention occurring up to 2 weeks after discontinuation of diuretic therapy.[56]

NEUROHUMORAL RESPONSES TO DIURETICS

Neurohumoral activation by diuretics remains an important consideration in the sustained effectiveness of diuretic therapy in HF. The neurohumoral response to a diuretic is dependent on both its route of administration and the level of drug exposure. Intravenous loop diuretics have an immediate (within minutes) stimulatory effect on the renin-angiotensin-aldosterone system that is independent of volume depletion. This may diminish the effectiveness of a diuretic for a short time. A second-phase response is initiated within 15 minutes of intravenous loop diuretic administration, which is the result of an increase in the renal production of prostaglandins. This second response offers a probable explanation for the reduction in preload and ventricular filling pressures that take place shortly after intravenous loop diuretic administration. The next stage of neurohumoral activation occurs with excess volume removal, and can occur with either intravenous or oral diuretics. Volume removal can chronically activate the renin-angiotensin-aldosterone system and increase circulating concentrations of both angiotensin-II and aldosterone, which, in turn, can promote Na^+ absorption in proximal and distal tubular locations, respectively.[22]

ADVERSE EFFECTS OF DIURETICS

Diuretic-related side effects can be separated into several categories, including those with well worked out mechanisms, such as electrolyte defects or metabolic abnormalities, and occurrences that are less well understood mechanistically, such as impotence. In addition, various drug–drug interactions are recognized to occur with diuretics. Diuretic-related side effects are dose-dependent as well as being more common and of greater intensity with loop diuretics. Thiazide-related side effects tend to be more common with longer-acting compounds, such as chlorthalidone and metolazone.[57]

Hyponatremia

Mild hyponatremia is not uncommon in untreated HF and can either improve or worsen with diuretic therapy. Thiazide diuretics are more likely to cause hyponatremia than are loop diuretics. Loop diuretics inhibit Na^+ transport in the renal medulla and preclude the generation of a maximal osmotic gradient. Thus, urinary concentrating ability is impaired with loop diuretics. Alternatively, thiazide-type diuretics increase Na^+ excretion and prevent maximal urine dilution while preserving the kidney's innate concentrating capacity. Diuretic-related hyponatremia is of little immediate clinical consequence if serum Na^+ values are R130 mEq/L. However, HF management becomes more complex in that both diuretic therapy and free water intake must be at least temporarily reduced.[57] Heretofore, serum Na^+ values lower than 130 mEq/L in diuretic-treated patients with HF were especially difficult to treat. Therapy of such patients may be simplified soon with the availability of orally administered selective vasopressin-receptor antagonists.[58]

Acid–Base Changes

Mild metabolic alkalosis is not uncommon with thiazide-type diuretic therapy.

Severe metabolic alkalosis is much less frequent and, when it occurs, it does so in association with the use of loop diuretics. The generation of a metabolic alkalosis with diuretic therapy is primarily due to contraction of the extracellular fluid space caused by urinary losses of a relatively bicarbonate-free fluid. Diuretic-induced metabolic alkalosis is best managed by administration of K^+ or Na^+ chloride, although the latter is oftentimes ill-advised in patients with HF. In such cases, a carbonic anhydrase inhibitor, such as acetazolamide, may be considered. Metabolic alkalosis also impairs the natriuretic response to loop diuretics and may contribute to diuretic resistance in the patient with HF.[59] All K^+-sparing diuretics can cause hyperkalemic metabolic acidosis, which in elderly patients, especially those with HF, can represent a serious complication.[60]

Hyperuricemia

Xanthine oxidoreductase activity is upregulated in patients with HF, leading to increased free radicals and hyperuricemia, independent of renal impairment or the effects of diuretics. A beneficial effect of targeted inhibition of xanthine oxidoreductase with allopurinol, and hence reduction of free radical load and uric acid production, has been suggested in a number of studies.[61] In fact, in patients with mild-to-moderate HF, hyperuricemia predicts exercise intolerance and inflammatory activation and is strongly and independently related to a worse prognosis.[62] If a gouty attack occurs in a diuretic-treated patient (unusual unless serum urate concentrations exceed 12 mg/dL), the diuretic should be at least temporarily discontinued. If diuretic discontinuation is not practical, then the lowest effective dose should be given with careful attention to maintaining an euvolemic state. An additional alternative in the gouty patient requiring diuretic therapy is the use of the xanthine oxidase inhibitor, allopurinol.[63] Allopurinol should be used cautiously (dose-adjusted according to level of renal function) in patients receiving a thiazide-type diuretic (and probably a loop diuretic as well), because allopurinol hypersensitivity reactions are more frequent with this combination than with allopurinol alone.

Hypokalemia and Hyperkalemia

A serum K^+ value of less than 3.5 mEq/L, which is the most common criterion for a diagnosis of hypokalemia, is not uncommon in patients with HF treated with loop or thiazide diuretics.[64] It is unusual, however, for serum K^+ values to remain less than 3.0 mEq/L in diuretic-treated outpatients unless there is a high dietary Na^+ intake, high-dose diuretic therapy is in play, or hypomagnesemia is present. Mechanisms that contribute to the onset of hypokalemia during diuretic use include increased flow-dependent distal nephron K^+ secretion (more commonly observed with a high Na^+ intake), a fall in distal tubule luminal Cl^- concentration, metabolic alkalosis, or secondary hyperaldosteronism.[65]

The risk from diuretic-related hypokalemia is most apparent in patients with left ventricular hypertrophy, HF, or myocardial ischemia, particularly when they become acutely ill and require hospitalization.[65,66] Logically, arrhythmia-related event rates should be coupled to the degree of hypokalemia. However, this is in no way a clear-cut relationship, at least in the outpatient setting. Several factors complicate the relationship. These factors include the variable correlation between serum K^+ concentrations and total body K^+ deficits in the setting of diuretic therapy. The range of serum K^+ values most commonly associated with increased ventricular ectopy is narrow, typically between 3.0 and 3.5 mEq/L. Uncertainty continues to surround the issue of whether hypokalemia caused by transcellular shifts of K^+ bears the same risk as a value seen on the basis of body losses.[65]

K^+-sparing diuretics (such as triamterene and amiloride) and ARAs (such as spironolactone and eplerenone) may treat diuretic-related hypokalemia just as well as they cause significant hyperkalemia.[67] Hyperkalemia is more likely to develop in K^+-sparing diuretic-treated patients in the setting of a reduction in the glomerular filtration rate (especially elderly individuals); in patients also receiving K^+ chloride supplements or salt substitutes (60 mEq/teaspoonful); in patients on an ACE inhibitor, an angiotensin-receptor blocker, or an NSAID; or in other situations that predispose to hyperkalemia, such as metabolic acidosis, hyporeninemic hypoaldosteronism, or heparin therapy (including subcutaneous heparin regimens).[67]

Hypomagnesemia

Both thiazide and loop diuretics increase urine Mg^{++} excretion. Conversely, all K^+-sparing diuretics reduce urinary Mg^{++} losses. Prolonged therapy with thiazide or loop diuretics decreases plasma Mg^{++} concentration on average by 5% to 10%, although some patients can develop more severe hypomagnesemia. Cellular Mg^{++} depletion occurs in up to 50% of patients during diuretic therapy, and can be present regardless of normal serum Mg^{++} concentrations. Hypomagnesemia occurs more often in elderly individuals and in those receiving continuous high-dose diuretic therapy, as is the case for patients with HF.

Although a low serum Mg^{++} level is helpful in making the diagnosis, and is in general indicative of low intracellular stores, normal serum Mg^{++} values can still be observed in the face of a significant body deficiency of Mg^{++}. Thus, serum Mg^{++} determinations are an unreliable measure of total body Mg^{++} balance. Hypomagnesemia often coexists with hyponatremia and hypokalemia, with one study finding 42% of patients with hypokalemia to also have low serum Mg^{++} concentrations.[68] Hypokalemia or hypocalcemia occurring in the presence of hypomagnesemia typically cannot be corrected until the underlying Mg^{++} deficit is put right.

Diuretic-related hypomagnesemia should be treated (beyond simple empiric correction to normalize a laboratory value) for several theoretical reasons. Such treatment can lead, for example, to improved control of blood pressure, fewer arrhythmias, or resolution of coexisting electrolyte or neuromuscular symptoms. Mg^{++} deficiency should be sought and treated in patients with HF, ischemic heart disease, or established arrhythmia patterns.[69] In mild-deficiency states,

Mg^{++} balance can often be reestablished by simply controlling the contributing factors (eg, by limiting diuretic use and Na^{+} intake) and allowing dietary Mg^{++} to correct the deficit. Parenteral Mg^{++}, however, is the most efficient way to correct hypomagnesemia and always should be the mode of administration when replacement is more urgent. Total body Mg^{++} deficits are typically in the order of 1 to 2 mEq/kg body weight in the depleted patient.

A variety of Mg^{++} salts are available for oral use. Mg^{++} oxide is a commonly used Mg^{++} salt, but is not very water-soluble and has a major cathartic effect. Thus, its use can unpredictably influence Mg^{++} concentrations. Mg^{++} gluconate is the preferred therapy for oral use. This salt form is very soluble and causes minimal diarrhea. Mg^{++} carbonate also is not very water-soluble and is not as effective as the gluconate salt in correcting hypomagnesemia.

SUMMARY

Diuretic therapy remains a cornerstone of HF therapy.[70] In the treatment of volume-overloaded patients, diuretics clearly improve symptoms and quality of life. Despite the acceptance of diuretic therapy for treatment of symptoms, considerable debate has ensued for many decades about the impact of this class of agent on mortality, cardiac function, and disease progression. Accordingly, diuretics should be used judiciously in the patient with HF, at the minimum effective dose, with careful monitoring of electrolyte balance, and continued only if there is a demonstrable ongoing clinical need. ARAs should be distinguished from both loop and thiazide-type diuretics in that outcomes data support their routine use in advanced systolic HF and in patients post myocardial infarction with clinical HF symptoms and a left ventricular ejection fraction 40%. ARAs also can be considered for use in patients with diastolic HF and a normal ejection fraction less than 40%.

REFERENCES

1. James PA, Oparil S, Carter BL, et al. 2014 evidence-based guideline for the management of high blood pressure in adults: report from the panel members appointed to the Eighth Joint National Committee (JNC8). JAMA 2014;311:507–20.
2. Yancy CW, Jessup M, Bozkurt B, et al. ACCF/AHA guideline for the management of heart failure: a report of the American College of Cardiology Foundation/American Heart Association Task Force of Practice Guidelines. J Am Coll Cardiol 2013;62:e147–239.
3. Ponikowski P, Voors AA, Anker SD, et al. ESC guidelines for the diagnosis and treatment of acute and chronic heart failure of the European Society of Cardiology (ESC). Developed with the special contribution of the Heart Failure Association (HFA) of the ESC. Eur J Heart Fail 2016;18:891–975.
4. Moe GW, Ezekowit JA, O'Meara E, et al. The 2014 Canadian Cardiovascular Society Heart Failure Management Guidelines Focus Update: anemia, biomarkers, and recent trial implications. Can J Cardiol 2014;31:3–16.
5. Writing Committee Members: ACC/AHA Task Force Members. 2016 ACC/AHA/HFSA focused update on new pharmacological therapy for heart failure: an update of the 2013 ACCF/AHA guideline for the management of heart failure: a Report of the American College of Cardiology/American Heart Association Task Force on Clinical Practice Guidelines and the Heart Failure Society of America. J Card Fail 2016;22:659–69.
6. Aronow WS. Current treatment of heart failure with reduction of left ventricular ejection fraction. Expert Rev Clin Pharmacol 2016;9:1619–31.
7. Faris R, Flather MD, Purcell H, et al. Diuretics for heart failure. Cochrane Database Syst Rev 2016;(1):CD003838.
8. Aurigemma GP, Gaasch WH. Diastolic heart failure. N Engl J Med 2004;351:1097–105.
9. de Giuli F, Khaw KT, Cowie MR, et al. Incidence and outcome of persons with a clinical diagnosis of heart failure in a general practice population of 696,884 in the United Kingdom. Eur J Heart Fail 2005;7:295–302.
10. Kitzman DW. Diastolic heart failure in the elderly. Heart Fail Rev 2002;7:17–27.
11. Sun WY, Reiser IW, Chou SY. Risk factors for acute renal insufficiency induced by diuretics in patients with congestive heart failure. Am J Kidney Dis 2006;47:798–808.
12. Rejnmark L, Vestergaard P, Mosekilde L. Fracture risk in patients treated with loop diuretics. J Intern Med 2006;259:117–24.
13. Paik JM, Rosen HN, Gordon CM, et al. Diuretic use and risk of vertebral fracture in women. Am J Med 2016;129:1299–306.
14. Eshaghian S, Horwich TB, Fonarow GC. Relation of loop diuretic dose to mortality in advanced heart failure. Am J Cardiol 2006;97:1759–64.
15. Krum H, Cameron P. Diuretics in the treatment of heart failure: mainstay of therapy or potential hazard? J Card Fail 2006;12:333–5.
16. Domanski M, Tian X, Haigney M, et al. Diuretic use, progressive heart failure, and death in patients in the DIG study. J Card Fail 2006;12:327–32.
17. Galve E, Mallol A, Catalan R, et al. Clinical and neurohumoral consequences of diuretic withdrawal in patients with chronic, stabilized heart failure and systolic dysfunction. Eur J Heart Fail 2005;7:892–8.

18. Mazur JE, Devlin JW, Peters MJ, et al. Single versus multiple doses of acetazolamide for metabolic alkalosis in critically ill medical patients: a randomized, double-blind trial. Crit Care Med 1999;27:1257–61.
19. Shankar SS, Brater DC. Loop diuretics: from the Na-K-2Cl transporter to clinical use. Am J Physiol Renal Physiol 2003;284:F11–21.
20. Brater DC. Diuretic therapy. N Engl J Med 1998;339: 387–95.
21. Andreasen F, Hansen U, Husted SE, et al. The pharmacokinetics of frusemide are influenced by age. Br J Clin Pharmacol 1983;16:391–7.
22. Sica DA, Gehr TWB. Diuretic combinations in refractory edema states: pharmacokinetic- pharmacodynamic relationships. Clin Pharmacokinet 1996;30: 229–49.
23. Murray MD, Haag KM, Black PK, et al. Variable furosemide absorption and poor predictability of response in elderly patients. Pharmacotherapy 1997;17:98–106.
24. Vargo DL, Kramer WG, Black PK, et al. Bioavailability, pharmacokinetics, and pharmacodynamics of torsemide and furosemide in patients with congestive heart failure. Clin Pharmacol Ther 1995; 57:601–9.
25. Cocco G, Iselin HU, Strozzi C, et al. Magnesium depletion in patients on long-term chlorthalidone therapy for essential hypertension. Eur J Clin Pharmacol 1987;32:335–8.
26. Sica DA. Metolazone and its role in edema management. Congest Heart Fail 2003;9:100–5.
27. Carter BL, Ernst ME, Cohen JD. Hydrochlorothiazide versus chlorthalidone: evidence supporting their interchangeability. Hypertension 2004;43:4–9.
28. Sica DA. Chlorthadilone: has it always been the best thiazide-type diuretic? [editorial comment]. Hypertension 2006;47:321–2.
29. Davis BR, Piller LB, Cutler JA, et al. Role of diuretics in the prevention of heart failure. The antihypertensive and lipid-lowering treatment to prevent heart attack trial. Circulation 2006;113:2201–10.
30. Davis BR, Piller LB, Cutler JA, et al, Antihypertensive and Lipid-Lowering Treatment to Prevent Heart Attack Trial Collaborative Research Group. Role of diuretics in the prevention of heart failure: the Antihypertensive and Lipid-Lowering Treatment to Prevent Heart Attack Trial. Circulation 2006;113:2201–10.
31. Gardiner P, Schrode K, Quinlan D, et al. Spironolactone metabolism: steady-state serum levels of the sulfur-containing metabolites. J Clin Pharmacol 1989;29:342–7.
32. Sica DA. Pharmacokinetics and pharmacodynamics of mineralocorticoid blocking agents and their effects on potassium homeostasis. Heart Fail Rev 2005;10:23–9.
33. Ravis WR, Reid S, Sica DA, et al. Pharmacokinetics of eplerenone after single and multiple dosing in subjects with and without renal impairment. J Clin Pharmacol 2005;45:810–21.
34. van Vliet AA, Donker AJ, Nauta JJ, et al. Spironolactone in congestive heart failure refractory to high-dose loop diuretic and low-dose angiotensin-converting enzyme inhibitor. Am J Cardiol 1993;71: 21A–8A.
35. Masoudi FA, Gross CP, Wang Y, et al. Adoption of spironolactone therapy for older patients with heart failure and left ventricular systolic dysfunction in the United States, 1998–2001. Circulation 2005; 112:39–47.
36. Wang TY, Vora AN, Peng SA, et al. Effectiveness and safety of aldosterone antagonist therapy use among older patients with reduced ejection fraction after acute myocardial infarction. J Am Heart Assoc 2016;5:1–10.
37. Soberman JE, Weber KT. Spironolactone in congestive heart failure. Curr Hypertens Rep 2000;2:451–6.
38. Pitt B, Remme W, Zannad F, et al. Eplerenone, a selective aldosterone blocker, in patients with left ventricular dysfunction after myocardial infarction. N Engl J Med 2003;348:1309–21.
39. Pitt B, Zannad F, Remme WJ, et al. The effect of spironolactone on morbidity and mortality in patients with severe heart failure. N Engl J Med 1999;341: 709–17.
40. Pitt B, White H, Nicolau J, et al. Eplerenone reduces mortality 30 days after randomization following acute myocardial infarction in patients with left ventricular systolic dysfunction and heart failure. J Am Coll Cardiol 2005;46:425–31.
41. Pitt B, Reichek N, Willenbrock R, et al. Effects of eplerenone, enalapril, and eplerenone/enalapril in patients with essential hypertension and left ventricular hypertrophy: the 4E-left ventricular hypertrophy study. Circulation 2003;108:1831–8.
42. Bianchi S, Bigazzi R, Campese VM. Antagonists of aldosterone and proteinuria in patients with CKD: an uncontrolled pilot study. Am J Kidney Dis 2005; 46:45–51.
43. Iraqi W, Rossignol P, Angioi M, et al. Extracellular cardiac matrix biomarkers in patients with acute myocardial infarction complicated by left ventricular dysfunction and heart failure: insites from the Eplerenone Post-Acute Myocardial Infarction Heart Failure Efficacy and Survival Study (EPHESUS) study. Circulation 2009;119:2471–9.
44. Stier CT Jr, Koenig S, Lee DY, et al. Aldosterone and aldosterone antagonism in cardiovascular disease. Focus on eplerenone (Inspra). Heart Dis 2003;5: 102–18.
45. Pfeffer MA, Claggett B, Assmann SF, et al. Regional variation in patients and outcomes in the treatment of preserved cardiac function heart failure with an aldosterone antagonist (TOPCAT) trial. Circulation 2015;131:34–42.

46. Neuberg GW, Miller AB, O'Connor CM, et al. Diuretic resistance predicts mortality in patients with advanced heart failure. Am Heart J 2002;144:31–8.
47. Abildgaard U, Aldershvile J, Ring-Larsen H, et al. Bed rest and increased diuretic treatment in chronic congestive heart failure. Eur Heart J 1985;6:1040–6.
48. Tsuyuki RT, McKelvie RS, Arnold JM, et al. Acute precipitants of congestive heart failure exacerbations. Arch Intern Med 2001;161:2337–42.
49. De Pasquale CG, Dunne JS, Minson RB, et al. Hypotension is associated with diuretic resistance in severe chronic heart failure, independent of renal function. Eur J Heart Fail 2005;7:888–91.
50. McLay JS, McMurray JJ, Bridges AB, et al. Acute effects of captopril on the renal actions of furosemide in patients with chronic heart failure. Am Heart J 1993;126:879–86.
51. Sica DA. Drug absorption in the management of congestive heart failure: loop diuretics. Congest Heart Fail 2003;9:287–92.
52. Bleske BE, Welage LS, Kramer WG, et al. Pharmacokinetics of torsemide in patients with decompensated and compensated congestive heart failure. J Clin Pharmacol 1998;38:708–14.
53. Feenstra J, Heerdinck ER, Grobbee DE, et al. Association of nonsteroidal anti-inflammatory drugs with first occurrence of heart failure and with relapsing heart failure. Arch Intern Med 2002;162:262–70.
54. Kelly RA, Wilcox CS, Mitch WE, et al. Response of the kidney to furosemide. I. Effect of captopril on sodium balance. Kidney Int 1983;24:233–9.
55. Ellison DH, Velazquez H, Wright FS. Adaptation of the distal convoluted tubule of the rat. Structural and functional effects of dietary salt intake and chronic diuretic infusion. J Clin Invest 1989;83:113–26.
56. Loon NR, Wilcox CS, Unwin RJ. Mechanism of impaired natriuretic response to furosemide during prolonged therapy. Kidney Int 1989;36:682–9.
57. Sica DA. Diuretic-related side effects: development and treatment. J Clin Hypertens (Greenwich) 2004;6:532–40.
58. Gheorghiade M. The clinical effects of vasopressin receptor antagonists in heart failure. Cleve Clin J Med 2006;73(Suppl 2):S24–9.
59. Loon NR, Wilcox CS. Mild metabolic alkalosis impairs the natriuretic response to bumetanide in normal human subjects. Clin Sci (Lond) 1998;94:287–92.
60. O'Connell JE, Colledge NR. Type IV renal tubular acidosis and spironolactone therapy in the elderly. Postgrad Med J 1993;69:887–9.
61. Cappola TP, Kass DA, Nelson GS, et al. Allopurinol improves myocardial efficiency in patients with idiopathic dilated cardiomyopathy. Circulation 2001;104:2407–11.
62. Niizeki T, Takeishi Y, Arimoto T, et al. Hyperuricemia associated with high cardiac event rates in the elderly with chronic heart failure. J Cardiol 2006;47:219–28.
63. Gurwitz JH, Kalish SC, Bohn RL, et al. Thiazide diuretics and the initiation of anti-gout therapy. J Clin Epidemiol 1997;50:953–9.
64. Morgan DB, Davidson C. Hypokalemia and diuretics: an analysis of publications. BMJ 1980;280:905–8.
65. Sica DA, Struthers AD, Cushman WC, et al. Importance of potassium in cardiovascular disease. J Clin Hypertens 2003;4:198–206.
66. Macdonald JE, Struthers AD. What is the optimal serum potassium level in cardiovascular patients? J Am Coll Cardiol 2004;43:155–61.
67. Sica DA, Hess M. Aldosterone receptor antagonism: interface with hyperkalemia in heart failure. Congest Heart Fail 2004;10:259–64.
68. Whang R, Oei TO, Aikawa JK, et al. Predictors of clinical hypomagnesemia. Hypokalemia, hypophosphatemia, hyponatremia, and hypocalcemia. Arch Intern Med 1984;144:1794–6.
69. Sica DA, Frishman WH, Cavusoglu E. Magnesium, potassium, and calcium as potential cardiovascular disease therapies. In: Frishman W, Sonnenblick E, Sica DA, editors. Cardiovascular pharmacotherapeutics. 2nd edition. New York: McGraw-Hill; 2003. p. 177–90.
70. Sica DA, Gehr TWB, Frishman WH. Diuretic therapy in cardiovascular disease. In: Frishman WH, Sica DA, editors. Cardiovascular pharmacotherapeutics. 3rd edition. Minneapolis (MN): Cardiotext Publishing; 2012. p. 157–75.

Heart Failure Complicating Acute Mtyocardial Infarction

Wilbert S. Aronow, MD

KEYWORDS

• Heart failure • Myocardial infarction • Beta blockers • Angiotensin-converting enzyme inhibitors • Nitrates • Aldosterone antagonists • Digoxin • Positive inotropic drugs

KEY POINTS

- Factors predisposing the older person with acute myocardial infarction (MI) to develop heart failure (HF) include increased prevalence of prior MI and multivessel coronary artery disease, decreased left ventricular (LV) contractile reserve, impairment of LV diastolic relaxation, and an increased prevalence of hypertension, LV hypertrophy, diabetes mellitus, valvular heart disease, and renal insufficiency.
- The American College of Cardiology/American Heart Association (ACC/AHA) guidelines state that class I indications for the use of angiotensin-converting enzyme (ACE) inhibitors during acute MI are (1) patients within the first 24 hours of a suspected acute MI with ST-segment elevation in 2 or more anterior precordial leads, or with clinical HF in the absence of significant hypotension or known contraindications to the use of ACE inhibitors or (2) patients with MI and an LV ejection fraction 40% or less or patients with clinical HF based on systolic pump dysfunction during and after convalescence from acute MI.
- The ACC/AHA class I indications for use of early intravenous beta blockade in patients with acute MI are (1) patients without a contraindication to beta-blockers who can be treated within 12 hours of onset of MI, (2) patients with continuing or recurrent ischemic pain, and (3) patients with tachyarrhythmias, such as atrial fibrillation with a rapid ventricular rate, or hypertension.

Factors predisposing the older person with acute myocardial infarction (MI) to develop heart failure (HF) include an increased prevalence of prior MI and multivessel coronary artery disease, decreased left ventricular (LV) contractile reserve, impairment of LV diastolic relaxation, and an increased prevalence of hypertension, LV hypertrophy, diabetes mellitus, valvular heart disease, and renal insufficiency.[1–4] Women with acute MI are more likely to be older and to develop HF than men with acute MI.[5–8] Prior HF was present in 12% of 124 subjects younger than 70 years of age and in 17% of 137 subjects 70 years of age and older with acute MI.[5] HF occurred during acute MI in 33% of the 124 subjects younger than 70 years of age and in 56% of the 137 subjects 70 years of age and older.[5] Dyspnea due to HF was the initial clinical manifestation of acute MI in 35% of 110 subjects older than 62 years of age (mean age: 82 years) with acute MI.[9]

HF complicating acute MI is associated with a high mortality.[10] HF occurred during acute MI in 40% of 30 subjects who died at 1-year follow-up and in 9% of 202 subjects who were alive at

This is an updated version of an article that appeared in *Heart Failure Clinics*, Volume 3, Issue 4.
Disclosure Statement: The author has nothing to disclose.
Division of Cardiology, Department of Medicine, Westchester Medical Center, New York Medical College, Macy Pavilion, Room 141, Valhalla, NY 10595, USA
E-mail address: wsaronow@aol.com

Heart Failure Clin 13 (2017) 513–525
http://dx.doi.org/10.1016/j.hfc.2017.02.007

1-year follow-up.[5] In the Multicenter Postinfarction Program, the 1-year mortality rate was 28% in 123 subjects with pulmonary congestion occurring during acute MI versus 5.5% in 744 subjects with no pulmonary congestion occurring during acute MI.[11] An analysis of 790 surviving subjects from the Multicenter Postinfarction Program and 1060 placebo-treated subjects from the Multicenter Diltiazem Postinfarction Trial showed at 2-year follow-up that the cardiac mortality hazard ratios were 1.43 for subjects with mild or moderate pulmonary congestion occurring during acute MI and 4.20 for subjects with severe pulmonary congestion during acute MI.[12] Of 86, 771 subjects with acute MI, HF was present at admission or developed during hospitalization in 15.2% of men and 16.8% of women aged 55 to 74 years, and in 25.6% of men and 27.1% of women aged 75 to 85 years.[13] Of 63,853 subjects discharged alive without HF, 8058 subjects (12.6%) were hospitalized with or died of HF at 3.2-year median follow-up.[13]

Pulmonary venous hypertension with pulmonary congestion and a low cardiac output may complicate acute MI. Pulmonary congestion occurs when the pulmonary capillary wedge pressure exceeds 18 mm Hg.[14] Peripheral hypoperfusion occurs when the cardiac index falls below 2.2 L/min/m^2.[14] The greater the extent of injury to the left ventricle, the lower the LV ejection fraction and the higher the incidence of clinical manifestations of HF. At follow-up, a low LV ejection fraction is an independent predictor of mortality in subjects with HF associated with acute MI.[5,12,15]

Older patients with prior MI and HF have a higher mortality at follow-up if they have an abnormal LV ejection fraction than if they have a normal LV ejection fraction.[16,17] **Table 1** shows the mortality rates in older men and in older women with prior MI and HF at 1-year, 2-year, 3-year, 4-year, and 5-year follow-up.[17] The mortality rates were similar in men versus women with normal or abnormal LV ejection fraction.[17] Older patients with an abnormal LV ejection fraction had a 2.2 times higher mortality rate than older patients with a normal LV ejection fraction after controlling other prognostic variables.[17]

Table 1
Mortality rates in older men and women who have congestive heart failure and prior myocardial infarction

Mortality (y)	Normal LV Ejection Fraction (n = 276) (%)	Abnormal LV Ejection Fraction (n = 340) (%)
1	19	41
2	39	65
3	49	78
4	56	86
5	74	92

Data from Aronow WS, Ahn C, Kronzon I. Prognosis of congestive heart failure after prior myocardial infarction in older men and women with abnormal versus normal left ventricular ejection fraction. Am J Cardiol 2000;85:1382–4.

GENERAL MEASURES

In general, management of HF complicating acute MI is similar in older and younger patients. Underlying causes of HF should be treated when possible.[18,19] Precipitating factors of HF should be identified and treated.[18,19] The LV ejection fraction must be measured in patients with HF associated with acute MI to guide therapy.[18] Echocardiography with Doppler may be helpful in determining the presence and severity of valvular heart disease, such as aortic stenosis or mitral regurgitation; LV diastolic dysfunction due to LV hypertrophy; LV wall-motion abnormalities caused by acute myocardial ischemia; and complications of acute MI, including ventricular rupture, ventricular septal rupture, papillary muscle rupture, ruptured chordae tendineae, papillary muscle dysfunction, LV aneurysm, intracardiac thrombi, pericardial effusion with and without cardiac tamponade, and right ventricular infarction.[5,19–23]

HEMODYNAMIC MONITORING

Invasive hemodynamic monitoring may be necessary to guide the therapy for some patients with acute MI and a pulmonary capillary wedge pressure of 18 mm Hg or a cardiac index !2.2 L/min/m^2. The American College of Cardiology/American Heart Association (ACC/AHA) guidelines state that class I indications for balloon flotation right-heart catheter monitoring during acute MI include (1) severe or progressive HF or pulmonary edema, (2) progressive hypotension when unresponsive to fluid administration or when fluid administration may be contraindicated, and (3) suspected mechanical complications of acute MI, such as ventricular septal defect, papillary muscle rupture, or pericardial tamponade if an echocardiogram has not been performed.[24]

OXYGEN

Experimental data have shown that breathing oxygen may limit ischemic myocardial injury.[25] Patients with acute MI and HF may have hypoxemia due to pulmonary vascular congestion, pulmonary interstitial edema, and ventilation–perfusion mismatch.[26] Respiratory depression from narcotic analgesics can also contribute to hypoxemia. The ACC/AHA guidelines state that the class I indications for using oxygen during acute MI are (1) overt pulmonary congestion or (2) arterial oxygen desaturation (oxygen saturation !90%).[24]

Supplemental oxygen administered by nasal prongs may not correct significant hypoxemia in patients with severe HF, pulmonary edema, or a mechanical complication of acute MI. Continuous positive-pressure breathing or endotracheal intubation and mechanical ventilation is often needed in these patients.[27] The preferred modes of administering oxygen in patients who are capable of initiating spontaneous ventilation are intermittent mandatory ventilation, assist control, or pressure-support ventilation.[28] If wheezing complicates pulmonary congestion, bronchodilators that act primarily on beta(2)-adrenoceptors, such as albuterol, are preferable to bronchodilators, such as isoproterenol, which can increase myocardial ischemia by increasing myocardial oxygen demand.

MORPHINE

Intravenous morphine should be used to treat acute pulmonary edema associated with acute MI. Intravenous morphine provides beneficial effects in pulmonary edema by decreasing systemic vascular resistance, by increasing venodilation, and by reducing the work of breathing through inducing central nervous system euphoria.[29,30] Morphine should be avoided in patients with bronchospastic pulmonary disease or hypotension. The initial intravenous dose of morphine is 2 to 4 mg. This dose should be repeated every 10 to 15 minutes as necessary. The blood pressure should be checked before each dose because morphine can cause significant hypotension.

DIURETICS

Older persons with HF associated with acute MI should be treated with a loop diuretic, such as furosemide. These persons should not take nonsteroidal anti-inflammatory drugs because they may inhibit the induction of diuresis by furosemide. If severe HF is present, furosemide should be administered intravenously, initially in a dose of 20 to 40 mg with the dose doubled if there is no significant clinical improvement.[31] In addition to its diuretic effect, intravenous furosemide causes venodilation with a clinical benefit occurring within several minutes.[32,33]

Older persons with severe HF or concomitant renal insufficiency may need the addition of metolazone to the loop diuretic. Continuous intravenous infusion of furosemide may be necessary in some patients with severe HF. Older patients with HF treated with diuretics need close monitoring of serum electrolytes. Hypokalemia and hypomagnesemia may occur, both of which may precipitate ventricular arrhythmias and digitalis toxicity. Hyponatremia with activation of the renin-angiotensin-aldosterone system may develop.[18]

Older patients with HF are especially sensitive to volume depletion. Dehydration and prerenal azotemia may develop if excessive doses of diuretics are given. Therefore, the minimum effective dose of diuretics should be administered. Older patients with HF and abnormal LV ejection fraction tolerate higher doses of diuretics than do older patients with HF and normal LV ejection fraction. Older patients with HF associated with LV diastolic dysfunction with normal LV ejection fraction often need high LV filling pressures to maintain an adequate stroke volume and cardiac output, and cannot tolerate intravascular depletion.[18] (See discussion of use of diuretics in the treatment of patients with HF, in this issue.)

NITROGLYCERIN

In patients with acute MI, intravenous nitroglycerin reduces LV filling pressure and systemic vascular resistance.[34] Intravenous nitroglycerin is principally a venodilator at infusion rates of less than 50 mg per minute and causes more balanced venous and arterial dilating effects at higher infusion rates.[34] Intravenous nitroglycerin improves LV hemodynamics, LV geometry, and myocardial blood flow and perfusion in patients with acute MI.[35]

In 5124 subjects older than 70 years of age in the Gruppo Italiano per lo Studio della Sopravvivenza nell'Infarto Miocardico (GISSI)-3 trial, administration of transdermal nitroglycerin within 24 hours of symptom onset was associated with an 11% insignificant reduction in 6-week mortality and with a 9% insignificant decrease in the 6-week combined endpoint of death, HF, or severe LV dysfunction.[15] When data from all randomized control trials of nitrate use in the treatment of acute MI are combined, there is a 6% significant decrease in mortality, with 4 lives saved per 1000 subjects treated.[24,36] The ACC/AHA guidelines state that class I indications for using intravenous nitroglycerin in patients with acute MI are (1) for relief of ongoing ischemic discomfort, (2) for control of hypertension, or (3) for managing pulmonary congestion.[24]

Nitroglycerin should not be used if the systolic blood pressure is !90 mm Hg or if marked bradycardia (!50 beats per minute) or tachycardia is present.[37] Nitroglycerin should also be avoided in patients with right ventricular infarction.[38]

Long-acting oral nitrate preparations should not be used in the management of acute MI.[24] Sublingual or transdermal nitroglycerin can be used.[24] However, intravenous infusion of nitroglycerin is preferred because of its rapid onset and offset of action. Intravenous nitroglycerin can be titrated by frequent measurements of cuff blood pressure and heart rate. However, invasive hemodynamic monitoring should be used if high doses of vasodilators are administered, if there is an unstable blood pressure, or if there is doubt about the LV filling pressure.[39]

A bolus injection of 12.5 to 25.0 mg of intravenous nitroglycerin should be administered with a pump-controlled infusion of 10 to 20 mg per minute and the dosage increased by 5 to 10 mg every 5 to 10 minutes.[24] The endpoints are control of clinical symptoms or reduction in mean arterial pressure of 10% in normotensive patients or 30% in hypertensive patients, an increase in heart rate of 10 beats per minute, or reduction in pulmonary artery end-diastolic pressure of 10% to 30%.[24] The systolic blood pressure should not be allowed to fall below 90 mm Hg or the heart rate to exceed 110 beats per minute.[24] The nitroglycerin infusion should be slowed or temporarily discontinued if the systolic blood pressure falls below 90 mm Hg. The maximum dose infused should not exceed 200 mg per minute.

Nesiritide should be avoided in patients with HF complicating acute MI. In a study of 7141 subjects, median age 67 years, with acute decompensated congestive HF (CHF) randomized to intravenous nesiritide or to placebo, compared with placebo, nesiritide caused no significant effect on dyspnea at 6 hours or at 24 hours, caused no significant effect on rehospitalization for HF or death within 30 days, and caused a significant increase in hypotension (26.6% for nesiritide vs 15.3% for placebo).[40]

ANGIOTENSIN-CONVERTING ENZYME INHIBITORS

Angiotensin-converting enzyme (ACE) inhibitors should not be administered intravenously early in the course of acute MI.[41] The Cooperative New Scandinavian Enalapril Survival Study II was stopped due to a higher frequency of adverse outcomes in subjects receiving enalapril.[41] Subjects older than 70 years of age in this study also had an increased incidence of serious hypotension.[41]

However, all randomized trials investigating the use of oral ACE inhibitors early in the course of acute MI showed that ACE inhibitors reduced mortality.[15,36,42–46] Small but statistically significant decreases in mortality were reported in subjects treated with captopril[36] or lisinopril[15] within 24 hours of onset of acute MI in the Fourth International Study of Infarct Survival[36] and in the GISSI-3 trial.[15] Subjects aged 70 years and older treated with lisinopril in the GISSI-3 trial had a 14% significant decrease in the combined endpoint of death or severe LV dysfunction at 6-month follow-up.[47]

In the Acute Infarction Ramipril Efficacy Study, 2006 subjects with acute MI and HF were randomized to ramipril or placebo on day 3 to 10 after acute MI.[48] At 15-month follow-up, compared with placebo, ramipril 5 mg twice daily significantly reduced mortality by 27% overall and by 36% in persons 65 years of age and older.[48] At 42-month follow-up in the Survival and Ventricular Enlargement Trial, asymptomatic subjects with an LV ejection fraction of 40% or less treated with captopril 3 to 16 days after MI had, compared with placebo, a 19% decrease in mortality, a 21% reduction in death from cardiovascular requiring hospitalization, and a 25% decrease in recurrent MI.[48] Captopril reduced mortality 8% in subjects 55 years of age and younger, 13% in subjects aged 56 to 64 years, and 25% in subjects aged 65 years and older.[48]

An observational prospective study was performed in 477 subjects (mean age: 79 years) with prior MI and a low LV ejection fraction (mean LV ejection fraction: 31%).[49] Compared with no ACE inhibitor or beta-blocker therapy, at 34-month follow-up, ACE inhibitors alone significantly reduced new coronary events by 17% and new HF by 32%.[49] Compared with no ACE inhibitor or beta-blocker therapy, ACE inhibitors plus beta-blockers significantly reduced new coronary events by 37% and new HF by 61%.[49]

The ACC/AHA guidelines state that class I indications for the use of ACE inhibitors during acute MI are (1) patients within the first 24 hours of a suspected acute MI with ST-segment elevation in 2 or more anterior precordial leads, or with clinical HF in the absence of significant hypotension or known contraindications to the use of ACE inhibitors, or (2) patients with MI and an LV ejection fraction of 40% or less, or patients with clinical HF based on systolic pump dysfunction during and after convalescence from acute MI.[50]

ACE inhibitors should be started within the first 24 hours in patients with acute MI and HF after the blood pressure has stabilized.[24,50] ACE inhibitors should not be used if the systolic blood pressure is !100 mm Hg if renal failure is present, if there is a history of bilateral renal artery stenosis, or if there is known allergy to ACE inhibitors.[24,50] The initial dose should be low, such as captopril 6.25 mg, and the dose gradually increased to achieve a maintenance dose within 24 to 48 hours.[24,50] The patient's blood pressure, renal function, and serum potassium level should be monitored closely. Intravenous ACE inhibitors should be avoided, especially in elderly patients.[51]

The ACC/AHA guidelines recommend administering ACE inhibitors to all patients after MI without contraindications to their use and continuing their use indefinitely.[24] ACE inhibitors are effective in the treatment of postinfarction patients with HF associated with abnormal LV ejection fraction[42,43,52,53] or normal LV ejection fraction.[54,55]

Asymptomatic hypotension (systolic blood pressure 80–90 mm Hg) and a small increase in serum creatinine to a level of !2.5 mg/dL are side effects of ACE-inhibitor therapy that should not necessarily cause cessation of therapy in postinfarction patients with HF but should cause the physician to reduce the dose of diuretics, if the jugular venous pressure is normal, and to consider decreasing the dose of ACE inhibitor.[18] Symptomatic hypotension, progressive azotemia, intolerable cough, angioneurotic edema, hyperkalemia, and rash are contraindications to treatment with ACE inhibitors.

ANGIOTENSIN II RECEPTOR BLOCKERS

Angiotensin II receptor blockers (ARBs) should be used for treating HF with a class I indication if the patient cannot tolerate ACE inhibitors because of cough, angioneurotic edema, rash, or altered taste sensation.[56–62] ARBs are reasonable to use as an alternative to ACE inhibitors in patients with mild-to-moderate HF and reduced LV ejection fraction, especially in patients taking ARBs for other reasons, with a class IIa indication.[56]

ALDOSTERONE ANTAGONISTS

Patients with severe HF associated with an abnormal LV ejection fraction treated with diuretics, ACE inhibitors, and digoxin who received spironolactone 25 mg daily instead of placebo had a 30% significant reduction in mortality and a 35% significant decrease in hospitalization for HF at 2-year follow-up.[63] At 16-month follow-up of 6632 subjects (mean age 64 years) with acute MI complicated by HF and a low LV ejection fraction treated with diuretics, ACE inhibitors, and 75% with beta-blockers, eplerenone 50 mg daily significantly reduced mortality 15% and death from cardiovascular causes or hospitalization for cardiovascular events by 13%.[64] At 21-month median follow-up 2737 subjects, mean age 69 years, with class II HF and an LV ejection fraction of 35% or lower, randomized to eplerenone 50 mg daily or placebo, compared with placebo, eplerenone significantly reduced cardiovascular death or hospitalization for HF 37% and all-cause mortality 24%.[65]

The ACC/AHA guidelines recommend with a class I indication the addition of an aldosterone antagonist in selected patients with class II to IV HF and reduced LV ejection fraction who can be carefully monitored for preserved renal function and normal serum potassium concentration.[56] Patients should have a serum creatinine 2.5 mg/dL or lower in men and 2.0 mg/dL or lower in women, and the serum potassium should be less than 5.0 mEq/L.[56]

BETA-BLOCKERS

In the Göteborg Metoprolol Trial, intravenous metoprolol was given within 48 hours of acute MI and followed by therapy with oral metoprolol for 90 days.[66] In the Metoprolol in Acute Myocardial Infarction Trial, intravenous metoprolol was administered within 24 hours of acute MI and followed by treatment with oral metoprolol for 15 days.[67] In the First International Study of Infarct Survival, intravenous atenolol was given within 12 hours of acute MI and followed by treatment with oral atenolol for 7 days.[68] If the results of these 3 studies in which thrombolytic therapy was not used are pooled, the younger persons had a 5% nonsignificant decrease in mortality, and the older persons had a 23% significant reduction in mortality. Data from the Thrombolysis in Myocardial Infarction II-B Study[69] and the Global Utilization of Streptokinase and Tissue Plasminogen Activator for Occluded Coronary Arteries (GUSTO-I) Trial[70] support the use of early intravenous beta-blockade in patients with acute MI treated with thrombolytic therapy.

In the Göteborg Metoprolol Trial, 262 of 1395 randomized subjects had mild-to-moderate HF before randomization.[71] The 1-year mortality was significantly reduced in subjects treated with metoprolol (14%) compared with subjects treated with placebo (27%).[71]

The ACC/AHA class I indications for use of early intravenous beta-blockade in patients with acute MI are (1) patients without a contraindication to beta-blockers who can be treated within 12 hours of onset of MI, (2) patients with continuing or recurrent ischemic pain, and (3) patients with tachyarrhythmias, such as atrial fibrillation with a rapid ventricular rate, or hypertension.[24,50] Intravenous beta-blockers should not be administered to older patients with severe HF complicating acute MI and the dose should be reduced in older patients with mild-to-moderate HF.

Intravenous atenolol and metoprolol are the 2 beta-blockers that have been approved by the US Food and Drug Administration for use in patients with acute MI. The dose of atenolol used in the First International Study of Infarct Survival was 5 mg intravenously given twice at 10-minute intervals followed by oral atenolol 50 mg every 12 hours.[68] The dose of metoprolol used in the studies cited was 5 mg administered intravenously at 5-minute intervals for 3 doses, followed by oral metoprolol 50 mg every 6 hours with 100 mg given twice daily after 24 to 48 hours.[66,67,69–71] Lower doses may need to be used in older persons.

An analysis of 55 randomized controlled trials investigating the use of beta-blockers after MI demonstrated that beta-blockers caused a 19% significant decrease in mortality.[72] High-risk survivors of acute MI at 12 Norwegian hospitals randomized to treatment with propranolol for 1 year had a 52% significant reduction in sudden cardiac death.[73]

At 17-month follow-up in the Norwegian Multicenter Study, timolol administered in a dose of 10 mg twice daily, compared with placebo, caused a 31% significant decrease in mortality in persons younger than 65 years of age and a 43% significant reduction in mortality in persons aged 65 to 74 years.[74] At 61-month follow-up in this study, timolol caused a 13% nonsignificant decrease in mortality in persons younger than 65 years of age and a 19% significant reduction in mortality in persons aged 65 to 74 years.[75] At 25-month follow-up in the Beta Blocker Heart Attack Trial, propranolol administered in a dose of 80 mg 3 times daily caused a 19% nonsignificant decrease in mortality in persons younger than 60 years of age and a 33% significant reduction in mortality in persons aged 60 to 69 year old.[76] A retrospective cohort study also showed that persons aged 60 to 89 years treated after MI with metoprolol had an age-adjusted mortality decrease of 76% compared with a control group that did not receive beta-blockers.[77]

In the Beta Blocker Heart Attack Trial, propranolol caused a 27% significant reduction in mortality and a 47% significant decrease in sudden cardiac death in subjects with a history of CHF.[78] In the Beta-Blocker Pooling Project, data from 9 studies involving 3519 subjects with CHF at the time of acute MI demonstrated that beta-blockers caused a 25% significant decrease in mortality.[79] Beta-blockers have also been shown to reduce mortality in subjects with CHF due to coronary artery disease associated with an LV ejection fraction of 35% or lower[80–84] or 40% and higher.[84,85]

In a prospective study of 158 persons (mean age: 81 years) with HF, prior MI, and an LV ejection fraction 40% or higher treated with diuretics plus ACE inhibitors, persons randomized to treatment with propranolol had a 35% significant reduction in mortality at 32-month follow-up.[85] The reduction in mortality in persons treated with propranolol was similar in women and men, and in persons older and younger than 80 years.[85]

A retrospective analysis of the use of beta-blockers after MI found that persons 65 years and older had a 43% significant decrease in 2-year mortality and a 22% significant reduction in 2-year cardiac hospital readmissions compared with older persons who were not receiving beta-blockers.[86] Use of a calcium channel blocker instead of a beta-blocker after MI doubled the risk of mortality in this elderly population.[86] Beta-blockers were associated with a significant decrease in mortality after MI in persons 65 to 74 years, 75 to 84 years, and 85 years of age and older.[86] At 17-month follow-up, in 166 subjects, mean age 70 years with HF and abnormal LV ejection fraction treated with cardiac resynchronization therapy (CRT), compared with no beta-blocker, carvedilol significantly reduced all-cause mortality 86%, and metoprolol controlled-release/extended-release (CR/XL) significantly reduced all-cause mortality 81% (statistical probability not significant between the 2 beta blockers).[87]

In 477 subjects (mean age 79 years) with prior MI and a low LV ejection fraction, compared with no ACE inhibitor or beta-blocker therapy, at 34-month follow-up, beta-blockers alone significantly reduced new coronary events by 25% and new HF by 41%.[49] Compared with no ACE inhibitor or beta-blocker therapy, beta blockers plus ACE inhibitors significantly reduced new coronary events by 37% and new HF by 61%.[49]

A meta-analysis of trials also showed that the use of beta-blockers after non–Q-wave MI was likely to reduce mortality and recurrent MI by 25%.[87] All older patients with Q-wave MI or non–Q-wave MI, with or without HF, and without contraindications to beta-blockers, should be treated with beta-blockers indefinitely after MI. Propranolol, metoprolol, timolol, and carvedilol have been approved by the US Food and Drug Administration for long-term treatment after acute MI.

The ACC/AHA guidelines recommend that persons without contraindications to beta-blockers should receive beta-blockers within a few days of acute MI (if not initiated acutely) and continue them indefinitely.[24,50] Contraindications to the use of beta-blockers for long-term treatment after MI include severe HF, severe peripheral arterial disease with the threat of gangrene, greater than first-degree atrioventricular block, hypotension, severe bradycardia, lung disease with bronchospasm, and bronchial asthma.

CALCIUM CHANNEL BLOCKERS AND MAGNESIUM

The ACC/AHA guidelines state that there are no class I indications for using calcium channel blockers or magnesium during acute MI.[24,50] These guidelines also state that there are no class I indications for using calcium channel blockers after MI.[24,50]

Based on the available data, calcium channel blockers should not be used in treating patients during or after MI[72,86,88–92] or in treating patients with HF associated with an abnormal LV ejection fraction.[78,90,93] However, the author would treat postinfarction patients who have persistent angina pectoris despite nitrates and beta-blockers, and who are not candidates for coronary revascularization, with verapamil or diltiazem if the LV ejection fraction is normal, and with amlodipine or felodipine if the LV ejection fraction is abnormal.

DIGOXIN

Although mortality is higher in patients treated with digoxin after MI, it is not clear whether this increase in mortality is due to digoxin.[94] In the Digitalis Investigation Group trial, a recent MI was an exclusion criterion.[95] Although the overall trial showed at 37-month follow-up a similar mortality in subjects treated with digoxin or placebo, there was a reduction in deaths due to HF but a trend toward increased deaths due to presumed arrhythmia or MI in the digoxin-treated group.[95] Digitalis toxicity increased with age.[96] Digoxin may be used together with beta-blockers in treating supraventricular tachyarrhythmias, such as atrial fibrillation with a rapid ventricular rate, during and after acute MI. To reduce hospitalization for HF with a class IIa indication, a low dose of digoxin (0.125 mg daily in elderly patients) may be given to postinfarction patients with sinus rhythm and with persistent HF associated with an abnormal LV ejection fraction despite diuretics plus ACE inhibitors plus beta-blockers.[19,58] Elderly persons are at increased risk for developing digitalis toxicity.[95,96] The serum digoxin level should be below 1.2 ng/mL to avoid an increase in mortality caused by digoxin.[97] The LV ejection fraction should be below 35% in women with HF for a reduction in HF hospitalization.[97]

POSITIVE INOTROPIC DRUGS

If patients with acute MI have HF associated with severe LV systolic dysfunction and a low cardiac output with marked hypotension, intravenous norepinephrine should be administered until the systolic arterial pressure increases to at least 80 mm Hg.[24,50] These patients need balloon flotation right-heart catheter monitoring. Intravenous dopamine may then be administered in a dose of 5 to 15 mg/kg/min.[24,50] After the systolic arterial pressure increases to 90 mm Hg, intravenous dobutamine may be given simultaneously in an attempt to reduce the dosages of the norepinephrine and dopamine infusions.[24,50] Intravenous milrinone administered in a dose of 0.25 to 0.75 mg/kg/min is reserved for patients who do not respond to catecholamines or who have significant arrhythmias, tachycardia, or ischemia induced by catecholamines.[24,50]

Arrhythmic events are common in older persons with HF receiving intravenous dobutamine.[98] Patients needing intravenous inotropic support should receive these drugs for as short a time as possible.[24,50] Whenever possible, afterload-reducing drugs and intra-aortic balloon pumping should be substituted for positive inotropic drugs.[24,50] Long-term intermittent therapy with intravenous dobutamine has been associated with increased ventricular arrhythmias and mortality.[99,100] The 2013 ACCF/AHA HF guidelines recommend temporary intravenous inotropic support in patients with cardiogenic shock until definitive therapy, such as coronary revascularization, mechanical circulatory support (MCS), or heart transplantation, is begun to maintain systemic perfusion and preserve end-organ performance (class I indication).[56] With a class IIa indication, these guidelines recommend continuous intravenous inotropic support as bridge therapy in patients with stage D HF refractory to guided directed medical therapy and device therapy in those who are eligible for and awaiting MCS or cardiac transplantation.[56]

TREATMENT OF ARRHYTHMIAS

Patients with acute MI and HF who develop ventricular fibrillation or sustained ventricular tachycardia should be treated with direct-current electric shock.[24,50] Beta-blockers reduce mortality in postinfarction patients with complex ventricular arrhythmias and an LV ejection fraction of 40% or less[101] or of 40% or higher[102] and should be administered to postinfarction patients with complex ventricular arrhythmias and no contraindications to beta-blockers.

Patients with acute MI and HF who develop bradyarrhythmias may need temporary pacing.[24,50] The ACC/AHA has developed recommendations for permanent pacing after acute MI.[103]

Both atrial fibrillation and HF are associated with increased mortality.[104] When HF occurs during acute MI because of a rapid ventricular rate or loss of atrial contraction associated with atrial fibrillation, immediate direct-current cardioversion should be performed.[24,50,105] Heparin should be given. In treating postinfarction patients with chronic atrial fibrillation, the author prefers long-term warfarin therapy plus ventricular rate control with a beta-blocker plus digoxin, adding verapamil or diltiazem if necessary to slow the ventricular rate during exercise.[105] The dose of oral warfarin administered should achieve an international normalized ratio of 2.0 to 3.0.[105] Newer oral anticoagulants, such as dabigatran,[106] rivaroxaban,[107] apixaban,[108] or edoxaban,[109] may be used instead of warfarin to prevent thromboembolic events in patients with CHF who have nonvalvular atrial fibrillations.

MECHANICAL COMPLICATIONS

Sudden or progressive hemodynamic deterioration with low cardiac output or pulmonary edema in patients with acute MI may be due to acute mitral valve regurgitation, postinfarction ventricular septal defect, LV free-wall rupture, or ventricular aneurysm.[24,50,110–113] Transthoracic or transesophageal echocardiography can usually establish the diagnosis. A balloon flotation catheter is helpful for the diagnosis and monitoring of therapy. Coronary angiography to detect the presence of surgically correctable coronary artery disease should be performed unless the patient is severely unstable hemodynamically from the mechanical defect alone.[24,50,114] Insertion of an intra-aortic balloon pump can help stabilize the patient.

Prompt surgical repair of these mechanical defects is usually indicated because medical treatment alone is associated with a 90% mortality.[24,50,111] The ACC/AHA guidelines state that class I indications for emergent or urgent cardiac repair of mechanical defects caused by an acute MI are (1) papillary muscle rupture with severe acute mitral insufficiency (emergent); (2) postinfarction ventricular septal defect or free-wall rupture, and pulmonary edema or cardiogenic shock (emergent or urgent); and (3) postinfarction ventricular aneurysm associated with intractable ventricular tachyarrhythmias or pump failure (urgent).[24,50] Surgical repair may be deferred in patients with postinfarction ventricular septal defect if they are hemodynamically stable.[24,50,114]

CARDIAC RESYNCHRONIZATION THERAPY AND IMPLANTABLE CARDIOVERTER-DEFIBRILLATORS

Implantable cardioverter-defibrillator (ICD) therapy has a class I indication in selected patients with HF at least 40 days after acute MI with an LV ejection fraction of 35% or less and New York Heart Association class II or III symptoms on chronic guided directed medical therapy with a reasonable expectation of meaningful survival for more than 1 year.[56,115,116] ICD therapy also has a class I indication in selected patients with HF at least 40 days after acute MI with an LV ejection fraction of 30% or less and New York Heart Association class I symptoms on chronic guided directed medical therapy with a reasonable expectation of meaningful survival for more than 1 year.[56,117] (See discussion of ICD therapy, in this issue.)

CRT has a class I indication for patients with HF, an LV ejection fraction of 35% or less, class II, III, or ambulatory IV symptoms on guided directed medical therapy, sinus rhythm, and left bundle branch block (LBBB) with a QRS duration of 150 ms or greater.[56,118–121] CRT has a class IIa indication for patients with HF, an LV ejection fraction of 35% or less, class III or ambulatory IV symptoms on guided directed medical therapy, sinus rhythm, and a non-LBBB pattern with a QRS duration of 150 ms or greater.[56,119,121] CRT has a class IIa indication for patients with HF; an LV ejection fraction of 35% or less; class II, III, or ambulatory IV symptoms on guided directed medical therapy; sinus rhythm; and an LBBB pattern with a QRS duration of 120 to 149 ms.[56,119–122] CRT has a class IIa indication in patients with HF, atrial fibrillation, an LV ejection fraction of 35% or less on guided directed medical therapy if (1) the patient needs ventricular pacing or otherwise meets CRT criteria and (2) atrioventricular nodal ablation or pharmacologic rate control will allow near 100% ventricular pacing with CRT.[56,123] CRT also has a class IIa indication in patients with HF on guided directed medical therapy, an LVEF of 35% or less, and who are undergoing placement of a new or replacement device with anticipated need for more than 40% ventricular pacing.[56,124] (See discussion of CRT therapy, in this issue.)

REFERENCES

1. Aronow WS. Epidemiology, pathophysiology, prognosis, and treatment of systolic and diastolic heart failure in elderly patients. Cardiol Rev 2006;14:108–24.
2. Aronow WS, Ahn C, Kronzon I. Normal left ventricular ejection fraction in older persons with congestive heart failure. Chest 1998;113:867–9.

3. Aronow WS, Ahn C. Incidence of heart failure in 2,737 older persons with and without diabetes mellitus. Chest 1999;115:867–8.
4. Aronow WS, Ahn C, Kronzon I. Comparison of incidences of congestive heart failure in older African-Americans, Hispanics, and whites. Am J Cardiol 1999;84:611–2.
5. Rich MW, Bosner MS, Chung MK, et al. Is age an independent predictor of early and late mortality in patients with acute myocardial infarction? Am J Med 1992;92:7–13.
6. Bueno H, Vidan MT, Almazan A, et al. Influence of sex on the short-term outcome of elderly patients with a first acute myocardial infarction. Circulation 1995;92:1133–40.
7. Kober L, Torp-Pedersen C, Ottesen M, et al. Influence of gender on short- and long-term mortality after acute myocardial infarction. Am J Cardiol 1996;77:1052–6.
8. Weaver WD, White HD, Wilcox RG, et al. Comparisons of characteristics and outcomes among women and men with acute myocardial infarction treated with thrombolytic therapy. JAMA 1996; 275:777–82.
9. Aronow WS. Prevalence of presenting symptoms of recognized acute myocardial infarction and of unrecognized healed myocardial infarction in elderly patients. Am J Cardiol 1987;60:1182.
10. Wolk MJ, Scheidt S, Killip T. Heart failure complicating acute myocardial infarction. Circulation 1972;45:1125–38.
11. Dwyer EM Jr, Greenberg HM, Steinberg G, et al. Clinical characteristics and natural history of survivors of pulmonary congestion during acute myocardial infarction. Am J Cardiol 1989;63: 1423–8.
12. Gottlieb S, Moss AJ, McDermott M, et al. Interrelation of left ventricular ejection fraction, pulmonary congestion and outcome in acute myocardial infarction. Am J Cardiol 1992;69:977–84.
13. Sulo G, Igland J, Vollset SE, et al. Heart failure complicating acute myocardial infarction; burden and timing of occurrence: a nation-wide analysis including 86,771 patients from the Cardiovascular Disease in Norway (CVDNOR) Project. J Am Heart Assoc 2016;5(1). http://dx.doi.org/10.1161/JAHA.115.002667.
14. Forrester J, Diamond G, Chatterjee K, et al. Medical therapy of acute myocardial infarction by the application of hemodynamic subsets. N Engl J Med 1976;295:1356–62.
15. GISSI-3: effects of lisinopril and transdermal glyceryl trinitrate singly and together on 6-week mortality and ventricular function after acute myocardial infarction. Gruppo Italiano per lo Studio della Sopravvivenza nell'Infarto Miocardico. Lancet 1994; 343:1115–22.
16. Aronow WS, Ahn C, Kronzon I. Prognosis of congestive heart failure in elderly patients with normal versus abnormal left ventricular systolic function associated with coronary artery disease. Am J Cardiol 1990;66:1257–9.
17. Aronow WS, Ahn C, Kronzon I. Prognosis of congestive heart failure after prior myocardial infarction in older men and women with abnormal versus normal left ventricular ejection fraction. Am J Cardiol 2000;85:1382–4.
18. Aronow WS. Treatment of systolic and diastolic heart failure in elderly persons. J Gerontol A Biol Sci Med Sci 2006;60A:1597–605.
19. Rich MW, Aronow WS. Therapy of acute myocardial infarction. In: Aronow WS, Fleg JL, Rich MW, editors. Tresch and Aronow's cardiovascular disease in the elderly. 5th edition. Boca Raton (FL); London; New York: CRC Press; 2013. p. 238–72.
20. Aronow WS. Echo in the elderly. Cardio 1990;8: 81–90.
21. Harrison MR, MacPhail B, Gurley JC, et al. Usefulness of color Doppler flow imaging to distinguish ventricular septal defect from acute mitral regurgitation complicating acute myocardial infarction. Am J Cardiol 1989;64:697–701.
22. Butman S, Olson HG, Aronow WS. Remote right ventricular infarction mimicking pericardial constriction. Am Heart J 1982;103:912–4.
23. Smyllie JH, Sutherland GR, Geuskens R, et al. Doppler color flow mapping in the diagnosis of ventricular septal rupture and acute mitral regurgitation after myocardial infarction. J Am Coll Cardiol 1990;15:1449–55.
24. Antman EM, Anbe DT, Armstrong PW, et al. ACC/AHA guidelines for the management of patients with ST-elevation myocardial infarction—executive summary. J Am Coll Cardiol 2004;44:671–719.
25. Maroko PR, Radvany P, Braunwald E, et al. Reduction of infarct size by oxygen inhalation following acute coronary occlusion. Circulation 1975;52: 360–8.
26. Fillmore SJ, Shapiro M, Killip T. Arterial oxygen tension in acute myocardial infarction: serial analysis of clinical state and blood gas changes. Am Heart J 1970;79:620–9.
27. Aubier M, Trippenbach T, Roussos C. Respiratory muscle fatigue during cardiogenic shock. J Appl Physiol Respir Environ Exerc Physiol 1981;51: 499–508.
28. Hyzy R, Popovich J. Mechanical ventilation and weaning. In: Carlson RW, Geheb MA, editors. Principles and practice of medical intensive care. Philadelphia: WB Saunders; 1993. p. 924–33.
29. Zelis R, Mansour EJ, Capone RJ, et al. The cardiovascular effects of morphine: the peripheral capacitance and resistance vessels in human subjects. J Clin Invest 1974;54:1247–58.

30. Vismara LA, Leaman DM, Zelis R. The effects of morphine on venous tone in patients with acute pulmonary edema. Circulation 1976;54:335–7.
31. Butman S, Aronow WS. Updated treatment for left ventricular failure and acute cardiogenic pulmonary edema. ER Rep 1981;2:53–8.
32. Biddle TL, Yu PN. Effect of furosemide on hemodynamics and lung water in acute pulmonary edema secondary to myocardial infarction. Am J Cardiol 1973;43:86–90.
33. Dikshit K, Vyden MB, Forrester JS, et al. Renal and extrarenal hemodynamic effects of furosemide in congestive heart failure after acute myocardial infarction. N Engl J Med 1973;288:1087–90.
34. Flaherty JT. Role of nitrates in acute myocardial infarction. Am J Cardiol 1992;70:73B–81B.
35. Jugdutt BI. Role of nitrates after acute myocardial infarction. Am J Cardiol 1992;70:82B–7B.
36. ISIS-4: a randomised factorial trial assessing early oral captopril, oral mononitrate, and intravenous magnesium sulphate in 58,050 patients with suspected acute myocardial infarction. ISIS-4 (Fourth International Study of Infarct Survival) Collaborative Group. Lancet 1995;345:669–85.
37. Come PC, Pitt B. Nitroglycerin-induced severe hypotension and bradycardia in patients with acute myocardial infarction. Circulation 1976;54:624–8.
38. Kinch JW, Ryan TJ. Right ventricular infarction. N Engl J Med 1994;330:1211–7.
39. Gunnar RM, Lambrew CT, Abrams W, et al. Task force IV: pharmacologic interventions. Emergency cardiac care. Am J Cardiol 1982;50:393–408.
40. O'Connor CM, Starling RC, Hernandez PW, et al. Effect of nesiritide in patients with acute decompensated heart failure. N Engl J Med 2011;365: 32–43.
41. Swedberg K, Held P, Kjekhus J, et al. Effects of the early administration of enalapril on mortality in patients with myocardial infarction. N Engl J Med 1992;327:678–84.
42. Cohn JN, Johnson G, Ziesche S, et al. A comparison of enalapril with hydralazine-isosorbide dinitrate in the treatment of chronic congestive heart failure. N Engl J Med 1991;325:303–10.
43. Effect of ramipril on mortality and morbidity of survivors of acute myocardial infarction with clinical evidence of heart failure. The Acute Infarction Ramipril Efficacy (AIRE) Study Investigators. Lancet 1993;342:821–8.
44. Ambrosioni E, Borghi C, Magnani B, et al. The effect of the angiotensin-converting-enzyme inhibitor zofenopril on mortality and morbidity after anterior myocardial infarction. N Engl J Med 1995;332: 80–5.
45. Kober L, Torp-Pedersen C, Carlsen JE, et al. A clinical trial of the angiotensin-converting-enzyme inhibitor trandolapril in patients with left ventricular dysfunction after myocardial infarction. N Engl J Med 1995;333:1670–6.
46. Lisheng L, Liu LS, Wang W, et al. Oral captopril versus placebo among 13,364 patients with suspected acute myocardial infarction: interim report from the Chinese Cardiac Study (CCS-1). Lancet 1995;345:686–7.
47. Six-month effects of early treatment with lisinopril and transdermal glyceryl trinitrate singly and together withdrawn six-weeks after acute myocardial infarction: the GISSI-3 trial. Gruppo Italiano per lo Studio della Sopravvivenza nell'Infarto Miocardico. J Am Coll Cardiol 1996;27:337–44.
48. Pfeffer MA, Braunwald E, Moye LA, et al. Effect of captopril on mortality and morbidity in patients with left ventricular dysfunction after myocardial infarction. Results of the Survival and Ventricular Enlargement Trial. N Engl J Med 1992;327:669–77.
49. Aronow WS, Ahn C, Kronzon I. Effect of beta blockers alone, of angiotensin-converting enzyme inhibitors alone, and of beta blockers plus angiotensin-converting enzyme inhibitors on new coronary events and on congestive heart failure in older persons with healed myocardial infarcts and asymptomatic left ventricular systolic dysfunction. Am J Cardiol 2001;88:1298–300.
50. Ryan TJ, Anderson JL, Antman EM, et al. ACC/AHA guidelines for the management of patients with acute myocardial infarction. A report of the American College of Cardiology/American Heart Association Task Force on Practice Guidelines (Committee on Management of Acute Myocardial Infarction). J Am Coll Cardiol 1996;28:1328–428.
51. Sigurdsson A, Swedberg K. Left ventricular remodelling, neurohormonal activation and early treatment with enalapril (CONSENSUS II) following myocardial infarction. Eur Heart J 1994;15(Suppl B):14–9.
52. Effects of enalapril on mortality in severe congestive heart failure. Results of the Cooperative North Scandinavian Enalapril Survival Study (CONSENSUS). The CONSENSUS Trial Study Group. N Engl J Med 1987;316:1429–35.
53. Effect of enalapril on survival in patients with reduced left ventricular ejection fractions and congestive heart failure. The SOLVD Investigators. N Engl J Med 1991;325:293–302.
54. Aronow WS, Kronzon I. Effect of enalapril on congestive heart failure treated with diuretics in elderly patients with prior myocardial infarction and normal left ventricular ejection fraction. Am J Cardiol 1993;71:602–4.
55. Philbin EF, Rocco TA Jr, Lindenmuth NW, et al. Systolic versus diastolic heart failure in community practice: clinical features, outcomes, and the use of angiotensin-converting enzyme inhibitors. Am J Med 2000;109:605–13.

56. Yancy CW, Jessup M, Bozkurt B, et al. 2013 ACCF/AHA guideline for the management of heart failure: a report of the American College of Cardiology Foundation/American Heart Association Task Force on Practice Guidelines. J Am Coll Cardiol 2013;62: e147–239.
57. Pitt B, Poole-Wilson PA, Segal R, et al. Effect of losartan compared with captopril on mortality in patients with symptomatic heart failure: randomised trial—the Losartan Heart Failure Survival Study ELITE II. Lancet 2000;355:1582–7.
58. Cohn JN, Tognoni G. A randomized trial of the angiotensin-receptor blocker valsartan in chronic heart failure. N Engl J Med 2001;345:1667–75.
59. Pfeffer MA, McMurray JJV, Velazquez EJ, et al. Valsartan, captopril, or both in myocardial infarction complicated by heart failure, left ventricular dysfunction, or both. N Engl J Med 2003;349: 1893–906.
60. Granger CB, McMurray JJV, Yusuf S, et al. Effects of candesartan in patients with chronic heart failure and reduced left-ventricular systolic function intolerant to angiotensin-converting-enzyme inhibitors: the CHARM-Alternative trial. Lancet 2003;362: 772–6.
61. McMurray JJV, Ostergren J, Swedberg K, et al. Effects of candesartan in patients with chronic heart failure and reduced left-ventricular systolic function taking angiotensin-converting-enzyme inhibitors: the CHARM-Added trial. Lancet 2003;362:767–71.
62. Yusuf S, Pfeffer MA, Swedberg K, et al. Effects of candesartan in patients with chronic heart failure and preserved left-ventricular ejection fraction: the CHARM-Preserved trial. Lancet 2003;362: 777–81.
63. Pitt B, Zannad F, Remme WJ, et al. The effect of spironolactone on morbidity and mortality in patients with severe heart failure. N Engl J Med 1999;341:709–17.
64. Pitt B, Remme W, Zannad F, et al. Eplerenone, a selective aldosterone blocker, in patients with left ventricular dysfunction after myocardial infarction. N Engl J Med 2003;348:1309–21.
65. Zannad F, McMurray JJV, Krun H, et al. Eplerenone in patients with systolic heart failure and mild symptoms. N Engl J Med 2011;364:11–21.
66. Hjalmarson A, Elmfeldt D, Herlitz J, et al. Effect on mortality of metoprolol in acute myocardial infarction. Lancet 1981;2:823–7.
67. Metoprolol in acute myocardial infarction (MIAMI). A randomised placebo-controlled international trial. The MIAMI Trial Research Group. Eur Heart J 1985;6:199–226.
68. Randomised trial of intravenous atenolol among 16 027 cases of suspected acutemyocardial infarction: ISIS-1. First International Study of Infarct Survival Collaborative Group. Lancet 1986;2:57–66.
69. Roberts R, Rogers WJ, Mueller HS, et al. Immediate versus deferred beta-blockade following thrombolytic therapy in patients with acute myocardial infarction. Results of the Thrombolysis in Myocardial Infarction (TIMI) II-B Study. Circulation 1991; 83:422–37.
70. Smith SC Jr. Drug treatment after acute myocardial infarction: is treatment the same for the elderly as in the young patient? Am J Geriatr Cardiol 1998; 7:60–4.
71. Herlitz J, Waagstein F, Lindqvist J, et al. Effect of metoprolol on the prognosis for patients with suspected acute myocardial infarction and indirect signs of congestive heart failure (a subgroup analysis of the Göteborg Metoprolol Trial). Am J Cardiol 1997;80:40J–4J.
72. Teo KK, Yusuf S, Furberg CD. Effects of prophylactic antiarrhythmic drug therapy in acute myocardial infarction. An overview of results from randomized controlled trials. JAMA 1993;270:1589–95.
73. Hansteen V. Beta blockade after myocardial infarction: the Norwegian Propranolol Study in high-risk patients. Circulation 1983;67(Suppl I):I57–60.
74. Gundersen T, Abrahamsen AM, Kjekshus J, et al. Timolol-related reduction in mortality and reinfarction in patients ages 65–75 years surviving acute myocardial infarction. Circulation 1982;66: 1179–84.
75. Pedersen TR. Six-year follow-up of the Norwegian Multicentre Study on Timolol after acute myocardial infarction. N Engl J Med 1985;313:1055–8.
76. Beta-Blocker Heart Attack Trial Research Group. A randomized trial of propranolol in patients with acute myocardial infarction. JAMA 1982;247: 1707–14.
77. Park KC, Forman DE, Wei JY. Utility of betablockade treatment for older postinfarction patients. J Am Geriatr Soc 1995;43:751–5.
78. Chadda K, Goldstein S, Byington R, et al. Effect of propranolol after acute myocardial infarction in patients with congestive heart failure. Circulation 1986;73:503–10.
79. The Beta-Blocker Pooling Project (BBPP): subgroup findings from randomized trials in post infarction patients. The Beta-Blocker Pooling Project Research Group. Eur Heart J 1988;9:8–16.
80. Packer M, Bristow MR, Cohn JN, et al. The effect of carvedilol on morbidity and mortality in patients with chronic heart failure. N Engl J Med 1996; 334:1349–55.
81. CIBIS-II Investigators and Committees. The Cardiac Insufficiency Bisoprolol Study II (CIBIS-II): a randomised trial. Lancet 1999;353:9–13.
82. MERIT-HF Study Group. Effect of metoprolol CR/XL in chronic heart failure: Metoprolol CR/XL Randomised Intervention Trial in Congestive Heart Failure (MERIT-HF). Lancet 1999;353:2001–7.

83. Packer M, Coats AJS, Fowler MB, et al. Effect of carvedilol on survival in chronic heart failure. N Engl J Med 2001;344:651–8.
84. van Veldhuisen DJ, Cohen-Solal A, Bohm M, et al. Beta-blockade with nebivolol in elderly heart failure patients with impaired and preserved left ventricular ejection fraction: data from SENIORS (Study of Effects of Nebivolol Intervention on Outcomes and Rehospitalization in Seniors With Heart Failure). J Am Coll Cardiol 2009;53:2159–61.
85. Aronow WS, Ahn C, Kronzon I. Effect of propranolol versus no propranolol on total mortality plus nonfatal myocardial infarction in older patients with prior myocardial infarction, congestive heart failure, and left ventricular ejection fraction R40% treated with diuretics plus angiotensin-converting-enzyme inhibitors. Am J Cardiol 1997;80:207–9.
86. Soumerai SB, McLaughlin TJ, Spiegelman D, et al. Adverse outcomes of underuse of beta-blockers in elderly survivors of acute myocardial infarction. JAMA 1997;277:115–21.
87. Shen X, Nair CK, Aronow WS, et al. Effect of carvedilol versus metoprolol CR/XL on mortality in patients with heart failure treated with cardiac resynchronization therapy: a Cox multivariate regression analysis. Am J Ther 2013;20:247–53.
88. Yusuf S, Wittes J, Probstfield J. Evaluating effects of treatment subgroups of patients within a clinical trial: the case of non-Q-wave myocardial infarction and beta blockers. Am J Cardiol 1990;60:220–2.
89. The effect of diltiazem on mortality and reinfarction after myocardial infarction. The Multicenter Diltiazem Postinfarction Trial Research Group. N Engl J Med 1988;319:385–92.
90. Goldstein RE, Boccuzzi SJ, Cruess D, et al. Diltiazem increases late-onset congestive heart failure in postinfarction patients with early reduction in ejection fraction. Circulation 1991;83:52–60.
91. Furberg CD, Psaty BM, Meyer JV. Nifedipine: dose-related increase in mortality in patients with coronary heart disease. Circulation 1995;92:1321–6.
92. Yusuf S, Held P, Furberg C. Update of effects of calcium antagonists in myocardial infarction or angina in light of the second Danish Verapamil Infarction Trial (DAVIT-II) and other recent studies. Am J Cardiol 1991;67:1295–7.
93. Elkayam U, Amin J, Mehra A, et al. A prospective, randomized, double-blind, crossover study to compare the efficacy and safety of chronic nifedipine therapy with that of isosorbide dinitrate and their combination in the treatment of chronic congestive heart failure. Circulation 1990;82:1954–61.
94. Aronow WS. Digoxin or angiotensin converting enzyme inhibitors for congestive heart failure in geriatric patients. Which is the preferred treatment? Drugs Aging 1991;1:98–103.
95. The Digitalis Investigation Group. The effect of digoxin on mortality and morbidity in patients with heart failure. N Engl J Med 1997;336:525–33.
96. Rich MW, McSherry F, Williford WO, et al. Effect of age on mortality, hospitalizations and response to digoxin in patients with heart failure: the DIG Study. J Am Coll Cardiol 2001;38:806–13.
97. Ahmed A, Aban IB, Weaver MT, et al. Serum digoxin concentration and outcomes in women with heart failure: a bi-directional effect and a possible effect modification by ejection fraction. Eur J Heart Fail 2006;8:409–19.
98. Rich MW, Woods WL, Davila-Roman VG, et al. A randomized comparison of intravenous amrinone versus dobutamine in older patients with decompensated congestive heart failure. J Am Geriatr Soc 1995;43:271–4.
99. Dies F, Krell MJ, Whitlow P, et al. Intermittent dobutamine in ambulatory out-patients with chronic cardiac failure [abstract]. Circulation 1986;74(Suppl II). II-38.
100. O'Connor CM, Gattis WA, Uretsky BF, et al. Continuous intravenous dobutamine is associated with an increased risk of death in patients with advanced heart failure: insights from the Flolan International Randomized Survival Trial (FIRST). Am Heart J 2000;138:78–86.
101. Kennedy HL, Brooks MM, Barker AH, et al. Beta-blocker therapy in the Cardiac Arrhythmia Suppression Trial. Am J Cardiol 1994;74:674–80.
102. Aronow WS, Ahn C, Mercando AD, et al. Effect of propranolol versus no antiarrhythmic drug on sudden cardiac death, total cardiac death, and total death in patients R62 years of age with heart disease, complex ventricular arrhythmias, and left ventricular ejection fraction R40%. Am J Cardiol 1994;74:267–70.
103. Tracy CM, Epstein AE, Darbar D, et al. 2012 ACCF/AHA/HRS focused update of the 2008 guidelines for device-based therapy of cardiac rhythm abnormalities. A report of the American College of Cardiology Foundation/American Heart Association Task Force on Practice Guidelines. Developed in collaboration with the American Association for Thoracic Surgery, Heart Failure Society of America, and Society of Thoracic Surgeons. J Am Coll Cardiol 2012;60:1297–313.
104. Bajaj NS, Bhatia V, Sanam K, et al. Impact of atrial fibrillation and heart failure, independent of each other and in combination, on mortality in community-dwelling older adults. Am J Cardiol 2014;114:909–13.
105. Aronow WS. Management of atrial fibrillation in the elderly. Minerva Med 2009;100:3–24.
106. Connolly SJ, Ezekowitz MD, Yusuf S, et al. Dabigatran versus warfarin in patients with atrial fibrillation. N Engl J Med 2009;361:1139–51.

107. Patel MR, Mahaffey KW, Garg J, et al. Rivaroxaban versus warfarin in nonvalvular atrial fibrillation. N Engl J Med 2011;365:883–91.
108. Granger CB, Alexander JH, McMurray JJ, et al. Apixaban versus warfarin in patients with atrial fibrillation. N Engl J Med 2011;365:981–92.
109. Giugliano RP, Ruff CT, Braunwald E, et al. Edoxaban versus warfarin in patients with atrial fibrillation. N Engl J Med 2013;369:2093–104.
110. Nunez L, de La Llana R, Lopez Sendon J, et al. Diagnosis of treatment of subacute free wall ventricular rupture after infarction. Ann Thorac Surg 1983;35:525–9.
111. Labovitz AJ, Miller LW, Kennedy HL. Mechanical complications of acute myocardial infarction. Cardiovasc Rev Rep 1984;5:948–52.
112. Bolooki H. Surgical treatment of complications of acute myocardial infarction. JAMA 1990;263: 1237–40.
113. Lemery R, Smith HC, Giuliani ER, et al. Prognosis in rupture of the ventricular septum after acute myocardial infarction and role of early surgical intervention. Am J Cardiol 1992;70:147–51.
114. O'Gara PT, Kushner FG, Ascheim DD, et al. 2013 ACCF/AHA guideline for the management of ST-elevation myocardial infarction. A report of the American College of Cardiology Foundation/American Heart Association Task Force on Practice Guidelines. Developed in collaboration with the American College of Emergency Physicians and Society for Cardiovascular Angiography and Interventions. Circulation 2013;127:e362–425.
115. Bardy GH, Lee KL, Mark DB, et al. Amiodarone or an implantable cardioverter-defibrillator for congestive heart failure. N Engl J Med 2005;352: 225–37.
116. Moss AJ, Zareba W, Hall WJ, et al. Prophylactic implantation of a defibrillator in patients with myocardial infarction and reduced ejection fraction. N Engl J Med 2002;346:877–83.
117. Moss AJ, Hall WJ, Cannom DS, et al. Improved survival with an implanted defibrillator in patients with coronary disease at high risk for ventricular arrhythmia. N Engl J Med 1996;335:1933–40.
118. Aronow WS. CRT plus ICD in congestive heart failure. Use of cardiac resynchronization therapy and an implantable cardioverter-defibrillator in heart failure patients with abnormal left ventricular dysfunction. Geriatrics 2005;60(2):24–8.
119. Cleland JGF, Daubert J-C, Erdmann E, et al. The effect of cardiac resynchronization on morbidity and mortality in heart failure. N Engl J Med 2005;352: 1539–49.
120. Moss AJ, Hall WJ, Cannom DS, et al. Cardiac- resynchronization therapy for the prevention of heart-failure events. N Engl J Med 2009;361:1329–38.
121. Tang AS, Wells GA, Talajic M, et al. Cardiac-resynchronization therapy for mild-to-moderate heart failure. N Engl J Med 2010;363:2385–95.
122. Linde C, Abraham WT, Gold MR, et al. Randomized trial of cardiac resynchronization in mildly symptomatic heart failure patients and in asymptomatic patients with left ventricular dysfunction and previous heart failure symptoms. J Am Coll Cardiol 2008;52:1834–43.
123. Brignole M, Botto G, Mont L, et al. Cardiac resynchronization therapy in patients undergoing atrioventricular junction ablation for permanent atrial fibrillation: a randomized trial. Eur Heart J 2011;32:2420–9.
124. Vatankulu MA, Goktekin O, Kaya MG, et al. Effect of long-term resynchronization therapy on left ventricular remodeling in pacemaker patients upgraded to biventricular devices. Am J Cardiol 2009;103:1280–4.

The Role of Positive Inotropic Drugs in the Treatment of Older Adults with Heart Failure and Reduced Ejection Fraction

Daniel J. Dooley, MD[a,b,1], Phillip H. Lam, MD[a,b,1], Ali Ahmed, MD, MPH[a,c,d], Wilbert S. Aronow, MD[e,*]

KEYWORDS

• Heart failure • Inotropic drugs • Older adults • Mortality • Hospitalization

KEY POINTS

- Except for digoxin, the use of positive inotropes has been shown to be associated with higher risk of death and should not be used on a long-term basis.
- Therapy with short-term intravenous positive inotropes may be considered to maintain systemic perfusion until acute precipitating causes are resolved or a more definitive therapy may be considered, such as coronary revascularization, mechanical circulatory support, or heart transplantation.
- Therapy with short-term intravenous positive inotropes may be considered in patients with low blood pressure and hypoperfusion.
- Therapy with short-term intravenous positive inotropes may be considered as bridge therapy when patients are refractory to other evidence-based therapy and are waiting for mechanical circulatory support or heart transplantation.
- Therapy with long-term intravenous positive inotropes may be considered for patients with endstage heart failure enrolled into palliative and hospice care who are symptomatic despite other evidence-based therapy and are not candidates for mechanical circulatory support or heart transplantation.

INTRODUCTION

Heart failure (HF) is the most common cause for hospital admission in the United States among individuals 65 years of age and older, and is a significant burden on the health care system. It has been projected that by 2030, the total cost of HF will be $69.7 billion, an increase from the $30.7 billion spent in 2012.[1] About half of HF admissions derive from patients with HF and reduced

Disclosure Statement: The authors have nothing to disclose.
Conflict of Interest: None.

[a] Center for Health and Aging, Veterans Affairs Medical Center, 50 Irving Street NW, Washington, DC 20422, USA; [b] MedStar Heart and Vascular Institute, Georgetown University/MedStar Washington Hospital Center, 110 Irving Street NW, Washington, DC 20010, USA; [c] Department of Medicine, George Washington University, 2150 Pennsylvania Avenue, NW Suite 8-416, Washington, DC 20037, USA; [d] Department of Medicine, University of Alabama at Birmingham, 933 19th Street South, CH19 201, Birmingham, AL 35294, USA; [e] Cardiology Division, Westchester Medical Center, New York Medical College, Macy Pavilion, Room 141, Valhalla, NY 10595, USA
[1] Equal contribution.
* Corresponding author.
E-mail address: wsaronow@aol.com

Heart Failure Clin 13 (2017) 527–534
http://dx.doi.org/10.1016/j.hfc.2017.02.008
1551-7136/17/

ejection fraction (HFrEF), defined as left ventricular ejection fraction less than 40%.[1] One of the most common modes of death in patients with HFrEF is pump failure, an outcome preceded by deteriorating hemodynamics.[2] Several positive inotropic drugs have been studied in the treatment of HFrEF patients with low cardiac output who are unable to tolerate the standard guideline-directed medical therapies used in the treatment of HFrEF. The purpose of this article is to review these agents in the treatment of patients who have HFrEF, with a focus on older adults.

POSITIVE INOTROPIC DRUGS

Positive inotropic drugs have been shown to improve hemodynamics in patients with HFrEF in the acute decompensation setting in whom they are efficacious in improving symptoms. However, long-term use of these drugs has been associated with higher mortality. Except for digoxin, none of the positive inotropes are recommended for routine use in chronic HFrEF.[3] Many randomized clinical trials have been conducted to measure the clinical impact of these drugs on HFrEF (**Table 1**).[4–12] Evidence for increased mortality risk in studies of most positive inotropic drugs in patients with HFrEF suggests that the decision to initiate these drugs should be individualized.

ADRENERGIC AGONISTS

The adrenergic agonists stimulate the heart through the autonomic nervous system pathway. Most adrenergic agonists (dopamine, epinephrine, isoproterenol, norepinephrine, and phenylephrine) are not commonly used in the treatment of HF because of their vasoconstrictive and proarrhythmic properties, and their association with a higher risk of death. Although dobutamine is a more commonly used adrenergic agonist in HFrEF, its use is also associated with a higher risk of death.[13] However, when carefully used, dobutamine and dopamine may play a role in the management HFrEF patients who are refractory to other HF therapy.[3]

Dobutamine

Dobutamine stimulates beta-1 and beta-2 adrenergic receptor subtypes, thus increasing contractility through its beta-1 effect and vasodilation because of its beta-2 effect. At higher doses, dobutamine stimulates alpha-1 receptors and causes vasoconstriction.

Dobutamine has been evaluated in several clinical trials.[10,11,13–19] The Dobutamine Infusion in Severe Heart Failure (DICE) trial was designed to evaluate intermittent low-dose dobutamine.[11] In the trial, 38 subjects with an average age of 65 years were randomized to receive optimized oral therapy and intermittent ambulatory low-dose dobutamine versus optimized oral therapy alone. Although it did not achieve statistical significance, there was a trend toward a reduction in the primary outcome of reduced HF hospitalizations.[11] Although no significant impact on mortality in subjects who received dobutamine was observed,[11] an earlier study investigating the effects of intermittent dobutamine infusion in HF subjects was stopped early due to increased rates of death in the dobutamine group.[20] Subsequently, the effect of continuous dobutamine use was studied in a post hoc analysis of the Flolan International Randomized Survival Trial (FIRST), which analyzed 80 subjects receiving continuous dobutamine at the time of randomization compared with 391 who were not receiving this drug.[13] In that study, the use of continuous dobutamine was associated with an increase in 6-month all-cause mortality rate ($P = .001$). Some studies have shown association of dobutamine use with improved 6-minute walk tests and cardiac function[17,19] but large-scale randomized trials displaying these benefits are lacking.

Although specific investigations of the impact of dobutamine in older subjects with HF are limited to case series,[19] subjects in the relatively small (sample size 38) randomized controlled DICE trial had a mean age of approximately 65 years.[11] In that study, although there were no significant between-group differences in all-cause and HF hospitalizations, likely due to small sample size, these events were numerically lower in the dobutamine group.[11] Similarly, there were no significant between-group differences in all-cause mortality but these events were numerically higher in the dobutamine group.[11] Taken together with findings from other studies,[11,13,15,16,20] this suggests that dobutamine use does not prolong life and may be associated with a higher risk of mortality in patients with advanced HFrEF.

Dopamine

Dopamine stimulates not only alpha-adrenergic and beta-adrenergic receptors, which allows for vascular, inotropic, and chronotropic support, but also dopaminergic receptors. Stimulation of dopaminergic receptors results in proportionately greater increases in splanchnic and renal perfusion relative to other vasoactive drugs.[21]

Dopamine's use in the treatment of shock has been well studied.[22–24] Several studies have also examined the role dopamine in HF.[25–30] In older subjects (mean age, 75.7 years) hospitalized for acute decompensated HF, a low dose of IV

Table 1
Randomized controlled trials of positive inotropes in patients with heart failure and reduced ejection fraction

Study	Year	Study Drug	Mean Age (y)	Number of Subjects	Results
PROMISE	1991	Oral milrinone	64	1088	Higher risk of all-cause mortality (*P* = .038)[a] and CV mortality (*P* = .016) with milrinone compared with placebo
PICO	1996	Oral low-dose pimobendan	65	317	Improved exercise tolerance for 2.5 mg/d (*P* = .03) and 5 mg/d (*P* = .05) compared with placebo[a]
DIG Trial	1997	Oral digoxin	63	6800	No significant difference in all-cause mortality (*P* = .80)[a]; decrease in number of all-cause hospitalizations per subject with digoxin compared with placebo (*P* = .01)
DICE	1999	Intermittent low-dose dobutamine	65	38	No significant difference in HF hospitalizations[a] or mortality
OPTIME-CHF	2002	Short-term intravenous milrinone	65	951	No significant difference in days hospitalized at 60-d follow up (*P* = .71)[a]; higher risk of sustained hypotension (*P*<.001) and new atrial arrhythmias (*P* = .004) with milrinone compared with placebo
EPOCH	2002	Oral low-dose pimobendan	64	298	Lower risk of adverse cardiac events with pimobendan compared with placebo (*P* = .035) and no significant difference in combined death and hospitalization for cardiac causes (*P* = .202)[a]
SURVIVE	2007	Short-term intravenous levosimendan vs dobutamine	67	1327	No difference in risk of all-cause mortality at 180 d follow-up (*P* = .40)[a]
ESSENTIAL	2009	Oral enoximone	62	1854	No difference in composite of time to all-cause mortality or hospitalization (*P* = .71)[a]
REVIVE	2013	Short-term intravenous levosimendan	63	700	Improved rapid symptomatic relief and lower likelihood of clinical worsening (*P* = .015)[a] for levosimendan compared with placebo

Abbreviations: CV, cardiovascular; DICE, Dobutamine Infusion in Severe Heart Failure; DIG, Digitalis Investigation Group; EPOCH, Effects of Pimobendan on Chronic Heart Failure; ESSENTIAL, Studies of Oral Enoximone Therapy in Advanced HF; OPTIME-CHF, Outcomes of a Prospective Trial of Intravenous Milrinone for Exacerbations of Chronic Heart Failure; PICO, Pimobendan in Congestive Heart Failure; PROMISE, Prospective Randomized Milrinone Survival Evaluation; REVIVE, Randomized Multicenter Evaluation of Intravenous Levosimendan Efficacy versus Placebo in the Short-term Treatment of Acute Heart Failure; SURVIVE, Survival of Subjects with Acute Heart Failure in Need of Intravenous Inotropic Support.
[a] Outcomes reported in the original study as either primary or coprimary endpoint.

dopamine, when combined with low-dose intravenous (IV) furosemide, was equally effective in reducing length of stay and 60-day mortality or rehospitalization rates (all-cause, cardiovascular, and worsening HF) when compared with a high dose of IV furosemide alone.[29] However, in that study, subjects receiving low doses of both furosemide and dopamine had improved renal function compared with high-dose furosemide alone (P = .042). This study, along with a prior small study revealing improved renal function in 13 subjects with chronic HFrEF who received IV dopamine,[28] led to a class IIb recommendation from the 2013 the American College of Cardiology Foundation/American Heart Association Heart Failure guidelines for the use of low-dose IV dopamine in addition to a loop diuretic therapy to improve diuresis and better preserve renal blood flow.[3] The guidelines also recommend that dopamine, along with dobutamine and milrinone, may be considered in patients with HFrEF who have low cardiac index and evidence of systemic hypoperfusion and/or congestion.[3]

PHOSPHODIESTERASE INHIBITORS

The phosphodiesterase III (PDE III) enzyme is present in the cardiac muscle closely associated with the sarcoplasmic reticulum. This enzyme degrades cyclic adenosine monophosphate (cAMP) to adenosine monophosphate (AMP) and is involved in the release of calcium. PDE III inhibition in low doses results in increasing contractility without increasing heart rate. PDE III also is present in vascular smooth muscle and its inhibition enhances vasodilation through nitric oxide-dependent pathways. This inotrope-vasodilator property of PDE increases contractility, reduces preload, and reduces afterload, all of which are beneficial effects for the failing heart.

Milrinone

Milrinone, a PDE III inhibitor, was used in several studies to examine its benefits in patients with HFrEF in both the outpatient and hospitalized setting.[4,6] In the Prospective Randomized Milrinone Survival Evaluation (PROMISE) Trial, subjects with symptomatic chronic HFrEF were randomized to receive oral milrinone on top of the standard medical therapy at that time, which included digoxin, an angiotensin-converting enzyme inhibitor, and a diuretic.[6] Those who received oral milrinone had a 28% (P = .038) increase in all-cause mortality and a 34% (P = .016) increase in cardiovascular mortality compared with those who did not take oral milrinone,[6] regardless of age. Notably, the greatest increase in risk for mortality with milrinone use was observed in subjects with New York Heart Association (NYHA) class IV symptoms, suggesting that those with the most severe disease and most likely to be considered for inotropic therapy may be at greatest risk.[6]

The Outcomes of a Prospective Trial of Intravenous Milrinone for Exacerbations of Chronic Heart Failure (OPTIME-CHF) was designed to evaluate the use of IV milrinone in subjects admitted for acute decompensated HF.[4] Subjects with HFrEF randomized to receive IV milrinone did not show a significant decrease in the total number of days hospitalized for cardiovascular causes within the 60 days following randomization compared with those who did not receive the drug (P = .71). There was, however, a higher incidence of atrial arrhythmias (P = .004) and hypotension (P<.001) in the subjects who received IV milrinone compared with placebo.[4] The more recent analysis from the Acute Decompensated Heart Failure National Registry (ADHERE) also showed an increased mortality in subjects admitted for decompensated HF receiving IV milrinone when compared with receiving IV nitroglycerin (P<.005) or IV nesiritide (P<.005).[31] As with dobutamine, the totality of available evidence strongly suggests that milrinone increases the risk of mortality despite the resultant hemodynamic improvement. Although the mechanism of this deleterious effect is not entirely clear, elevated mortality risk in the absence of significant difference in hospitalizations compared with placebo may indicate that sudden cardiac death, perhaps due to lethal arrhythmias, may be a factor.

Enoximone

Enoximone is a highly specific PDE III inhibitor. Earlier studies have demonstrated an improvement in exercise capacity in subjects with HFrEF receiving low doses of oral enoximone,[32] although higher doses have been associated with an increase in mortality.[33] In the more recent Studies of Oral Enoximone Therapy in Advanced HF (ESSENTIAL) trial, subjects with chronic HFrEF and NYHA class III or IV symptoms were randomized to receive either oral enoximone in addition to optimal medical therapy or optimal medical therapy alone.[34] There was no difference in all-cause mortality (P = .73) or the combined endpoint of all-cause mortality or cardiovascular mortality (P = .71) in subjects who received enoximone compared with those who did not receive the therapy. Subgroup analyses suggested no difference in mortality outcomes in subjects older than 65 years. There was also no benefit in exercise capacity such as 6-minute walk test in the enoximone group, regardless of age. The lack of significant beneficial or adverse effect observed in the ESSENTIAL I and II trials may be an indication that the low dose, although shown to affect exercise capacity in subjects with less severe symptoms,[32] may not have been sufficient to produce effect in subjects with more severe disease.[34] Currently, enoximone is approved for IV use in several countries in Europe but not in the United States.

PHOSPHODIESTERASE INHIBITORS WITH CALCIUM SENSITIZATION

The inotropic actions of PDE inhibitors with calcium sensitization are believed to be primarily attributable to calcium sensitization.[35] These drugs stabilize the conformational change in troponin-C when it binds to calcium. They are more effective in systole when calcium is abundant and less effective in diastole; hence, they increase contractility but do not affect relaxation. The inotropic effects are attributable to PDE III inhibition at higher concentrations. Because these drugs increase contractility without increasing calcium concentration, their arrhythmogenic potential is low. Activation of adenosine triphosphate (ATP)-sensitive potassium channels results in a potent vasodilator effect, simultaneously increasing coronary blood flow.

Pimobendan

Pimobendan has a weak calcium sensitization action and its major inotropic activity is attributable to PDE III inhibition. The drug was evaluated in several trials, including the Pimobendan in Congestive Heart Failure (PICO) trial, which showed an improvement in exercise tolerance in subjects receiving pimobendan at doses of 2.5 mg and 5 mg per day ($P = .03$ and $P = .05$, respectively) but a trend toward increased all-cause mortality.[36] Although the Effects of Pimobendan on Chronic Heart Failure (EPOCH) Study assessing long-term outcomes in subjects with NYHA class II and III symptoms revealed a lower risk of adverse cardiac events with pimobendan (15.9%) compared with placebo (26.3%) over 52 weeks of follow-up ($P = .035$) with no significant difference in death and hospitalization for cardiac causes ($P = .202$).[37] Notably, randomized subjects in the pimobendan group were younger (mean age, 62.0 years vs 65.8 years in the placebo group).[37] The use of pimobendan has only been approved in Japan.[38]

Levosimendan

Levosimendan has been evaluated in 2 large-scale randomized control trials: Randomized Multicenter Evaluation of Intravenous Levosimendan Efficacy versus Placebo in the Short-term Treatment of Acute Heart Failure (REVIVE) I and II and Survival of Subjects with Acute Heart Failure in Need of Intravenous Inotropic Support (SURVIVE).[9,12] In the sequential REVIVE I and II trials, use of levosimendan in subjects with acute decompensated HF was associated with rapid symptomatic relief and a lower likelihood of clinical worsening ($P = .015$).[12] However, subjects receiving levosimendan experienced higher adverse cardiovascular risks such as hypotension and cardiac arrhythmias across both trials ($P<.05$) and had a non-statistically significant elevation in all-cause mortality ($P = .29$) across both studies. In the SURVIVE trial, there was no significant difference in long-term outcome between dobutamine and levosimendan during 180 days following randomization.[9] Although it is approved for IV use in several countries in Europe, levosimendan is currently not approved for use in the United States.

CARDIAC GLYCOSIDES

Digoxin

Although often considered separately from other drugs with positive inotropic effects, digoxin, a cardiac glycoside, works by inhibiting sodium-potassium (Na^+/K^+)-ATPase. The subsequent rise in concentration of intracellular calcium (Ca^{++}) results in increased myocardial contractility. Although cardiac glycosides have a long history of use dating back to the 1785 publication by William Withering,[39] rigorous studies demonstrating the deleterious effects of digoxin withdrawal in subjects with HF provided the impetus for further investigation on a larger scale.[7,8]

The landmark Digitalis Investigation Group (DIG) study was a randomized, double-blind, controlled trial conducted to evaluate the effect of digoxin in subjects with HFrEF on all-cause mortality.[5] The main study randomized 6800 participants with ejection fraction less than 45% to digoxin 0.25 mg per day or placebo.[5] Although digoxin had no effect on mortality (34.8% vs 35.1% for digoxin vs placebo, respectively; $P = .81$), it did reduce hospitalization attributable to HFrEF (26.8% vs 34.7% for digoxin vs placebo, respectively; $P<.001$).[5] Digoxin at low (0.5–0.9 ng/mL) and high ($\geq$1 ng/mL) serum concentrations has been shown to be associated with lower risk of HF hospitalization.[40] This benefit of digoxin has also been observed among patients 65 years and older.[41] A recent analysis of the DIG data has suggested that digoxin at serum concentrations 0.5 to 0.7 ng/mL is also associated with reduced death from worsening HF.[42] Another analysis of the DIG data suggested that the use of digoxin is associated with a higher risk of death in women.[43] Although the association of digoxin at low serum digoxin concentration on mortality was not examined in that study, digoxin should be used in low doses in older women with HFrEF who are symptomatic despite other evidence-based therapy.[44]

SUMMARY

Most studies of inotropic drugs have been conducted in subjects with a mean age of 65 years. Although few reported subgroup analyses for subjects 65 years and older, evidence based on these studies may be extrapolated to use in older subjects with the general geriatric principle: start low, go slow. Except for digoxin, the use of positive inotropes has been shown to be associated with higher risk of death and should not be used on a long-term basis. See later discussion of special situations in which it may be reasonable to consider short-term use of positive inotropes in older patients with HFrEF.[3] IV positive inotropic drugs should not be used in patients with HFrEF without these specific indications (class III recommendation based on level of evidence B).[3]

INPATIENT SETTINGS

Cardiogenic Shock

Therapy with short-term IV positive inotropes may be considered to maintain systemic perfusion until acute precipitating causes are resolved or a more definitive therapy may be considered, such as coronary revascularization, mechanical circulatory support, or heart transplantation (class I recommendation based on level of evidence C).[3]

Therapy with short-term IV positive inotropes may be considered in patients with low blood pressure and hypoperfusion (class IIb recommendation based on level of evidence B).[3]

OUTPATIENT SETTING

Stage D Refractory Heart Failure

Therapy with short-term IV positive inotropes may be considered as bridge therapy when patients are refractory to other evidence-based therapy and are waiting for mechanical circulatory support or heart transplantation (class IIa recommendation based on level of evidence B).[3]

Palliative Care

Therapy with long-term IV positive inotropes may be considered for patients with endstage HF enrolled into palliative and hospice care who are symptomatic despite other evidence-based therapy and are not candidates for mechanical circulatory support or heart transplantation (class IIb recommendation based on level of evidence C).[3]

REFERENCES

1. Mozaffarian D, Benjamin EJ, Go AS, et al. Heart disease and stroke statistics-2016 update: a report from the American Heart Association. Circulation 2016;133:e38–360.
2. Carson P, Anand I, O'Connor C, et al. Mode of death in advanced heart failure: the comparison of medical, pacing, and defibrillation therapies in heart failure (COMPANION) trial. J Am Coll Cardiol 2005;46:2329–34.
3. Yancy CW, Jessup M, Bozkurt B, et al. 2013 ACCF/AHA guideline for the management of heart failure: a report of the American College of Cardiology Foundation/American Heart Association Task Force on Practice Guidelines. J Am Coll Cardiol 2013;62:e147–239.
4. Cuffe MS, Califf RM, Adams KF Jr, et al. Short-term intravenous milrinone for acute exacerbation of chronic heart failure: a randomized controlled trial. JAMA 2002;287:1541–7.
5. DIG Investigators. The effect of digoxin on mortality and morbidity in patients with heart failure. N Engl J Med 1997;336:525–33.
6. Packer M, Carver JR, Rodeheffer RJ, et al. Effect of oral milrinone on mortality in severe chronic heart failure. The PROMISE Study Research Group. N Engl J Med 1991;325:1468–75.
7. Uretsky BF, Young JB, Shahidi FE, et al. Randomized study assessing the effect of digoxin withdrawal in patients with mild to moderate chronic congestive heart failure: results of the PROVED trial. PROVED investigative group. J Am Coll Cardiol 1993;22:955–62.
8. Packer M, Gheorghiade M, Young JB, et al. Withdrawal of digoxin from patients with chronic heart failure treated with angiotensin-converting-enzyme inhibitors. RADIANCE Study. N Engl J Med 1993;329:1–7.
9. Mebazaa A, Nieminen MS, Packer M, et al. Levosimendan vs dobutamine for patients with acute decompensated heart failure: the SURVIVE Randomized Trial. JAMA 2007;297:1883–91.
10. Oliva F, Gronda E, Frigerio M, et al. Outpatient intermittent dobutamine therapy in congestive heart failure. Z Kardiol 1999;88:S028–32.
11. Oliva F, Latini R, Politi A, et al. Intermittent 6-month low-dose dobutamine infusion in severe heart failure: DICE multicenter trial. Am Heart J 1999;138:247–53.
12. Packer M, Colucci W, Fisher L, et al. Effect of levosimendan on the short-term clinical course of patients with acutely decompensated heart failure. JACC Heart Fail 2013;1:103–11.

13. O'Connor CM, Gattis WA, Uretsky BF, et al. Continuous intravenous dobutamine is associated with an increased risk of death in patients with advanced heart failure: insights from the Flolan International randomized survival trial (FIRST). Am Heart J 1999;138:78–86.
14. Levine TB, Levine AB, Elliott WG, et al. Dobutamine as bridge to angiotensin-converting enzyme inhibitor-nitrate therapy in endstage heart failure. Clin Cardiol 2001;24:231–6.
15. Applefeld MM, Newman KA, Sutton FJ, et al. Outpatient dobutamine and dopamine infusions in the management of chronic heart failure: clinical experience in 21 patients. Am Heart J 1987;114:589–95.
16. Krell MJ, Kline EM, Bates ER, et al. Intermittent, ambulatory dobutamine infusions in patients with severe congestive heart failure. Am Heart J 1986;112:787–91.
17. López-Candales A, Vora T, Gibbons W, et al. Symptomatic improvement in patients treated with intermittent infusion of inotropes: a double-blind placebo controled pilot study. J Med 2002;33:129–46.
18. Roffman DS, Applefeld MM, Grove WR, et al. Intermittent dobutamine hydrochloride infusions in outpatients with chronic congestive heart failure. Clin Pharm 1985;4:195–9.
19. Van den Brande P, Van Mieghem W, Demedts M. Intermittent dobutamine infusion in severe chronic heart failure in elderly patients. Gerontology 1990;36:49–54.
20. Dies F, Krell MJ, Whitlow P. Intermittent dobutamine in ambulatory outpatients with chronic cardiac failure (abstract). Circulation 1986;74:38.
21. Bertorello AM, Sznajder JI. The dopamine paradox in lung and kidney epithelia: sharing the same target but operating different signaling networks. Am J Respir Cell Mol Biol 2005;33:432–7.
22. De Backer D, Biston P, Devriendt J, et al. Comparison of dopamine and norepinephrine in the treatment of shock. N Engl J Med 2010;362:779–89.
23. Loeb HS, Winslow EB, Rahimtoola SH, et al. Acute hemodynamic effects of dopamine in patients with shock. Circulation 1971;44:163–73.
24. Marik PE, Iglesias J. Low-dose dopamine does not prevent acute renal failure in patients with septic shock and oliguria. NORASEPT II study investigators. Am J Med 1999;107:387–90.
25. Miller RR, Awan NA, Joye JA, et al. Combined dopamine and nitroprusside therapy in congestive heart failure. Greater augmentation of cardiac performance by addition of inotropic stimulation to afterload reduction. Circulation 1977;55:881–4.
26. Rajfer SI, Anton AH, Rossen JD, et al. Beneficial hemodynamic effects of oral levodopa in heart failure. Relation to the generation of dopamine. N Engl J Med 1984;310:1357–62.
27. van de Borne P, Oren R, Somers VK. Dopamine depresses minute ventilation in patients with heart failure. Circulation 1998;98:126–31.
28. Elkayam U, Ng TM, Hatamizadeh P, et al. Renal vasodilatory action of dopamine in patients with heart failure: magnitude of effect and site of action. Circulation 2008;117:200–5.
29. Giamouzis G, Butler J, Starling RC, et al. Impact of dopamine infusion on renal function in hospitalized heart failure patients: results of the Dopamine in acute decompensated heart failure (DAD-HF) trial. J Card Fail 2010;16:922–30.
30. Chen HH, Anstrom KJ, Givertz MM, et al. Low-dose dopamine or low-dose nesiritide in acute heart failure with renal dysfunction: the ROSE acute heart failure randomized trial. JAMA 2013;310:2533–43.
31. Abraham WT, Adams KF, Fonarow GC, et al. In-hospital mortality in patients with acute decompensated heart failure requiring intravenous vasoactive medications: an analysis from the Acute Decompensated Heart Failure National Registry (ADHERE). J Am Coll Cardiol 2005;46:57–64.
32. Lowes BD, Higginbotham M, Petrovich L, et al. Low-dose enoximone improves exercise capacity in chronic heart failure. Enoximone Study Group. J Am Coll Cardiol 2000;36:501–8.
33. Uretsky BF, Jessup M, Konstam MA, et al. Multicenter trial of oral enoximone in patients with moderate to moderately severe congestive heart failure. Lack of benefit compared with placebo. Enoximone Multicenter Trial Group. Circulation 1990;82:774–80.
34. Metra M, Eichhorn E, Abraham WT, et al. Effects of low-dose oral enoximone administration on mortality, morbidity, and exercise capacity in patients with advanced heart failure: the randomized, double-blind, placebo-controlled, parallel group ESSENTIAL trials. Eur Heart J 2009;30:3015–26.
35. Sorsa T, Pollesello P, Permi P, et al. Interaction of levosimendan with cardiac troponin C in the presence of cardiac troponin I peptides. J Mol Cell Cardiol 2003;35:1055–61.
36. Lubsen J, Just H, Hjalmarsson AC, et al. Effect of pimobendan on exercise capacity in patients with heart failure: main results from the Pimobendan in Congestive Heart Failure (PICO) trial. Heart 1996;76:223–31.
37. EPOCH Study Investigators. Effects of pimobendan on adverse cardiac events and physical activities in patients with mild to moderate chronic heart failure: the effects of pimobendan on chronic heart failure study (EPOCH study). Circ J 2002;66:149–57.
38. Kass DA, Solaro RJ. Mechanisms and use of calcium-sensitizing agents in the failing heart. Circulation 2006;113:305–15.
39. Withering W. An account of the foxglove and some of its medical uses. Birmingham (England): M. Swinney; 1785.
40. Ahmed A, Rich MW, Love TE, et al. Digoxin and reduction in mortality and hospitalization in heart

failure: a comprehensive post hoc analysis of the DIG trial. Eur Heart J 2006;27:178–86.
41. Ahmed A. Digoxin and reduction in mortality and hospitalization in geriatric heart failure: importance of low doses and low serum concentrations. J Gerontol A Biol Sci Med Sci 2007;62: 323–9.
42. Adams KF Jr, Butler J, Patterson JH, et al. Dose response characterization of the association of serum digoxin concentration with mortality outcomes in the Digitalis Investigation Group trial. Eur J Heart Fail 2016;18:1072–81.
43. Rathore SS, Wang Y, Krumholz HM. Sex-based differences in the effect of digoxin for the treatment of heart failure. N Engl J Med 2002;347:1403–11.
44. Ahmed A, Aban IB, Weaver MT, et al. Serum digoxin concentration and outcomes in women with heart failure: a bi-directional effect and a possible effect modification by ejection fraction. Eur J Heart Fail 2006;8:409–19.

Interventional Therapies for Heart Failure in Older Adults

Dhaval Kolte, MD, PhD[a], Jinnette Dawn Abbott, MD[a], Herbert D. Aronow, MD, MPH[b,*]

KEYWORDS

• Heart failure • Elderly • Percutaneous coronary intervention • Mechanical circulatory support • Transcatheter aortic valve replacement • MitraClip • Transcatheter valve therapies • Implantable hemodynamic monitors

KEY POINTS

- Several transcatheter and interventional therapies have evolved over the past decade for the treatment of heart failure (HF) in older adults.
- Percutaneous coronary intervention with newer drug-eluting stents, percutaneous mechanical circulatory support devices, transcatheter aortic valve replacement, and percutaneous mitral valve repair with MitraClip have emerged as safe and effective alternatives to surgery in older patients with HF.
- Careful selection of the appropriate patient population, including the elderly, and end points in future clinical trials will be crucial to show the potential efficacy of novel interventional HF therapies.

INTRODUCTION

Heart failure (HF) remains a global epidemic with an estimated prevalence of 40 million individuals worldwide.[1] In the United States, approximately 5.7 million people have HF, with an incidence of 870,000 new cases per year.[2] Epidemiologic data suggest that HF increasingly represents a disease of the elderly. The prevalence of HF is less than 1% in individuals less than 40 years of age and is greater than 10% in those greater than 80 years of age.[3] HF is the leading cause of hospitalization in patients more than 65 years of age, and more than half of patients hospitalized for HF are more than 75 years of age. Despite advances in guideline-directed medical therapy (GDMT), 5-year survival for HF is approximately 50%, and advanced age remains a strong predictor of poor outcomes.[3] The use of GDMT in the elderly is often complicated by the presence of comorbid conditions (eg, renal dysfunction) and polypharmacy, which increase the risk of drug-related adverse effects. Older adults with HF are often considered poor candidates for surgical therapies, such as coronary artery bypass grafting (CABG), valve replacement, or heart transplant, because of multiple comorbidities and frailty, and this has led to an unmet need for novel therapeutic approaches for the treatment of HF, particularly in older adults. As a result, several transcatheter and interventional HF therapies have evolved over the past decade as alternatives to surgery in the elderly. This article summarizes data on interventional HF therapies that are currently approved or under investigation.

Disclosures: None.
This is an updated version of an article that appeared in *Heart Failure Clinics*, Volume 3, Issue 4.
[a] Division of Cardiovascular Medicine, Brown University, 593 Eddy Street, Providence, RI 02903, USA; [b] Division of Cardiovascular Medicine, The Warren Alpert Medical School of Brown University, 593 Eddy Street, RIH APC 730, Providence, RI 02903, USA
* Corresponding author.
E-mail address: herbert.aronow@lifespan.org

Heart Failure Clin 13 (2017) 535–570
http://dx.doi.org/10.1016/j.hfc.2017.02.009
1551-7136/17/

INTERVENTIONAL THERAPIES FOR HEART FAILURE

Revascularization for Ischemic Cardiomyopathy

Coronary artery disease (CAD) is the most common cause of left ventricular dysfunction (LVD) and the underlying cause of HF with reduced ejection fraction (HFrEF) in 65% of patients.[4] In patients undergoing percutaneous coronary intervention (PCI) for a spectrum of indications, worsening LVD is an independent predictor of short-term and long-term mortality across all ages.[5,6] Nonetheless, revascularization has the potential to improve symptoms and also survival in this high-risk population. Recent data from the Surgical Treatment for Ischemic Heart Failure Extension Study (STICHES) showed that, at 10 years, the rates of all-cause death, cardiovascular death, and all-cause death or cardiovascular hospitalization were significantly lower with CABG plus medical therapy compared with medical therapy alone.[7] For a detailed discussion, see Sahil Khera and Julio A. Panza's article, "Surgical Revascularization in the Older Adult with Ischemic Cardiomyopathy," in this issue. This article reviews the current data and recommendations on PCI and the potential role of hybrid coronary revascularization (HCR) in patients with HF caused by ischemic cardiomyopathy.

Percutaneous coronary intervention

In contrast with CABG, data on PCI in patients with ischemic cardiomyopathy are scarce and the benefits less clear. In the past, most randomized controlled trials (RCTs) comparing PCI with medical therapy alone or with CABG have excluded patients with HFrEF. Three trials that included patients with left ventricle (LV) systolic dysfunction were BARI (Bypass Angioplasty Revascularization Investigation), AWESOME (Angina With Extremely Serious Operative Mortality Evaluation), and HEART (The Heart Failure Revascularisation Trial) (**Table 1**).[8–10] These studies showed no difference in long-term survival with PCI versus CABG. However, combined, these trials involve fewer than 500 patients with LV systolic dysfunction and include percutaneous transluminal coronary angioplasty or PCI with bare metal stents. The more contemporary trials comparing PCI versus CABG are also limited by the small number of patients with LV systolic dysfunction. Only 2% of patients enrolled in the SYNTAX (Synergy Between Percutaneous Coronary Intervention with Taxus and Cardiac Surgery) trial had left ventricular ejection fraction (LVEF) less than 30%.[11] The FREEDOM (Future Revascularization Evaluation in Patients with Diabetes Mellitus: Optimal Management of Multivessel Disease) trial reported similar outcomes with PCI with drug-eluting stents and CABG in patients with LVEF less than 40%, but only 32 patients (2.5%) were in this prespecified subgroup.[12]

In a systematic review and meta-analysis of 19 observational studies that included 4766 patients with LVEF less than or equal to 40%, among the 2981 who underwent PCI (mean age, 65 years; 95% confidence interval [CI], 62–68), in-hospital mortality was 1.8% (95% CI, 1.0%–2.9%) and 2-year mortality was 15.6% (95% CI, 11.0%–20.7%). Five studies compared PCI versus CABG and showed no difference in long-term mortality (relative risk, 0.98; 95% CI, 0.8–1.2; $P = .83$).[13] Recently, Bangalore and colleagues[14] compared outcomes of PCI with everolimus-eluting stents (EES) versus CABG in a propensity-matched cohort of 2126 patients with multivessel CAD and LVEF less than or equal to 35% included in the New York State PCI Reporting System and the Cardiac Surgery Reporting System registries (see **Table 1**). At a median follow-up of 2.9 years, PCI with EES had similar survival to CABG (hazard ratio [HR], 1.01; 95% CI, 0.81–1.28; $P = .91$) (**Fig. 1**). PCI was associated with a higher risk of myocardial infarction (in patients with incomplete revascularization) and repeat revascularization, and a lower risk of stroke compared with CABG. Although propensity analysis cannot be a substitute for RCT, this study represents the most contemporary evidence, suggesting that PCI with newer-generation drug-eluting stents may be an acceptable alternative to CABG in selected patients with LV dysfunction in whom complete revascularization is possible.

The 2014 European Society of Cardiology and the European Association of Cardio-Thoracic Surgery guidelines on myocardial revascularization give a class I recommendation for CABG and a class IIb recommendation for PCI in patients with chronic HF and LVEF less than or equal to 35%.[15] However, the American College of Cardiology Foundation (ACCF)/American Heart Association (AHA) stable ischemic heart disease guidelines give a class IIb recommendation for CABG for improving survival in patients with severe LV systolic dysfunction (LVEF <35%) with no recommendations for PCI.[16] The ACCF/AHA guideline state that, "the choice of revascularization in patients with CAD and LV systolic dysfunction is best based on clinical variables (eg, coronary anatomy, presence of diabetes mellitus, presence of CKD), magnitude of LV systolic dysfunction, patient preferences, clinical judgment, and consultation between the interventional cardiologist and the cardiac surgeon."[16]

Table 1
Selected studies comparing percutaneous coronary intervention versus coronary artery bypass grafting in patients with ischemic cardiomyopathy

	Study Design	Definition of Systolic LVD	Intervention	n	No of Older Adults	Follow-up (y)	Outcomes	Rates (%)
BARI	Substudy of RCT	LVEF <50%	PTCA vs CABG	131 vs 117	70 vs 72 (age >65 y)	7	Survival	72.5 vs 73.5
AWESOME	Substudy of RCT	LVEF <35%	PCI with BMS vs CABG	40 vs 54	25 (age >70 y)	3	Survival	69 vs 72
HEART	RCT[a]	LVEF ≤35%	PTCA vs CABG	15 vs 30	Median (IQR) age 65 y (58–70 y)	5	Survival	73 vs 70
FREEDOM	Prespecified subgroup analysis of RCT	LVEF <40%	PCI with SES/PES vs CABG	21 vs 11	—	5	MACE (all-cause death, nonfatal MI, nonfatal stroke)	62 vs 31 (*P* = NS)
NYS PCI and Cardiac Surgery Reporting System	Propensity analysis of observational data	LVEF ≤35%	PCI with EES vs CABG	1063 vs 1063	433 vs 412 (age >70 y)	4	Death MI Stroke Revascularization	25.2 vs 21.0 (*P* = .91) 11.3 vs 5.6 (*P* = .0003) 3.9 vs 5.9 (*P* = .04) 22.3 vs 11.5 (*P*<.0001)

Abbreviations: BMS, bare metal stent; EES, everolimus-eluting stent; FREEDOM, Future Revascularization Evaluation in Patients With Diabetes Mellitus: Optimal Management of Multivessel Disease; IQR, interquartile range; LVEF, left ventricular ejection fraction; MACE, major adverse cardiovascular events; MI, myocardial infarction; NS, nonsignificant; NYS, new york state; PES, paclitaxel-eluting stent; PTCA, percutaneous transluminal coronary angioplasty; SES, sirolimus-eluting stent.

[a] Terminated prematurely because of withdrawal of funding caused by slow recruitment.

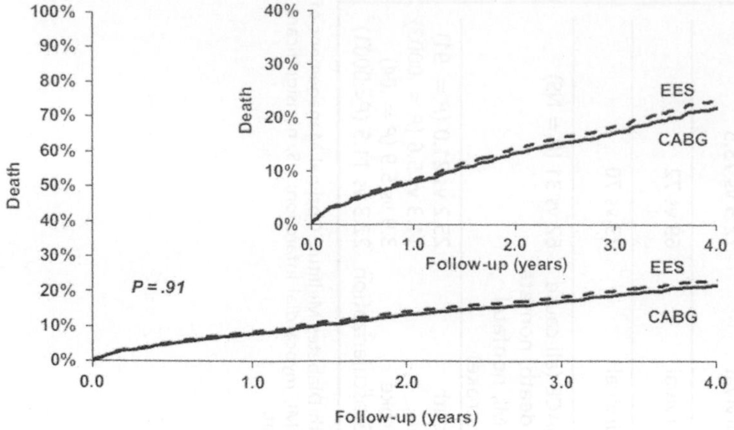

Fig. 1. All-cause mortality with PCI versus CABG in patients with ischemic cardiomyopathy. In a propensity-matched cohort of 2126 patients with multivessel CAD and LVEF less than or equal to 35%, PCI with EES had similar survival compared with CABG (HR, 1.01; 95% CI, 0.81–1.28; *P* = .91). (*From* Bangalore S, Guo Y, Samadashvili Z, et al. Revascularization in patients with multivessel coronary artery disease and severe left ventricular systolic dysfunction: everolimus-eluting stents versus coronary artery bypass graft surgery. Circulation 2016;133:2135; with permission.)

Hybrid coronary revascularization

Combining the off-pump minimally invasive direct coronary artery bypass technique for left internal mammary artery to left anterior descending (LAD) coronary artery graft with PCI of the non-LAD coronary arteries has emerged as an attractive option in patients with significant left main and/or multivessel CAD. Several observational studies, a meta-analysis of 6 observational studies, and a small pilot RCT have all shown similar short-term and long-term outcomes with HCR versus CABG, even in patients 65 years of age and older.[17–21] However, the proportion of patients with HF in these studies was small, with most patients having preserved LVEF. Recently, data from a multicenter observational study showed that, in 298 patients with multivessel CAD (mean age, 64.2 ± 11.5 years; and mean SYNTAX score, 19.7 ± 9.6), rates of major adverse cardiac and cerebrovascular events (MACCE) were similar between HCR and multivessel PCI at 12 months and during a median 17.6 months' follow-up.[22] However, patients with LVEF less than 30% were excluded in this study. Thus, further studies are needed to determine the role of HCR, especially in older adults with LV systolic dysfunction.

Percutaneous Mechanical Circulatory Support

High-risk percutaneous coronary intervention

PCI in older adults is often considered high risk because of the presence of more severe and complex CAD, including multivessel and left main disease, as well as severe LVD, compared with younger adults. The availability of percutaneous mechanical circulatory support (MCS) devices such as intra-aortic balloon pump (IABP), Impella (Abiomed, Danvers, MA), and TandemHeart (CardiacAssist, Inc, Pittsburgh, PA) has enabled interventionalists to perform complex, high-risk PCI in this group of patients with acceptable outcomes. The BCIS-1 (Balloon Pump–Assisted Coronary Intervention Study) trial showed no difference in rates of MACCE at discharge with or without elective insertion of IABP before high-risk PCI (LVEF <30% and BCIS-1 Jeopardy score ≥8) in 301 patients (mean age, 71 ± 9 years).[23] However, at a median follow-up of 51 months, elective IABP use was associated with a 34% relative reduction in all-cause mortality compared with unsupported PCI.[24] Similarly, in the PROTECT II (Prospective Randomized Clinical Trial of Hemodynamic Support with the Impella 2.5 vs Intra-Aortic Balloon Pump in Patients Undergoing High-Risk Percutaneous Coronary Intervention) trial, 30-day incidence of major adverse events (MAE) was similar with Impella 2.5 versus IABP support in nonemergent high-risk PCI (unprotected left main or last patent coronary vessel with LVEF ≤35%, or 3-vessel disease with LVEF ≤30%). However, there was a strong trend for improved outcomes at 90 days in the Impella-supported patients.[25] A post hoc analysis of PROTECT II showed similar rates of MAE and MACCE in patients greater than or equal to 80 years of age versus less than 80 years of age.[26] Impella 2.5 was independently associated with lower 90-day MAE rates (adjusted odds ratio, 0.60; 95% CI, 0.39–0.92; *P* = .02) irrespective of age ($p_{interaction}$ = 0.188). The SHIELD II (Coronary Interventions in High-Risk Patients Using a Novel Percutaneous Left Ventricular Support Device) US Investigational Device Exemption Clinical Trial is an ongoing prospective, randomized, multicenter, open-label study comparing a novel percutaneous ventricular assist device (pVAD), the HeartMate PHP (Thoratec Corp, Burlington, MA), with Impella 2.5 in patients aged 18 to 100 years undergoing high-risk PCI.[27]

Cardiogenic shock
The incidence of cardiogenic shock (CS) complicating acute myocardial infarction (AMI) in older adults is approximately 9.4%.[28] Older patients with CS are less likely to undergo early revascularization, and have a 2-fold higher in-hospital mortality, compared with younger adults.[28] Several studies have shown improved hemodynamics with the use of percutaneous MCS in patients with CS. However, this has not translated into improvement in outcomes in RCTs. The IABP-SHOCK II (Intraaortic Balloon Pump in Cardiogenic Shock II) trial showed no improvement in 30-day or 1-year mortality with IABP use in patients undergoing early revascularization for AMI complicated by CS.[29,30] Similar results were seen in patients more than 75 years of age in the prespecified subgroup analysis. Similarly, in an RCT comparing TandemHeart versus IABP in patients with AMI and CS, hemodynamic and metabolic parameters were reversed more effectively with TandemHeart; however, there was no difference in 30-day mortality.[31] The ISAR-SHOCK (Impella LP2.5 vs IABP in Cardiogenic SHOCK) trial showed that, in patients with AMI and CS (median age, 65 years), the use of pVAD was feasible and safe, and provided superior hemodynamic support compared with IABP. Overall 30-day mortality was 46% in both groups.[32] Recently, the IMPRESS in Severe Shock (Impella vs IABP reduces mortality in STEMI [ST-elevation myocardial infarction] patients treated with primary PCI in severe cardiogenic shock) trial compared Impella CP versus IABP in mechanically ventilated patients with CS (mean age, 58 years) after AMI. Thirty-day and 6-month mortalities were similar in both the groups.[33] The ISAR-SHOCK and IMPRESS are limited by the small number of patients as well as the fact that almost all patients enrolled in these studies received MCS therapy after revascularization. Data from 154 patients with CS included in the USpella registry showed that the use of Impella 2.5 pre-PCI was associated with significantly lower in-hospital and 30-day mortalities compared with Impella post-PCI.[34] However, in subgroup analysis, there was no difference in in-hospital mortality in patients 75 years of age or older (n = 34), which may be because of the small number of older patients. Larger, well-designed RCTs are therefore needed to determine whether the use of pVAD before revascularization is associated with improved outcomes in patients with CS, including in the elderly.

Right ventricular failure
Severe right ventricular failure (RVF) may occur as a complication of acute inferior myocardial infarction (MI) or open heart surgery, including transplant or surgical LV assist device (LVAD) placement, and is associated with poor outcomes. The recently US Food and Drug Administration (FDA)–approved Impella RP is the only percutaneous MCS specifically designed for right ventricle (RV) support. The RECOVER RIGHT (The Use of Impella RP Support System in Patients With Right Heart Failure) was a prospective, open-label, single-arm, nonrandomized, multicenter study that examined the safety and efficacy of the Impella RP in patients with RVF after LVAD implantation (n = 18; age, 55.8 ± 13.9 years) or after cardiotomy or AMI (n = 12; age, 64.3 ± 16.2 years).[35] The Impella RP was safe, easy to deploy, and provided immediate and sustained hemodynamic benefits with favorable outcomes at 30 and 180 days. Survival to discharge was 73.3% and at 6 months was 70% in this study.[35]

Interventional Therapies for Heart Failure Secondary to Valvular Heart Disease and Septal Defects

The prevalence of valvular heart disease (VHD) in the United States is estimated to be 2.5%.[2] The primary causes of VHD in the United States and Europe are age-associated calcific valve changes and inherited or congenital conditions such as bicuspid aortic valve or myxomatous mitral valve (V) disease. LVD and HF are common manifestations of VHD and portend a poor prognosis. The development of newer transcatheter techniques for the treatment of valve dysfunction along with the heart-team approach have revolutionized the management of patients with VHD and HF.

Transcatheter aortic valve replacement
Aortic stenosis (AS) is characterized by a long latent period during which patients remain asymptomatic. However, once even mild symptoms develop, progression is rapid, with an average survival of 2 years in patients with HF, 3 years in those with syncope, and 5 years in those with angina.[36] Surgical aortic valve replacement (SAVR) reduces symptoms and improves survival in patients with severe symptomatic AS, and, in the absence of serious coexisting conditions, is associated with low operative mortality. However, approximately 30% of patients with severe symptomatic AS do not undergo SAVR, owing to advanced age, LVD, or the presence of multiple comorbidities.[37]

Since 2002, when the first procedure was performed by Cribier and colleagues,[38] transcatheter aortic valve replacement (TAVR) has rapidly emerged as a safe and effective alternative to SAVR, not only in patients who are considered inoperable but also in those at high or intermediate risk for surgery. **Tables 2** and **3** summarize the landmark clinical trials and registry studies comparing TAVR versus standard therapy or SAVR.[39–60] Prespecified subgroup analyses of the PARTNER (Placement of Aortic Transcatheter Valves) trials have shown that TAVR may be safe and effective even in patients 85 years of age and older. The 2 devices currently approved in the United States are the balloon-expandable SAPIEN prosthesis (Edwards Lifesciences, Irvine, CA) and the self-expandable CoreValve revalving prosthesis (Medtronic, Inc, Minneapolis, MN), with several others being evaluated in clinical trials (**Fig. 2**).

Transcatheter mitral valve repair

Mitral regurgitation (MR) is a common comorbidity in HF, affecting greater than 50% of patients with LVEF less than 40%, and it is associated with high mortality and poor clinical outcomes.[61] MV surgery is recommended in patients with severe symptomatic MR. However, many patients with severe MR are at high surgical risk because of advanced age, LVD, or comorbidities. Recent data suggest that 53% of patients with functional or degenerative MR do not undergo surgery, and, among the unoperated patients, prognosis is poor, with a 5-year mortality of 50%, and high rate of HF hospitalization.[62]

Percutaneous MV repair based on the surgical Alfieri stitch technique has been developed using the MitraClip device (Abbott, Menlo Park, CA). The MitraClip device is a 4-mm-wide cobalt chromium and covered-polyester implant with 2 arms that are opened and closed by control mechanisms on the clip delivery system (**Fig. 3**). The clip may be repositioned or removed, and additional devices can be implanted to achieve adequate MR reduction, defined as less than or equal to 2+ as measured by echocardiography. **Tables 4** and **5** summarize data from nonrandomized studies and RCTs of MitraClip, respectively.[63–80] The Endovascular Valve Edge-to-Edge repair Study (EVEREST) II trial showed comparable outcomes with MitraClip vs surgical MV repair at 5 years, particularly in older patients (≥70 years of age) with functional MR and LVEF less than 60%.[79] Four ongoing RCTs will provide data on the efficacy of this treatment strategy for reducing HF hospitalizations and mortality compared with optimal medical therapy alone.[81–84]

Percutaneous mitral annuloplasty

Several percutaneous devices have been developed in the last decade as an alternative to surgical annuloplasty in high-risk patients with functional MR (**Fig. 4**). These devices are based on 1 of 2 approaches: indirect annuloplasty, which takes advantage of the proximity of the coronary sinus to the posterior and lateral mitral annulus, and direct annuloplasty, which more closely reproduces surgical annuloplasty by cinching the mitral annulus with sutures, anchors, or similar devices (**Table 6**).[85–96]

Transcatheter mitral valve replacement

The complex anatomy of the MV explains why the development of transcatheter mitral valve replacement (TMVR) devices has not been as rapid as that of TAVR. Nonetheless, there are at least 4 TMVR systems that have been tested in preclinical studies and the first-in-human data have been reported (**Fig. 5**).[97–100] The mean age of patients in these studies was greater than or equal to 60 years. However, subgroup analysis in older patients is not available.

Transcatheter tricuspid valve interventions

Untreated isolated severe tricuspid regurgitation (TR) is associated with increased mortality and morbidity, including RVF.[101] Although surgery is an effective treatment of the disease, less than 1% of eligible patients are treated annually in the United States, either because of the presence of multiple comorbidities or the high risks of reoperative surgery for severe TR that develops late after left-sided valve surgery.[102,103] Furthermore, recent data have shown that the presence of severe TR at baseline may adversely influence outcomes in patients undergoing TAVR and transcatheter MV repair. This finding has led to the development of various percutaneous approaches to the treatment of severe TR, which are currently being evaluated in clinical trials (**Table 7**).[102–109]

Percutaneous closure of atrial septal defect and paravalvular leak

Atrial septal defect (ASD) is the second most common congenital heart disease diagnosed in adult life. Secundum ASD is commonly associated with atrial fibrillation, HF, pulmonary hypertension, and paradoxic systemic embolism, and closure of hemodynamically significant defects is recommended irrespective of symptoms. Several studies have shown that, even in older adults, percutaneous ASD closure is safe and is associated with improvement in right ventricular size and hemodynamics, New York Heart Association (NYHA) functional class, and quality of life (QoL).[110–112] Moreover, long-term outcomes were similar in patients greater than or equal to 75 years of age compared with their younger

Table 2
Major clinical trials and registry studies of transcatheter aortic valve replacement in inoperable, high-risk, intermediate-risk, and low-risk patients

	Comparison	N	Major Exclusion Criteria	Age (y)	STS Score	Logistic EuroSCORE	Valve Used	Follow-up	Primary Outcome	Secondary Outcomes
Inoperable										
PARTNER 1B	TAVR vs standard therapy	179 vs 179	Bicuspid or noncalcified AV, MI within 30 d, CAD requiring revascularization, LVEF <20%, aortic annulus diameter <18 mm or >25 mm, preexisting prosthetic heart valve, >3+ MR or AI, TIA/stroke within 6 mo, ESRD or Cr >3 mg/dL, life expectancy <1 y, significant aortic disease	83.1 ± 8.6 vs 83.2 ± 8.3	11.2 ± 5.8 vs 12.1 ± 6.1	26.4 ± 17.2 vs 30.4 ± 19.1	SAPIEN	1, 2, 3 and 5 y	All-cause death; time to death from any cause of repeat hospitalization because of valve-related or procedure-related clinical deterioration	CV death, NYHA functional class, repeat hospitalization because of valve-related or procedure-related clinical deterioration, 6MWT distance, valve performance (assessed by echocardiography), MI, stroke, AKI, vascular complications, and bleeding
US CoreValve Extreme Risk Pivotal Trial	Nonrandomized (TAVR alone)	489	MI within 30 d, active GIB within 3 mo, major stroke within 6 mo, life expectancy <1 y, LVEF <20%, ESRD or CrCl <20 mL/min, bicuspid or unicuspid AV, aortic annular diameter <18 mm or >29 mm, preexisting prosthetic heart valve, >3+ MR or AI, 4+ TR, moderate to severe MS, dilated ascending aorta	83.2 ± 8.7	10.3 ± 5.5	22.6 ± 17.1	CoreValve	1, 2 y	All-cause death or major stroke	MACCE (all-cause death, MI, all stroke, AV reintervention), CV death, NYHA functional class, device success, procedure success, major or life-threatening bleeding, major vascular complications, AKI

(*continued on next page*)

Table 2
(continued)

	Comparison	N	Major Exclusion Criteria	Age (y)	STS Score	Logistic EuroSCORE	Valve Used	Follow-up	Primary Outcome	Secondary Outcomes
PARTNER 2B	SAPIEN vs SAPIEN XT	276 vs 284	Similar to PARTNER 1B	84.6 ± 8.6 vs 84.1 ± 8.7	11.0 ± 5.7 vs 10.3 ± 5.4	21.0 ± 17.0 vs 18.8 ± 14.6	SAPIEN or SAPIEN XT	1, 2 y	Composite of all-cause mortality, major stroke, or rehospitalization	CV death, rehospitalization, NYHA functional class, MI, stroke, AKI, vascular complications, bleeding, 6MWT distance, echocardiography-assessed valve performance, new PPM, AV reintervention
PARTNER 2 S3 Registry	Nonrandomized (TAVR alone)	199	Similar to PARTNER 2B	80.3 (55–100)	7.4 (4.6–10.4)	5.6 (3.2–10.6)	SAPIEN 3	1 y	Composite of death, all stroke, and AI	All-cause death, CV death, all stroke, major stroke, repeat hospitalization, >moderate AI, new PPM
High Risk										
PARTNER 1A	TAVR vs SAVR	348 vs 351	Similar to PARTNER 1B	83.6 ± 6.8 vs 84.5 ± 6.4	11.8 ± 3.3 vs 11.7 ± 3.5	29.3 ± 16.5 vs 29.2 ± 15.6	SAPIEN	1, 2, 5 y	All-cause death	Similar to PARTNER 1B
US CoreValve High-Risk Study	TAVR vs SAVR	390 vs 357	Similar to US CoreValve Extreme Risk Pivotal Trial	83.1 ± 7.1 vs 83.2 ± 6.4	7.3 ± 3.0 vs 7.5 ± 3.4	17.7 ± 13.1 vs 18.6 ± 13.0	CoreValve	1, 2 y	All-cause death	Similar to US CoreValve Extreme Risk Pivotal Trial
CoreValve Evolut R CE Mark Clinical Study	Nonrandomized (TAVR alone)	60	Similar to US CoreValve High-Risk Study	82.8 ± 6.1	7.0 ± 3.7	20.5 ± 12.5	CoreValve Evolut R	1 mo	All-cause death, any stroke, device success, ≤mild AI	Composite and individual components of VARC 2 safety end points; echocardiography-assessed valve performance
PARTNER 2 S3 Registry	Nonrandomized (TAVR alone)	384	Similar to PARTNER 2B, except aortic annulus diameter <16 mm or >28 mm	83.4 (46–98)	8.6 (7.5–9.9)	6.6 (4.1–11.0)	SAPIEN 3	1 y	Composite of death, all stroke, and AI	All-cause death, CV death, all stroke, major stroke, repeat hospitalization, >moderate AI, new PPM

REPRISE II	Nonrandomized (TAVR alone)	120	MI within 30 d, TIA/stroke within 3 mo, ESRD or Cr >3.0 mg/dL, unicuspid or bicuspid AV, ≥3+ AI or MR, LVEF <30%, unsuitable femoral anatomy	84.4 ± 5.3	7.1 ± 4.6	6.9 ± 5.8	LOTUS	1 y	Mean AV pressure gradient, all-cause mortality	VARC 2 safety end points, NYHA functional class
Intermediate Risk										
OBSERVANT Study (Propensity Analysis)	TAVR vs SAVR	133 vs 133	—	79.4 ± 7.4 vs 78.8 ± 6.9	—	8.8 ± 9.5 vs 9.4 ± 10.4	SAPIEN XT or CoreValve	1, 6 mo	All-cause death	In-hospital MACCE (stroke, vascular complications, MI, and red blood cell transfusion)
PARTNER 2A	TAVR vs SAVR	1011 vs 1021	Similar to PARTNER 2B, except aortic annulus diameter <18 mm or >27 mm	81.5 ± 6.7 vs 81.7 ± 6.7	5.8 ± 2.1 vs 5.8 ± 1.9	—	SAPIEN XT	1, 2 y	Composite of all-cause death or disabling stroke	Similar to PARTNER 2B
PARTNER 2 S3 (Propensity Analysis)	TAVR vs SAVR	1077 vs 944	Similar to PARTNER 2A	81.9 ± 6.6 vs 81.6 ± 6.8	5.2 (4.3–6.3) vs 5.4 (4.4–6.7)	—	SAPIEN 3	1 y	Composite of all-cause death, all strokes, >moderate AI)	Individual components of primary end point
Low Risk										
NOTION	TAVR vs SAVR	145 vs 135	Life expectancy <1 y, another severe valve disease, CAD requiring intervention, previous cardiac surgery, MI or stroke within 30 d, ESRD, FEV_1 or diffusion capacity <40% predicted	79.2 ± 4.9 vs 79.0 ± 4.7	2.9 ± 1.6 vs 3.1 ± 1.7	8.4 ± 4.0 vs 8.9 ± 5.5	CoreValve	1, 2 y	Composite of all-cause death, stroke, MI	Individual components of primary end point, CV death, prosthesis reintervention, CS, valve endocarditis, new PPM, atrial fibrillation or flutter, vascular, renal, and bleeding complications, NYHA functional class, echocardiography-assessed valve performance

(*continued on next page*)

Table 2
(continued)

	Comparison	N	Major Exclusion Criteria	Age (y)	STS Score	Logistic EuroSCORE	Valve Used	Follow-up	Primary Outcome	Secondary Outcomes
PARTNER 3[a]	TAVR vs SAVR	1228	Similar to PARTNER 2, except LVEF <45%, life expectancy <2 y, and ≥1 out of 4 on frailty scale	—	—	—	SAPIEN 3	1 y	Composite of all-cause death, all strokes, rehospitalization	Death or stroke, stroke, new atrial fibrillation, length of index hospitalization, death, KCCQ <45 or KCCQ decrease ≥10 points
US CoreValve low-risk study[a]	TAVR vs SAVR	1250	Similar to US CoreValve Extreme and High Risk, except life expectancy <2 y	—	—	—	CoreValve or CoreValve Evolut R	2 y	All-cause death or disabling stroke	Composite of death, disabling stroke, life-threatening bleed, major vascular complication, or AKI; new PPM, prosthetic valve endocarditis and thrombosis, all stroke, life-threatening bleed, valve reintervention, QoL (KCCQ), rehospitalization

Abbreviations: 6MWT, 6-minute walk test; AI, aortic insufficiency; AKI, acute kidney injury; AV, aortic valve; CAD, coronary artery disease; CE, Conformité Européene; Cr, creatinine; CrCl, creatinine clearance; CV, cardiovascular; ESRD, end-stage renal disease; FEV_1, forced expiratory volume in 1 second; GIB, gastrointestinal bleeding; KCCQ, Kansas City Cardiomyopathy Questionnaire; MACCE, major adverse cardiovascular and cerebrovascular events; MI, myocardial infarction; MR, mitral regurgitation; MS, mitral stenosis; NOTION, Nordic Aortic Valve Intervention; NYHA, New York Heart Association; PARTNER, Placement of Aortic Transcatheter Valves; PPM, permanent pacemaker; QoL, quality of life; SAVR, surgical aortic valve replacement; STS, Society of Thoracic Surgeons; TIA, transient ischemic attack; TR, tricuspid regurgitation; VARC, valve academic research consortium.

[a] Ongoing trials.

Table 3
Outcomes of transcatheter aortic valve replacement in clinical trials

	Follow-up	All-Cause Mortality (%)	CV Mortality (%)	Rehospitalization (%)	TIA/ Stroke (%)	AKI/Renal Failure (%)	Major Vascular Complications (%)	Major Bleeding (%)	New Atrial Fibrillation (%)	New PPM (%)	Paravalvular Regurgitation ≥ Moderate (%)
Inoperable											
PARTNER 1B	1 y	30.7	19.6	22.3	10.6	2.8	16.8	22.3	0.6	4.5	10.5
	2 y	43.3	31.0	35.0	13.8	4.3	NA	28.9	NA	6.4	10
	3 y	54.0	41.4	43.5	15.7	3.2	17.4	32.0	NA	7.6	4.5
	5 y	71.8	57.5	47.6	16.0	NA	NA	NA	NA	NA	NA
US CoreValve Extreme Risk Pivotal Trial	1 y	24.3	18.3	NA	8.1	11.8	8.4	28.5	NA	26.4	4.3
	2 y	36.6	26.2	NA	8.6	NA	8.4	21.1	NA	28.8	4.4
PARTNER 2B[a]	1 y	22.3	16.6	23.1	7.1	31.0	10.3	22.2	NA	8.1	27.5
PARTNER 2 S3 Registry	1 y	17.7	9.6	19.9	1.8	NA	NA	NA	NA	21.3	2.7
High Risk											
PARTNER 1A	1 y	24.2	14.3	18.2	8.3	5.4	11.3	14.7	12.1	5.7	6.8
	2 y	33.9	21.4	24.7	11.2	6.2	11.6	19.0	NA	7.2	6.9
	5 y	67.8	53.1	42.3	15.9	8.6	11.9	26.6	NA	9.7	NA
US CoreValve High-Risk Study	1 y	14.2	10.4	NA	10.4	6.0	6.2	29.5	15.9[b]	22.3	6.1
	2 y	22.2	15.4	NA	10.9	6.2	7.1	32.3	19.5	25.8	6.1
CoreValve Evolut R CE Mark Clinical Study	30 d	0	0	NA	0	1.7	8.3	NA	NA	11.7	3.3
PARTNER 2 S3 Registry	1 y	12.7	7.4	15.6	5.6	NA	NA	NA	NA	14.5	2.7
REPRISE II	1 y	10.9	6.7	NA	9.2	3.4	2.5	21.0	5.9	31.9	0
Intermediate Risk											
OBSERVANT Study (Propensity Analysis)	30 d	3.8	NA	NA	0	NA	5.3	NA	NA	12.0	6.1
PARTNER 2A	1 y	12.3	7.1	14.8	10.1	3.4	8.4	NA	10.1	9.9	0.5
	2 y	16.7	10.1	19.6	12.7	3.8	8.6	NA	11.3	11.8	1.3
PARTNER 2 S3 (Propensity Analysis)	1 y	7.4	4.5	11.4	6.4	NA	NA	NA	5.9	12.4	1.5
Low Risk											
NOTION	1 y	4.9	4.3	NA	5.0	NA	NA	NA	21.2[b]	38.0	15.7[c]
	2 y	8.0	6.5	—	9.7	—	—	—	22.7	41.3	15.4[c]

[a] Outcomes in the SAPIEN XT group.
[b] New or worsening atrial fibrillation.
[c] Total aortic regurgitation.

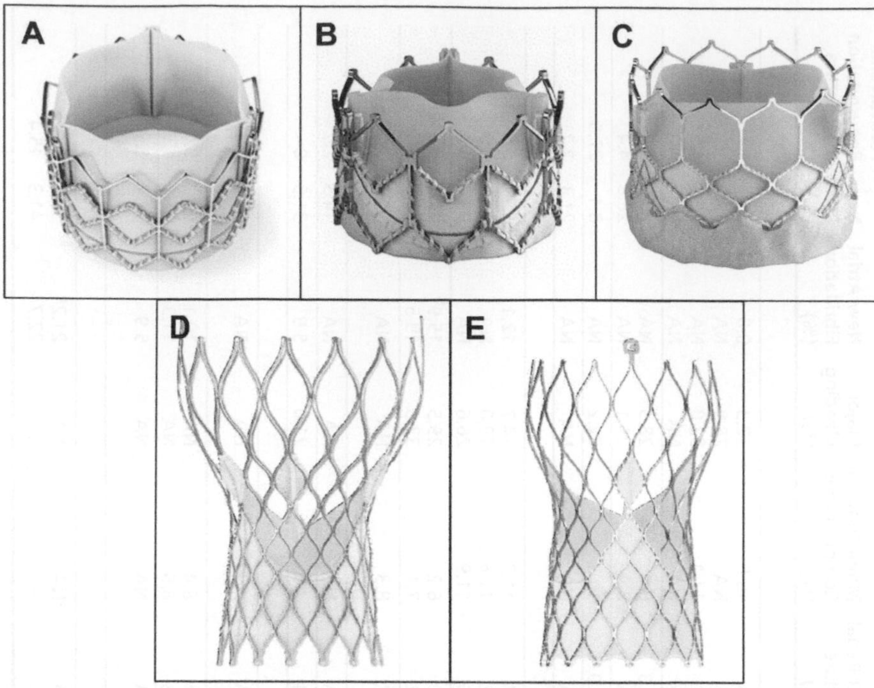

Fig. 2. Transcatheter aortic valve replacement prostheses. Edwards SAPIEN (*A*), SAPIEN XT (*B*), and SAPIEN 3 (*C*) valves. Medtronic CoreValve (*D*) and CoreValve Evolut R (*E*). (*Courtesy of* [*A–C*] Edwards Lifesciences LLC, Irvine, CA, with permission; and [*D, E*] Medtronic, Minneapolis, MN, with permission.)

counterparts, suggesting that transcatheter ASD closure can be considered a valuable therapeutic option in the elderly.[113]

Paravalvular leak (PVL) occurs in 7% to 17% of mitral valve replacements (MVRs) and 5% to 10% of aortic valve replacements (AVRs) and can be associated with disabling symptoms related to HF or hemolysis. Repeat surgery to repair PVL is associated with significant mortality and morbidity. Recent data suggest that percutaneous device closure of PVL represents an effective approach and compares favorably with surgical repair.[114–116] However, data on outcomes of PVL closure in the elderly are lacking.

Other Interventional Therapies for Heart Failure

Implantable hemodynamic monitors

Approximately 22% of older adults with HF are readmitted to the hospital within a month after discharge.[117] Approaches to monitoring patients with HF using noninvasive markers of clinical status have failed to improve QoL or to reduce hospitalization rates. This has led to the development of several implantable hemodynamic monitors (IHMs) to more accurately assess clinical status and adjust medical therapy in patients with HF.

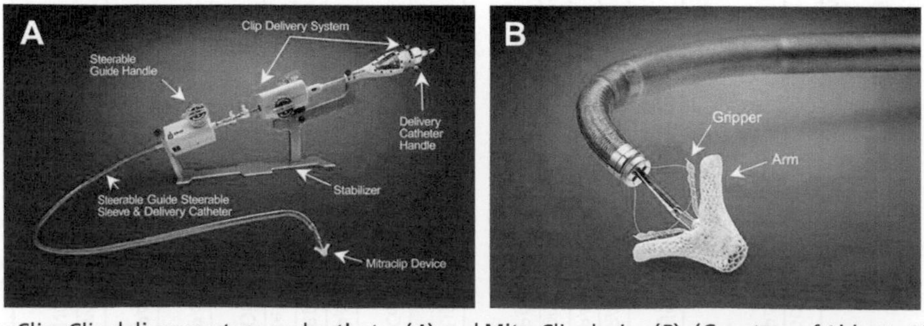

Fig. 3. MitraClip. Clip delivery system and catheter (*A*) and MitraClip device (*B*). (*Courtesy of* Abbott, Abbott Park, IL; with permission.)

Table 4
Outcomes in nonrandomized studies of MitraClip for the treatment of functional or degenerative mitral regurgitation

	No of Patients	Functional MR (%)	Age (y)	LVEF (%)	Logistic EuroSCORE (%)	Procedural Success (%)	Need for ≥2 Devices (%)	Residual MR ≤2+ at Discharge (%)	Mortality at 30 Days/ In-Hospital (%)[a]	Follow-Up (mo)	NYHA I–II at Follow-up (%)	LVEF at Follow-up (%)	Residual MR ≤2+ at Follow-up (%)	All-cause/ CV Death[b] at Follow-up (%)
EVEREST	107	21	71[c]	62[c]	NA	74	29	77	0.9[a]	12	92	NA	66	4.1
Franzen et al, 2011	50	100	70 ± 11	19 ± 5	34 ± 21	94	20	92	6[a]	6	72	25 ± 9	87	18.8
PERMIT-CARE	51	100	70 ± 9	27 ± 9	30 ± 19	96	49	>80	4.2	14[c]	>75	33	>90	18
EVEREST II HRR	78	59	76.7 ± 9.8	54.4 ± 13.7	STS Score 14.2 ± 8.2	96	NA	92	7.7	12	74.1	NA	77.8	24.4
Taramasso et al, 2012	52	100	68 ± 9	28 ± 10	22 ± 5	98	79	90	0[a]	8.5[c]	84	35 ± 11	NA	3.8[b]
ACCESS-EU	567	69.3	73.7 ± 9.6	53.7 (EF <40)	23.0 ± 18.3	91	39.9	91.2	3.4	12	71.4	NA	78.9	17.3
Conradi et al, 2013	95	100	73 ± 8	36 ± 13	34 ± 19	96	35	96	4.2	6.6	70	NA	88	13
Armoiry et al, 2013	62	72.6	72.7 ± 11.4	39.9 ± 14.8	18.7 ± 13.1	95.2	16.9	88.2	3.2[a]	6	90.9	NA	80	16.9
GRASP	117	76	72 ± 10	38 ± 13	12 ± 14	100	41	100	0.9	12	74	NA	84.4	14
Mitra-SWISS	74	62	72 ± 12	47 ± 19	21 ± 17	85	40	85	4[a]	24	53	47 ± 19	58	25
MARS	142	53.5	71.4 ± 11.9	47 ± 17	16.8 ± 14.6	93.7	50.7	93.7	4.2[a]	1	82.1	45 ± 17	76.8	5.6
Taramasso et al, 2014	109	100	69 ± 9	28 ± 11	22 ± 17	99	70	87	1.8	13	86	35 ± 10	NA	9.1[b]
EVERSEST II HRR + REALISM	351	70.1	75.7 ± 10.5	47.5 ± 14.2	STS Score >12	95.7	38.5	85.8	4.8	12	82.9	47.5 ± 13.4	83.6	22.8
TVT Sentinel Pilot Registry	628	72	74.2 ± 9.7	42.6	20.4 ± 16.7	95.4	37.5	98.2	2.9[a]	12	74.2	41.2	94	15.3
Lesevic et al, 2015	136	43	72.9 ± 12	45.2 ± 17.9	20.3 ± 19.9	88.4	29	92	4[a]	36	95	47 ± 13.8	85	12
TRAMI	749	71.3	76[c]	69 (EF <50)	20.0[c]	97.0	NA	96.7	4.5	12	63.3	NA	NA	20.3

Abbreviations: ACCESS-EU, ACCESS-Europe A Two-Phase Observational Study of the MitraClip System in Europe; EVEREST, Endovascular Valve Edge-to-Edge Repair Study; GRASP, getting reduction of mitral insufficiency by percutaneous clip implantation; HRR, high-risk registry; MARS, MitraClip Asia-Pacific Registry; NA, not available; PERMIT-CARE, percutaneous mitral valve repair in cardiac resynchronization therapy; REALISM, Real World Expanded Multicenter Study of the MitraClip System; TRAMI, transcatheter mitral valve interventions; TVT, transcatheter valve treatment.

[a] In-Hospital Mortality.
[b] CV Death.
[c] Median Values.

Table 5
Completed and ongoing clinical trials comparing MitraClip with surgery or optimal medical therapy

	EVEREST II	COAPT	RESHAPE-HF2	MITRA-CRT	MITRA-FR
ClinicalTrials.gov Identifier	NCT00209274	NCT01626079	NCT02444338	NCT02592889	NCT01920698
Design/Location	Multicenter RCT; United States and Canada	Multicenter RCT; United States	Multicenter RCT; Germany	Single center; Spain	Multicenter RCT; France
Patients (N)	279	555	380	30	288
Control Group	Surgery	Optimal standard of care therapy	Optimal standard of care therapy	Optimal medical therapy	Optimal standard of care therapy
Functional MR (%)	27	100	100	100	100
MR Grade Definition	≥3+	≥3+	Moderate to severe or severe MR	≥2+	Severe MR: regurgitation Volume >30 mL/beat and a regurgitant orifice area >20 mm^2
NYHA Functional Class	I–IV	II–IV	II–IV	II or III	II–IV
LVEF (%)	>25 (symptomatic) 25 to 60 (asymptomatic)	≥20 to ≤50	≥15 to ≤35 (if in NYHA class II) or ≥15 to ≤45 (if in NYHA class III or IV).	≥15 to ≤40	≥15 to ≤40
LV Measure	LVEDD ≤55 mm (symptomatic) LVESD 40–55 mm (asymptomatic)	LVESD ≤70 mm	—	LVEDD <75 mm	—

Other Inclusion Criteria	New-onset atrial fibrillation or pulmonary hypertension (in asymptomatic patients); candidate for MV repair or replacement surgery, including CPB; the primary regurgitant jet originates from malcoaptation of the A2 and P2 scallops of the MV	≥1 HF hospitalization in previous 12 mo, and NT-proBNP ≥1500 pg/mL or BNP ≥300 pg/mL	≥1 HF hospitalization in previous 12 mo, and NT-proBNP ≥1000 pg/mL or BNP ≥300 pg/mL	CRT implanted within 6 mo to 5 y, adequate CRT (correct stimulation in >98% heart beats), correct position of leads, wide QRS (>0.12) and LBBB pre-CRT	≥1 HF hospitalization in previous 12 mo
Major Exclusion Criteria	MI within 12 wk, endovascular or surgical procedure within 30 d, LVEF <25%, LVESD >55 mm, MVOA <4.0 cm^2, unfavorable leaflet anatomy, prior MV surgery or valvuloplasty	PCI, CABG, TAVR, carotid surgery/stenting, CRT, CRT-D, or stroke within 30 d; CAD requiring revascularization, COPD on home oxygen or chronic steroids, PASP >70 mm Hg, right-sided HF, nondilated CM, MVOA <4.0 cm^2, unfavorable leaflet anatomy, prior surgical or transcatheter MV procedure, life expectancy <12 mo	PCI, CABG, carotid surgery/stenting, CRT, CRT-D, ICD, TIA, stroke, or ACS within 90 d, degenerative MR, ESRD, 6MWT distance <475 m, MVOA <4.0 cm^2	Severe renal insufficiency, life expectancy <12 mo, anatomic contraindication to MitraClip, hemodynamic instability	Degenerative MR, MI, stroke, CABG, cardioversion, CRT within 3 mo, PCI within 1 mo, prior MV repair, ESRD
Primary Efficacy End point	Freedom from death, MV surgery, or ≥3+ MR 1 y: 55% vs 73% (P = .007) 4 y: 39.8% vs 53.4% (P = .070) 5 y: 44.2% vs 64.3% (P = .01)	Recurrent HF hospitalizations	CV death and composite of HF hospitalization and CV death	Freedom from adverse events (stroke, device embolization, emergent surgery/pericardiocentesis or procedure-related mortality); clinical improvement (>10% improvement in 6MWT and no readmission for HF, heart transplant or mortality)	Composite of all-cause mortality and recurrent HF hospitalizations

(*continued on next page*)

Table 5
(continued)

	EVEREST II	COAPT	RESHAPE-HF2	MITRA-CRT	MITRA-FR
Primary Safety End Point	MAE (composite of death, MI, reoperation for failed MV surgery, nonelective CV surgery for adverse events, stroke, renal failure, deep wound infection, mechanical ventilation >48 h, GI complication requiring surgery, new-onset permanent atrial fibrillation, septicemia, and transfusion of $\geq$2 units of blood) at 30 d 15% vs 48% (P<.001)	Composite of SLDA, device embolizations, endocarditis, or MS requiring surgery, and any device-related complications requiring nonelective CV surgery	—	—	—

Abbreviations: ACS, acute coronary syndrome; BNP, brain natriuretic peptide; COAPT, Cardiovascular Outcomes Assessment of the MitraClip Percutaneous Therapy for Heart Failure Patients With Functional Mitral Regurgitation; COPD, chronic obstructive lung disease; CPB, cardiopulmonary bypass; CRT, cardiac resynchronization therapy; CRT-D, cardiac resynchronization therapy implantable cardioverter defibrillator; ICD, implantable cardioverter-defibrillator; LBBB, left bundle branch block; LVEDD, left ventricular end-diastolic diameter; LVESD, left ventricular end-systolic diameter; MITRA-CRT, MitraClip in Non-Responders to Cardiac Resynchronization Therapy; MITRA-FR, Multicentre Study of Percutaneous Mitral Valve Repair MitraClip Device in Patients With Severe Secondary Mitral Regurgitation; MVOA, MV orifice area; NT-proBNP, N-terminal prohormone of brain natriuretic peptide; PASP, pulmonary artery systolic pressure; RESHAPE-HF, Randomized Study of the MitraClip Device in Heart Failure Patients With Clinically Significant Functional Mitral Regurgitation; SLDA, single leaflet device attachment.

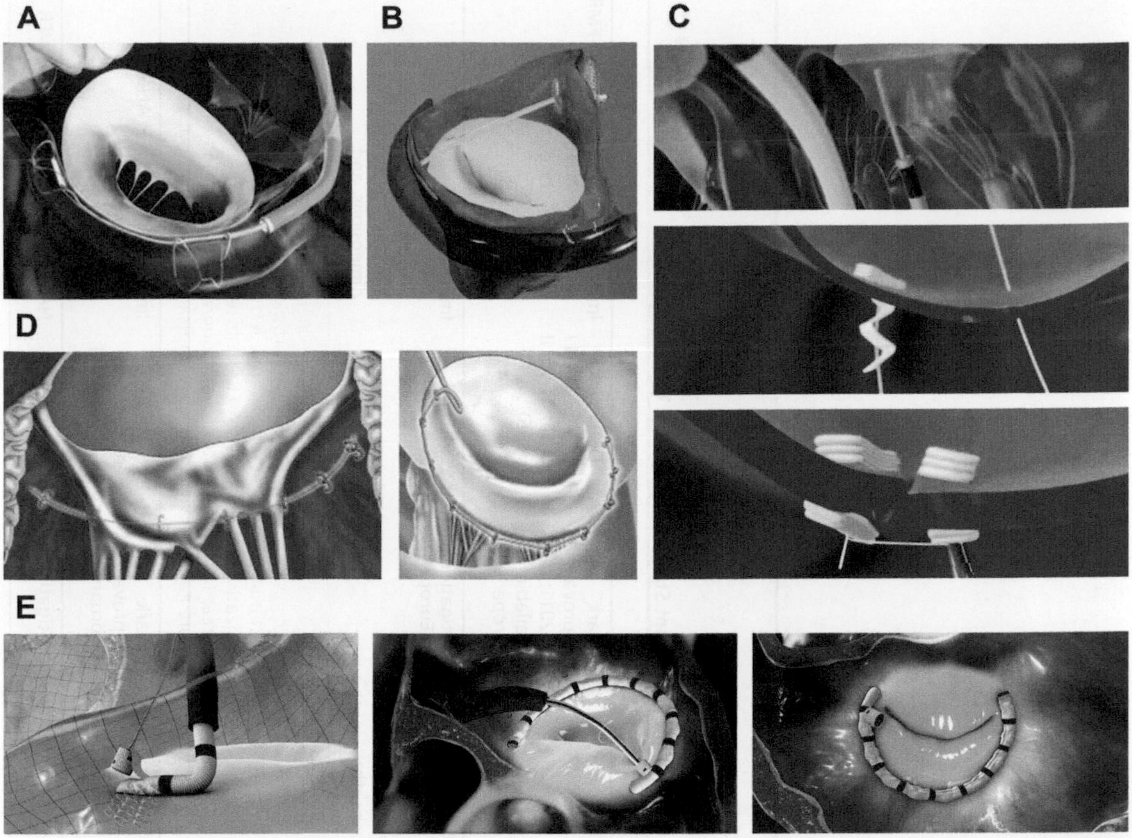

Fig. 4. Percutaneous mitral annuloplasty devices for the treatment of functional mitral regurgitation. Carillon mitral contour system (*A*). ARTO system (*B*). Mitralign system (*C*). Accucinch system (*D*). Cardioband system (*E*). (*Courtesy of* [*A*] Cardiac Dimensions, Kirkland, WA, with permission; [*B*] MVRx, Inc, Belmont, CA, with permission; [*C*] Mitralign, Inc, Tewksbury, MA, with permission; [*D*] *From* Feldman T, Cilingiroglu M. Percutaneous leaflet repair and annuloplasty for mitral regurgitation. J Am Coll Cardiol 2011;57:532, with permission, Figure illustration by Craig Skaggs; *Courtesy of* Guided Delivery Systems, Santa Clara, CA, with permission; and [*E*] "*Courtesy of* Edwards Lifesciences, Irvine, California, USA.")

Right ventricular pressure monitor The Chronicle (Medtronic, Inc, Minneapolis, MN) was the first IHM developed for patients with HF (**Table 8**).[118] The COMPASS-HF (Chronicle Offers Management to Patients with Advanced Signs and Symptoms of Heart Failure) trial showed a nonsignificant 21% reduction in rates of HF-related events (hospitalizations and emergency or urgent care visits requiring intravenous therapy) with Chronicle IHM compared with control.[119] Because of concerns regarding lack of clinical effectiveness based on the trial results, the device was not approved by the FDA.[120]

Left atrial pressure monitor The safety and efficacy of the HeartPOD (St. Jude Medical, Inc, Minneapolis, MN), a permanent implantable left atrial pressure (LAP) monitoring system (see **Table 8**), was evaluated in 40 patients with HF (mean age, 66 ± 10 years) in the HOMEOSTASIS (Hemodynamically Guided Home Self-Therapy in Severe Heart Failure Patients) trial.[121,122] The study device was successfully implanted in all patients and no MAE were recorded at 6 weeks (primary safety end point). Compared with the 3-month observation period, event (death or acute decompensated HF)-free survival was significantly higher over a median follow-up of 25 months during which treatment was targeted to achieve and maintain optimal LAP (HR, 0.16; 95% CI, 0.04–0.68; $P = .012$). Significant improvements in NYHA class and LVEF were also observed. The LAPTOP-HF (Left Atrial Pressure Monitoring to Optimize Heart Failure Therapy Study) was a prospective, multicenter RCT in NYHA class III patients randomized to LAP-guided therapy with HeartPOD or standard

Table 6
Percutaneous mitral annuloplasty devices for the treatment of functional mitral regurgitation

	Design	Placement Site	Mechanism	Access	Current Status	Completed Trials	Results	Ongoing Trials
Indirect Annuloplasty								
Carillon Mitral Contour System (Cardiac Dimension, I006Ec, Kirkland, WA)	Nitinol device with proximal and distal anchors connected by a ribbon	CS	Plication/cinching	9 F via internal jugular vein	CE mark approval in 2011; available in Europe	AMADEUS (n = 30), TITAN I (n = 36), TITAN II (n = 36)	Improvement in FMR grade, NYHA functional class, QoL, 6MWT	REDUCE-FMR
ARTO System (MVRx Inc, Belmont, CA)	Magnetic catheters placed in the CS and in left atrium (via transseptal puncture) linked behind the posterior mitral leaflet. CS and atrial septal anchors connected via a suture	CS and left atrium (atrial septum)	Anteroposterior septal-sinus shortening	16 F internal jugular vein and 16 F femoral vein sheaths	Investigational in Europe	MAVERIC FIM (n = 11)	Improvement in FMR grade, LV volumes, mitral annulus dimensions, and NYHA functional class	—
Direct Annuloplasty								
Mitralign System (Mitralign, Inc, Tewksbury, MA)	Wire delivery catheter, crossing wires and a bident catheter	P1 and P3 scallops	Pledgets	14 F, retrograde transfemoral approach	CE mark approval in February 2016	Mitralign Percutaneous Annuloplasty FIM (n = 71)	Improvement in FMR grade, NYHA functional class, QoL, 6MWT	ALIGN
Accucinch System (Guided Delivery	Series of anchors connected with a	Posterior mitral annulus	Drawstring to cinch the		Investigational	LVRESTORESA (n = 8)	NA	LVRECOVER

Systems, Santa Clara, CA)	polyethylene cable		annular circumference	18 F, retrograde transfemoral approach				
Cardioband System (Valtech Cardio Ltd, Or-Yehuda, Israel)	The implant is a polyester sleeve with radiopaque markers spaced 8 mm apart. Implantable stainless steel, 6-mm long anchors, used to fasten the Cardioband implant to the annulus. A contraction wire in the Cardioband is connected to an adjusting spool	Atrial side of the mitral annulus. The screw anchors are deployed from the posteromedial to the anterolateral commissure in a counterclockwise fashion	Cinching	25 F transseptal steerable sheath	CE mark approval in September 2015	Cardioband With Transfemoral Delivery System (n = 31)	Improvement in FMR grade, NYHA functional class, QoL, 6MWT	REPAIR

Abbreviations: ALIGN, Mitralign Percutaneous Annuloplasty System For Chronic Functional Mitral Valve Regurgitation; AMADEUS, The Carillon Mitral Annuloplasty Device European Union Study; CS, coronary sinus; FIM, first-in-man; FMR, functional mitral regurgitation; LVRECOVER, Feasibility of the AccuCinch System for Left Ventricular Reshaping of the Mitral Apparatus to Reduce Functional Mitral Regurgitation and Improve Left Ventricular Function; LVRESTORESA, A Study of Percutaneous Left Ventricular Reshaping of Mitral Apparatus to Reduce Functional Mitral Regurgitation and Improve LV Function Using the Accucinch System; MAVERIC, Mitral Valve Repair Clinical Trial; REDUCE FMR, Carillon Mitral Contour System for Reducing Functional Mitral Regurgitation; REPAIR, Transcatheter Repair of Mitral Insufficiency with Cardioband System; TITAN, Transcatheter Implantation of Carillon Mitral Annuloplasty Device.

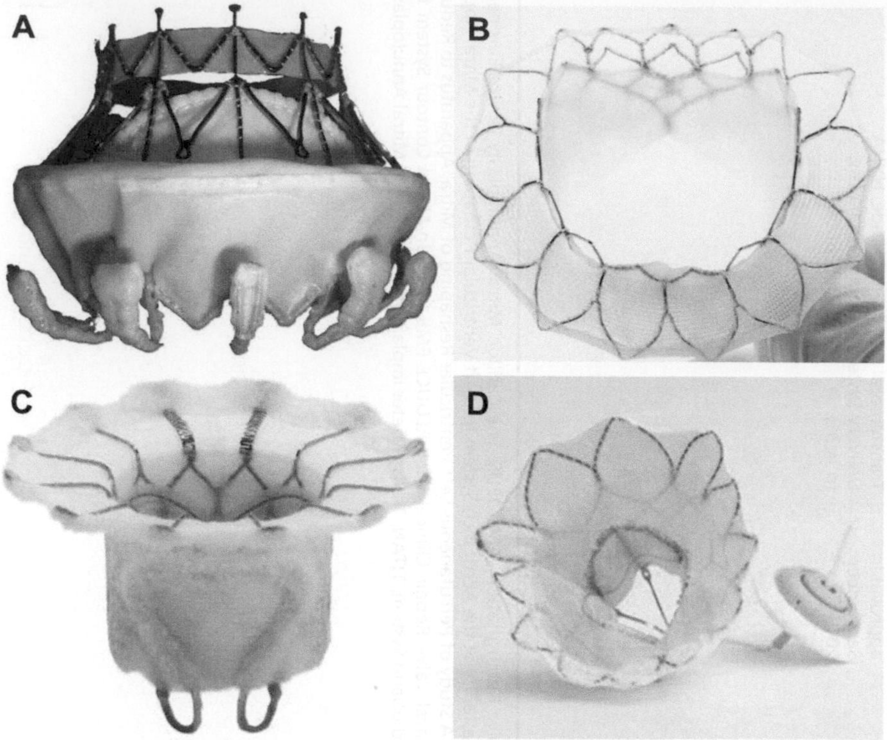

Fig. 5. Transcatheter MV replacement prostheses. CardiAQ valve (*A*). Tiara valve (*B*). Fortis valve (*C*). Tendyne valve (*D*). (*Courtesy of* [*A, C*] Edwards Lifesciences LLC, Irvine, CA, with permission; [*B*] Neovasc, New Brighton, MN, with permission; and [*D*] Tendyne, Roseville, MN, with permission.)

of care.[123] The trial, which planned to enroll 730 patients, was terminated prematurely (at 486 patients) because of excess procedure-related complications. The safety end point of freedom from major adverse cardiovascular and neurologic events at 12 months was 90.6% in the treatment group with a lower 95% CI of 86.7%, which met the prespecified performance criterion of 80%. There was a 41% reduction in HF hospitalizations with LAP-guided therapy compared with the standard of care (P = .005).

Pulmonary artery pressure monitor The CardioMEMS HF System (St. Jude Medical, Saint Paul, MN) is the only IHM currently approved by the FDA (see **Table 8**).[124] The CHAMPION (CardioMEMS Heart Sensor Allows Monitoring of Pressure to Improve Outcomes in NYHA Class III Heart Failure Patients) trial showed a 37% reduction in HF-related hospitalizations over a mean follow-up of 15 months in patients (mean age, 61 ± 13 years) randomized to wireless implantable hemodynamic monitor placement and daily pulmonary artery pressure (PAP)–guided HF management in addition to standard of care, compared with those receiving standard of care alone.[124] A prespecified subgroup analysis of patients with HF with preserved ejection fraction (HFpEF; n = 119) also showed a 50% reduction in HF hospitalizations over a mean follow-up of 17.6 months.[125] The 2016 European Society of Cardiology HF guidelines provide a class IIb (level of evidence, B) recommendation to the use of CardioMEMS in symptomatic patients with prior HF hospitalization to reduce the risk of recurrent HF hospitalization.[126]

Transcatheter interatrial shunt devices

Increased LAP or pulmonary capillary wedge pressure (PCWP), especially during exercise, is pathognomonic of HF and is associated with poor outcomes. This association, along with the observation that patients with Lutembacher syndrome (mitral stenosis plus ASD) are less symptomatic and have better outcomes compared with patients with pure mitral stenosis, forms the basis for development of interatrial shunt devices in the treatment of HF.

The interatrial septal device (IASD; Corvia Medical, Inc, Tewksbury, MA) system consists of a nitinol device (outer diameter, 19 mm) inserted percutaneously in the interatrial septum to produce a permanent 8-mm atrial septal communication (**Fig. 6**A). The REDUCE LAP-HF

Table 7
Ongoing clinical trials of transcatheter therapies for severe tricuspid regurgitation

Trial Acronym	Trial Name and Device	N	Inclusion	Exclusion	Primary End Points
PREVENT	Percutaneous Treatment of Tricuspid Valve Regurgitation with the TriCinch System	24	Functional symptomatic TR 2+ to 4+ on a scale of 4+ (moderate to severe), with annular dilatation >40 mm	At the heart team's judgment, patient IVC dimension not adequate for device implantation	Safety: MAE at 30 d, defined as death, Q-wave MI, cardiac tamponade, cardiac surgery for failed TriCinch implantation, stroke, or septicemia Efficacy: reduction in the degree of TR at discharge; ability to reduce TR by at least 1° immediately following implantation of the TriCinch device assessed by means of quantitative echocardiographic parameters
HOVER	Heterotopic Implantation of the Edwards SAPIEN XT Transcatheter Valve in the Inferior Vena Cava for the Treatment of Severe Tricuspid Regurgitation	30	TR should be functional, without anatomic abnormalities of the tricuspid valve leaflets	Mean PAPs ≥40 mm Hg and PVR >4 Wood units as assessed by right heart catheterization	Procedural success at 30 d, defined as device success and no device-related or procedure-related serious adverse events, including all death, all stroke, MI, acute kidney injury grade 3, life-threatening bleeding, major vascular complications, pericardial effusion or tamponade requiring drainage, vena cava syndrome Individual success at 1 y, defined as device success and no readmissions to hospital for right-sided HF or right-sided HF equivalents, including drainage of ascites or pleural effusions; new listing for heart transplant, VAD, or other mechanical support; and KCCQ improvement >10 vs baseline and 6MWT improvement >50 m vs baseline

(*continued on next page*)

Table 7
(*continued*)

Trial Acronym	Trial Name and Device	N	Inclusion	Exclusion	Primary End Points
TRICAVAL	Treatment of Severe Secondary Tricuspid Regurgitation in Patients with Advance Heart Failure with Caval Vein Implantation of the Edwards SAPIEN XT VALve	40	Severe symptomatic TR with a significant regurgitation jet into the caval and hepatic veins	IVC diameter >32 mm, severe LVD with LVEF <30%	Maximum relative Vo_2 uptake at 3 mo (difference of means in maximum relative Vo_2 uptake at 3 mo compared with control group)
Early Feasibility Study of the Edwards FORMA Tricuspid Transcatheter Repair System	Edwards FORMA Tricuspid Transcatheter Repair System	30	Clinically significant, symptomatic (NYHA functional class ≥II) functional or secondary TR (per applicable guidelines) requiring tricuspid valve repair or replacement as assessed by the heart team; high surgical risk for tricuspid valve repair or replacement	Tricuspid valve/right heart Anatomy not suitable for the study device	Procedural success defined as device success and freedom from device or procedure-related serious adverse events at 30 d

SPACER	Repair of Tricuspid Valve Regurgitation Using the Edwards Tricuspid Transcatheter Repair System	75	Clinically significant, symptomatic (NYHA functional class ≥II); TR (per applicable guidelines) requiring tricuspid valve repair or replacement as assessed by the heart team; functional TR as the primary cause	Tricuspid valve/right heart Anatomy not suitable for the study device	Cardiac mortality at 30 d
SCOUT	Early Feasibility of the Mitralign Percutaneous Tricuspid Valve Annuloplasty System	15	Chronic functional TR with a minimum of moderate TR	Tricuspid valve annular Diameter ≥40 mm (or 21 mm/m^2) and ≤55 mm (or 29 mm/m^2)	Technical success at 30 d defined as freedom from death with successful access, delivery, and retrieval of the device delivery system, and deployment and correct Positioning of the intended devices, and no need for additional unplanned or emergency surgery or reintervention related to the device or access procedure

Abbreviations: IVC, inferior vena cava; PVR, pulmonary vascular resistance; VAD, ventricular assist device; V_{O_2}, oxygen consumption.

Adapted from O'Neill BP, O'Neill WW. Tricuspid valve intervention: new direction and new hope. J Am Coll Cardiol 2016;68(10):1035; and Rodes-Cabau J, Taramasso M, O'Gara PT. Diagnosis and treatment of tricuspid valve disease: current and future perspectives. Lancet 2016;388(10058):2439, with permission.

Table 8
Implantable hemodynamic monitors for management of heart failure

Device	Manufacturer	Design	Implant Site	Parameters Monitored
Chronicle	Medtronic, Inc, Minneapolis, MN	Programmable device and a transvenous lead with a sensor at its tip	Device positioned subcutaneously in the pectoral area and the lead tip in the RV outflow tract or septum	Heart rate, body temperature, patient activity, RV systolic and diastolic pressure, maximal positive and negative rate of change in RV pressure (dP/dt), RV preejection and systolic time intervals, and ePAD[a]
HeartPOD	St. Jude Medical, Inc, Minneapolis, MN	Sensor lead coupled with a subcutaneous antenna coil, a patient advisory module, and the clinician's personal computer software. Sensor system comprises a 3 × 7 mm hermetically sealed sensor module with a titanium pressure-sensing membrane and circuitry	Sensor system implanted into the atrial septum via a transseptal puncture technique, and oriented to the left atrium	LAP[b], temperature, and intracardiac electrogram
CardioMEMS HF System	St. Jude Medical, Inc, Minneapolis, MN	Sensor that consists of a three-dimensional coil and a pressure-sensitive capacitor encased within a hermetically sealed, fused silica capsule completely covered in medical-grade silicone. Two wired nitinol loops avoid sensor distal migration. PAP changes are transmitted wirelessly using an external antenna, which is held against the patient's side or back in the approximate area of deployment of the sensor. The antenna provides power to the device and allows device calibration and daily waveform recording	Distal pulmonary artery	PAP

Abbreviations: ePAD, estimated pulmonary artery diastolic pressure; LAP, left atrial pressure; PAP, pulmonary artery pressure.
[a] ePAD is defined as the RV pressure at the time of pulmonary valve opening, which occurs at the time of maximal dP/dt, and correlates well with directly measured pulmonary artery diastolic pressure.
[b] LAP is calculated by subtracting the absolute pressure obtained by the implant from an atmospheric reference measured by a pressure sensor located in the patient advisory module.

(Reduce Elevated Left Atrial Pressure in Patients with Heart Failure) was a multicenter, prospective, nonrandomized, open-label, single-arm study that examined the safety and performance of IASD in 68 patients (mean age, 69 ± 8 years) with HFpEF, LVEF greater than 40%, NYHA functional class II to IV, and increased PCWP at rest (>15 mm Hg) or during exercise (>25 mm Hg).[127] Device placement was successful in 94% of patients and 71% of patients met the primary device performance end point of reduction in PCWP at rest or during exercise. No patient had periprocedural or MACCE during the 6-month follow-up. There were significant improvements in NYHA class, 6-minute walk test (6MWT) distance, and QoL at 6 months and these were sustained even at 1 year.[127,128] The REDUCE LAP-HF 1 is an ongoing multicenter, single (patient)-blinded RCT designed to assess the safety and efficacy of IASD in patients with HFpEF randomized to IASD System II implantation or control (intracardiac echocardiogram with examination of the interatrial septum and left atrial appendage).[129]

The V-Wave interatrial shunt (V-Wave Ltd, Caesarea, Israel) consists of an expanded polytetrafluoroethylene (ePTFE)–encapsulated hourglass-shaped nitinol frame that is implanted at the interatrial septum and contains 3 porcine pericardial leaflets sutured within to ensure unidirectional flow from the left to the right atrium if the pressure gradient exceeds 5 mm Hg (**Fig. 6**B). A safety and proof-of-principle cohort study was conducted at 1 center in Canada. The V-Wave device was successfully implanted in 10 patients aged 62 ± 8 years with chronic (>6 months) HFrEF (LVEF ≤40%) and NYHA functional class III or ambulatory class IV symptoms. PCWP was reduced from 23 ± 5 mm Hg at baseline to 17 ± 8 mm Hg at 3 months with significant improvement in NYHA class, 6MWT distance, and QoL at 3 months. The RELIEVE-HF (Reducing Lung Congestion Symptoms Using the V-Wave Shunt in Advanced Heart Failure) is an ongoing prospective, nonrandomized, open-label, single-arm multicenter study that will evaluate the performance and safety of the V-Wave interatrial shunt in 60 patients with HFpEF or HFrEF.[130]

Percutaneous left ventricle restoration devices Ischemic cardiomyopathy is characterized by LV remodeling as a result of myocardial injury and scarring, which results in progressive LV dilatation and systolic dysfunction and, ultimately, HF. The Surgical Treatment for Ischemic Heart Failure (STICH) (Hypothesis 2) trial showed that, in patients with CAD and LVEF less than or equal to 35%, the addition of surgical ventricular reconstruction (SVR) to CABG did not improve symptoms or exercise tolerance and did not reduce all-cause death or cardiovascular hospitalizations compared with CABG alone.[131] Although the methodology and results of this trial have been widely criticized, SVR has fallen into disfavor and is no longer performed.[132,133] However, the development of a percutaneous alternative to SVR has led to a renewed interest in mechanical LV restoration.

The Parachute (Cardiokinetix, Inc, Menlo Park, CA) is a ventricular partitioning device that is composed of a self-expanding nitinol frame, an ePTFE occlusive membrane, and a distal atraumatic (Pebax polymer) foot (**Fig. 7**). The nitinol frame is shaped like an umbrella with 16 struts. The tip of each strut ends in a 2-mm anchor. The PARACHUTE (Percutaneous Ventricular Restoration in Chronic Heart Failure due to Ischemic Heart Disease) first-in-human study was a prospective, nonrandomized, single-arm, multicenter study that enrolled 39 patients aged 56.4 ± 4.6 years with NYHA class II to IV

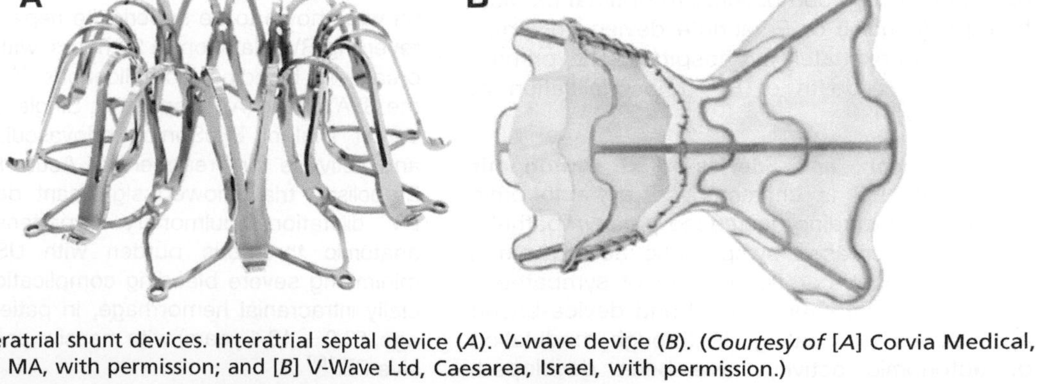

Fig. 6. Interatrial shunt devices. Interatrial septal device (*A*). V-wave device (*B*). (*Courtesy of* [*A*] Corvia Medical, Tewksbury, MA, with permission; and [*B*] V-Wave Ltd, Caesarea, Israel, with permission.)

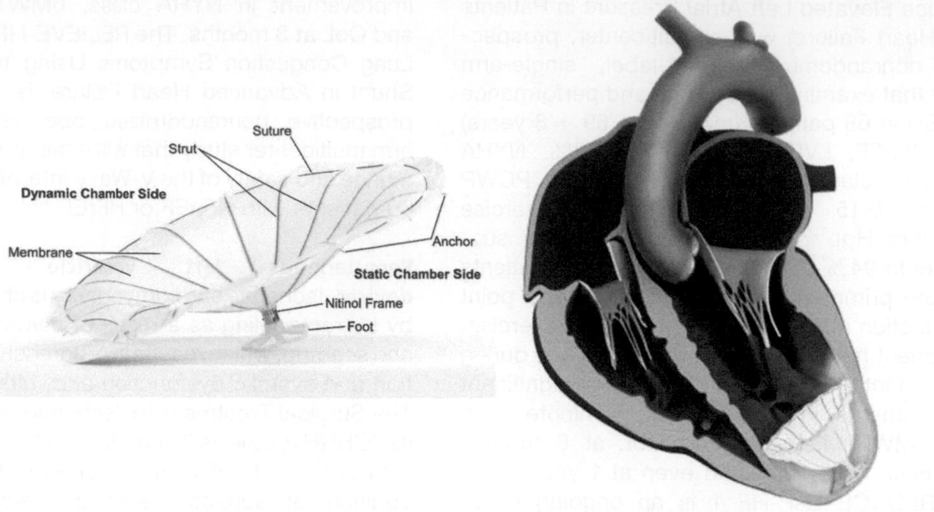

Fig. 7. Parachute left ventricular partitioning device. (*From* Ige M, Al-Kindi SG, Attizzani G, et al. Percutaneous left ventricular restoration. Heart Failure Clinics 2015;11(2):263–4, with permission; and *Courtesy of* CardioKinetix, Menlo Park, CA, with permission.)

ischemic HFrEF (LVEF 15%–40%), and dilated akinetic or dyskinetic anterior-apical wall without the need to be revascularized.[134] Device implantation was attempted in 34 patients and was successful in 31 (91%). The primary safety end point, defined as the successful delivery and deployment of the Parachute device and 6-month follow-up without the occurrence of major adverse cardiovascular events related to the investigational device was met in 29 of 34 patients (85.3%).[134] Improvements in LV volume indices and NYHA class were sustained through 1-year and 3-year follow-ups.[134,135] Similarly, in the PARACHUTE III study in Europe in 100 patients (mean age, 62.8 $\pm$ 10.4 years), the device was successfully implanted in 97%. One-year rates of the primary (procedure-related or device-related MACCE) and secondary (composite of mortality and morbidity) end points were 7% and 32.3%, respectively.[136] A US pivotal trial (PARACHUTE IV) is currently ongoing and will randomly assign 560 patients to optimal medical therapy (control) or Parachute device implantation in approximately 65 hospitals. The primary end point is death or HF rehospitalization at 12 months.[137]

Interventional and device-based autonomic modulation HF is characterized by autonomic imbalance, including decreased parasympathetic tone and increased sympathetic activity along with impaired baroreflex control of sympathetic activity. Several interventional and device-based approaches for treating HF through modulation of autonomic activity have been developed; however, the results to date have been disappointing (**Table 9**).[138–156]

Catheter-directed thrombolysis for acute right ventricular failure secondary to massive/submassive pulmonary embolism Acute RVF is common in patients with massive or submassive pulmonary embolism. Catheter-directed thrombolysis (CDT) has emerged as an effective therapy for such patients and has been shown to improve outcomes while minimizing the risk of major bleeding, compared with systemic thrombolysis.[157,158] Ultrasonography-accelerated catheter-directed thrombolysis (USAT) combines conventional CDT with high-frequency (2.2 MHz), low-power (0.5 W per element) ultrasonography, which causes reversible disaggregation and separation of un–cross-linked fibrin fibers, increasing thrombus permeability of thrombolytic drugs. In the ULTIMA (Ultrasound Accelerated Thrombolysis of Pulmonary Embolism) trial, USAT plus heparin was shown to be superior to heparin alone in reversing RV dilatation at 24 hours, without an increase in bleeding complications.[159] Recently, the SEATTLE II (A Prospective, Single-arm, Multicenter Trial of EkoSonic Endovascular System and Activase for Treatment of Acute Pulmonary Embolism) trial showed significant decrease in RV dilatation, pulmonary hypertension, and anatomic thrombus burden with USAT while minimizing severe bleeding complications, especially intracranial hemorrhage, in patients (mean age, 59.0 $\pm$ 16.1 years) with massive and submassive PE.[160]

Table 9
Completed and ongoing studies of interventional and device-based autonomic modulation for treatment of heart failure

Trial	Design	N	Main Inclusion Criteria	Follow-up	Primary End Point	Results/Event Rate
Spinal Cord Stimulation						
SCS Pilot Study	Prospective, randomized, double-blind, crossover study	9	LVEF ≤30%, NYHA class III, HF hospitalization or IV inotropic support at least once in prior year, walked <450 m on 6MHW	7	Composite of death, HF hospitalization, symptomatic Bradyarrhythmia, or tachyarrhythmia requiring cardioversion	Phase I: 3/9 Phase II (after crossover): 4/9
SCS HEART	Prospective, multicenter, pilot trial	21	LVEF 20%–35%, NYHA class III, implantable cardioverter-defibrillator	6	Safety: death caused by ventricular tachyarrhythmia or sudden unexpected death, MI, or HF hospitalization. Efficacy: Δ composite score based on 6 efficacy parameters (NYHA class, MLHFQ, Vo_{2max}, NT-proBNP, LVEF, and LVESV)	Safety: no events Efficacy: composite score improved by 4.2 ± 1.3, and 11 (73%) patients showed improvement in ≥4 of 6 efficacy parameters
DEFEAT-HF	Prospective, multicenter randomized (3:2), parallel, single-blind, controlled study	66	LVEF ≤35%, NYHA class III, QRS duration <120 ms, LVEDD ≥55 mm	6	ΔLVESV index	SCS off: −2.2 (95% CI, −9.1–4.6) vs SCS on: 2.1 (95% CI, −2.7–6.9); $P = .30$
Vagus Nerve Stimulation						
CardioFit	Single-arm, open-label interventional phase 2 study	32	LVEF ≤35%, NYHA class II–III, sinus rhythm with a 24-h Holter heart rate of 60–110 bpm	6	System-related or procedure-related SAE	26 SAE in 13 of 32 patients (40.6%)

(*continued on next page*)

Table 9
(continued)

Trial	Design	N	Main Inclusion Criteria	Follow-up	Primary End Point	Results/Event Rate
ANTHEM-HF	Multicenter, open-label, feasibility study	60	LVEF ≤40%, NYHA class II–III, LVEDD ≥50 mm to <80 mm, QRS duration ≤150 ms	6	Safety: procedure-related and device-related SAE Efficacy: ΔLVEF and ΔLVESV	Safety: 21 SAE in 16 of 60 patients (26.7%) Efficacy: ↑LVEF by 4.5% (95% CI, 2.4–6.6) and ↓LVESV by −4.1 mL (95% CI, −9.0–0.8)
NECTAR-HF	Phase 2, randomized controlled trial	96	LVEF ≤35%, LVEDD ≥55 mm, NYHA class II–III	6	ΔLVESD	VNS on, −0.04 ± 0.25 cm vs VNS off, −0.08 ± 0.32 cm (P = .60)
VANGUARD[a]	Phase 2, single-arm, open-label study	20	LVEF <40%, NYHA class II–III, sinus rhythm with heart rate ≥60 bpm	12	Freedom from procedure-related or device-related SAE	—
VITARIA Registry[a]	Observational patient registry	200	LVEF ≤40%, NYHA class II–III, implantation of VITARIA System (Cyberonics, Inc, Houston, TX)	12	Serious and nonserious adverse events, ΔLVEF	—
Baroreceptor Activation Therapy						
Gronda et al	Single center, open label	11	LVEF ≤40%, NYHA class III, 6MHW distance 140–450 m, heart rate 60–100 bpm, eGFR ≥30 mL/min/1.73 m^2	6	Δ in MSNA, 6MHW distance, QoL (MLHFQ), NYHA class, LVEF	ΔMSNA: −13.8 ± 1.4 (P<.001), improvement in 6MHW distance, MLHFQ, NYHA class, and LVEF (P<.05)
Barostim HOPE4HF	Multicenter, open-label, randomized controlled trial	146	LVEF ≤35%, NYHA class II, 6MHW distance 140–450 m, heart rate 60–100 bpm, eGFR ≥30 mL/min/1.73 m^2	6	Safety: event-free rate of system-related or procedure-related MANCE Efficacy: Δ in NYHA class, QoL, and 6MHW distance	Safety: 97.2% (lower 95% confidence bound 91.4%) Efficacy: improvement in NYHA class, QoL, and 6MHW distance, compared with control (P<.05)
Rheos Diastolic HF Trial[a]	Randomized, parallel assignment, double blind	6	LVEF ≥45%, clinical HF with increased BNP or NT-proBNP	6	Safety: all adverse events Efficacy: ΔLV mass index	—
Renal Sympathetic Nerve Denervation						
REACH-Pilot Study	Open-label, nonrandomized, FIM safety study	7	Chronic HF, NYHA class II–IV	6	Procedural complications or symptomatic adverse effects	No events

REACH[a]	Phase 3, double-blind, RCT	76	LVEF <40%, NYHA class II–III	12	Improvement in symptoms assessed using KCCQ	—
DIASTOLE[a]	Multicenter, open-label, RCT	60	LVEF ≥50%, HF symptoms, echo evidence of LV diastolic dysfunction, hypertension on at least 2 drugs, and BP <140/90 mm Hg)	12	Efficacy: Δ in E/E′, Ard-Ad, and LAVI Safety: major and minor adverse events	—
Renal Denervation in Patients with Chronic HF[a]	Prospective, multicenter, randomized, open-label, feasibility, safety and efficacy study	100	LVEF 10%–40%, NYHA class II–III, BNP >100 pg/mL or NT-proBNP >400 pg/mL, eGFR ≥30 mL/min/1.73 m^2	6	Complications associated with the delivery and/or use of the Symplicity Catheter (Medtronic, Inc, Minneapolis, MN)	—
RESPECT-HF[a]	Phase 2, open-label, RCT	144	LVEF ≥50%, NYHA class II–IV, echo evidence of LV diastolic dysfunction and/or NT-proBNP >220 pg/mL	6	Δ in LAVI and/or LVMI on cardiac MRI	—
RDT-PEF[a]	Phase 2, open-label, RCT	25	LVEF >40%, NYHA class II–III, evidence of HFpEF	12	Δ in QoL (MLHFQ), peak Vo_2, BNP, E/E′, LAVI, LVMI	—
DENRENIC[a]	Single arm, open label	12	LVEF <35%, NYHA class III–IV, eGFR >45 mL/min/1.73 m^2	6	Improvement in 6MHW, symptoms, BNP, Vo_{2max}, or pharmacologic therapy	—
Heart-RND[a]	Randomized, parallel assignment, open-label	40	LVEF <45%, NYHA class III–IV, 6MHW <440 m	24	6MHW	—

Abbreviations: 6MHW, 6-minute hallway walk; Ad, duration of the MV atrial wave flow; ANTHEM-HF, Autonomic Neural Regulation Therapy to Enhance Myocardial Function in Heart Failure; Ard, duration of reversed pulmonary vein arterial systolic flow; bpm, beats per minute; DEFEAT-HF, Determining the Feasibility of Spinal Cord Neuromodulation for the Treatment of Chronic Heart Failure; DENRENIC, Renal Denervation in Chronic Heart Failure d'Insuffisance Cardiaque; DIASTOLE, Denervation of the Renal Sympathetic Nerves in Heart Failure with normal LV Ejection Fraction; E, mitral peak velocity of early filling; E′, early diastolic mitral annular velocity; echo, echocardiography; eGFR, estimated glomerular filtration rate; HOPE4HF, Hope for Heart Failure; IV, intravenous; LAVI, left atrial volume index; LVESV, left ventricular end-systolic volume; LVMI, left ventricular mass index; MLHFQ, Minnesota Living with Heart Failure Questionnaire; MSNA, muscle sympathetic nerve activity; NECTAR-HF, Neural Cardiac Therapy for Heart Failure; NT-proBNP, N-terminal pro–brain natriuretic peptide; RDT-PEF, Renal Denervation in Heart Failure with Preserved Ejection Fraction; REACH, Renal Artery Denervation in Chronic Heart Failure; RESPECT-HF, Renal Denervation in Heart Failure Patients with Preserved Ejection Fraction; SAE, serious adverse events; SCS, spinal cord stimulation; VANGUARD, Vagal Nerve Stimulation: Safeguarding Heart Failure Patients; VNS, vagal nerve stimulation.

[a] Ongoing studies.

SUMMARY

HF remains the leading cause of hospitalization in older adults and is associated with increased morbidity and mortality despite the use of GDMT. The past decade has seen tremendous progress in the development of novel interventional therapies for HF designed to improve symptoms, reduce rehospitalizations, and/or decrease mortality. The evolution of structural heart disease interventions and interventional heart failure fields has led to a multidisciplinary heart team approach in the management of patients with HF, especially those with ischemic cardiomyopathy requiring high-risk PCI and MCS, or severe VHD requiring valve replacement. Although therapies such as TAVR and MitraClip have already become mainstream, many others are still in the investigational stages. Careful selection of the appropriate patient population (eg, HFrEF vs HFpEF, functional vs degenerative VHD) and end points in future RCTs will be crucial to show the potential efficacy of the novel interventional HF therapies.

REFERENCES

1. GBD 2015 Disease and Injury Incidence and Prevalence Collaborators. Global, regional, and national incidence, prevalence, and years lived with disability for 310 diseases and injuries, 1990–2015: a systematic analysis for the Global Burden of Disease Study 2015. Lancet 2016;388: 1545–602.
2. Mozaffarian D, Benjamin EJ, Go AS, et al. Heart disease and stroke statistics-2016 update: a report from the American Heart Association. Circulation 2016;133:e38–360.
3. Ziaeian B, Fonarow GC. Epidemiology and aetiology of heart failure. Nat Rev Cardiol 2016;13: 368–78.
4. Gheorghiade M, Sopko G, De LL, et al. Navigating the crossroads of coronary artery disease and heart failure. Circulation 2006;114:1202–13.
5. Kwok CS, Anderson SG, McAllister KS, et al. Impact of age on the prognostic value of left ventricular function in relation to procedural outcomes following percutaneous coronary intervention: insights from the British Cardiovascular Intervention Society. Catheter Cardiovasc Interv 2015;85: 944–51.
6. Mamas MA, Anderson SG, O'Kane PD, et al. Impact of left ventricular function in relation to procedural outcomes following percutaneous coronary intervention: insights from the British Cardiovascular Intervention Society. Eur Heart J 2014;35:3004–3312a.
7. Velazquez EJ, Lee KL, Jones RH, et al. Coronary-artery bypass surgery in patients with ischemic cardiomyopathy. N Engl J Med 2016;374:1511–20.
8. Berger PB, Velianou JL, Aslanidou VH, et al. Survival following coronary angioplasty versus coronary artery bypass surgery in anatomic subsets in which coronary artery bypass surgery improves survival compared with medical therapy. Results from the Bypass Angioplasty Revascularization Investigation (BARI). J Am Coll Cardiol 2001;38: 1440–9.
9. Sedlis SP, Ramanathan KB, Morrison DA, et al. Outcome of percutaneous coronary intervention versus coronary bypass grafting for patients with low left ventricular ejection fractions, unstable angina pectoris, and risk factors for adverse outcomes with bypass (the AWESOME Randomized Trial and Registry). Am J Cardiol 2004;94:118–20.
10. Cleland JG, Calvert M, Freemantle N, et al. The Heart Failure Revascularisation Trial (HEART). Eur J Heart Fail 2011;13:227–33.
11. Serruys PW, Morice MC, Kappetein AP, et al. Percutaneous coronary intervention versus coronary-artery bypass grafting for severe coronary artery disease. N Engl J Med 2009;360: 961–72.
12. Farkouh ME, Domanski M, Sleeper LA, et al. Strategies for multivessel revascularization in patients with diabetes. N Engl J Med 2012;367:2375–84.
13. Kunadian V, Pugh A, Zaman AG, et al. Percutaneous coronary intervention among patients with left ventricular systolic dysfunction: a review and meta-analysis of 19 clinical studies. Coron Artery Dis 2012;23:469–79.
14. Bangalore S, Guo Y, Samadashvili Z, et al. Revascularization in patients with multivessel coronary artery disease and severe left ventricular systolic dysfunction: everolimus-eluting stents versus coronary artery bypass graft surgery. Circulation 2016; 133:2132–40.
15. Windecker S, Kolh P, Alfonso F, et al. 2014 ESC/EACTS guidelines on myocardial revascularization: the Task Force on Myocardial Revascularization of the European Society of Cardiology (ESC) and the European Association for Cardio-Thoracic Surgery (EACTS) developed with the special contribution of the European Association of Percutaneous Cardiovascular Interventions (EAPCI). Eur Heart J 2014;35:2541–619.
16. Fihn SD, Gardin JM, Abrams J, et al. 2012 ACCF/AHA/ACP/AATS/PCNA/SCAI/STS Guideline for the diagnosis and management of patients with stable ischemic heart disease: a report of the American College of Cardiology Foundation/American Heart Association Task Force on Practice Guidelines, and the American College of Physicians, American Association for Thoracic Surgery, Preventive

Cardiovascular Nurses Association, Society for Cardiovascular Angiography and Interventions, and Society of Thoracic Surgeons. J Am Coll Cardiol 2012;60:e44–164.
17. Harskamp RE, Puskas JD, Tijssen JG, et al. Comparison of hybrid coronary revascularization versus coronary artery bypass grafting in patients ≥65 years with multivessel coronary artery disease. Am J Cardiol 2014;114:224–9.
18. Harskamp RE, Bagai A, Halkos ME, et al. Clinical outcomes after hybrid coronary revascularization versus coronary artery bypass surgery: a meta-analysis of 1,190 patients. Am Heart J 2014;167:585–92.
19. Harskamp RE, Vassiliades TA, Mehta RH, et al. Comparative effectiveness of hybrid coronary revascularization vs coronary artery bypass grafting. J Am Coll Surg 2015;221:326–34.
20. Rosenblum JM, Harskamp RE, Hoedemaker N, et al. Hybrid coronary revascularization versus coronary artery bypass surgery with bilateral or single internal mammary artery grafts. J Thorac Cardiovasc Surg 2016;151:1081–9.
21. Gasior M, Zembala MO, Tajstra M, et al. Hybrid revascularization for multivessel coronary artery disease. JACC Cardiovasc Interv 2014;7:1277–83.
22. Puskas JD, Halkos ME, DeRose JJ, et al. Hybrid coronary revascularization for the treatment of multivessel coronary artery disease: a multicenter observational study. J Am Coll Cardiol 2016;68:356–65.
23. Perera D, Stables R, Thomas M, et al. Elective intra-aortic balloon counterpulsation during high-risk percutaneous coronary intervention: a randomized controlled trial. JAMA 2010;304:867–74.
24. Perera D, Stables R, Clayton T, et al. Long-term mortality data from the balloon pump-assisted coronary intervention study (BCIS-1): a randomized, controlled trial of elective balloon counterpulsation during high-risk percutaneous coronary intervention. Circulation 2013;127:207–12.
25. O'Neill WW, Kleiman NS, Moses J, et al. A prospective, randomized clinical trial of hemodynamic support with Impella 2.5 versus intra-aortic balloon pump in patients undergoing high-risk percutaneous coronary intervention: the PROTECT II study. Circulation 2012;126:1717–27.
26. Pershad A, Fraij G, Massaro JM, et al. Comparison of the use of hemodynamic support in patients ≥80 years versus patients <80 years during high-risk percutaneous coronary interventions (from the Multicenter PROTECT II Randomized Study). Am J Cardiol 2014;114:657–64.
27. NCT02468778 Coronary Interventions in High-risk Patients Using a Novel Percutaneous Left Ventricular Support Device (SHIELD II). ClinicalTrials.gov. 8-23-2016. 11-26-2016.
28. Kolte D, Khera S, Aronow WS, et al. Trends in incidence, management, and outcomes of cardiogenic shock complicating ST-elevation myocardial infarction in the United States. J Am Heart Assoc 2014;3:e000590.
29. Thiele H, Zeymer U, Neumann FJ, et al. Intraaortic balloon support for myocardial infarction with cardiogenic shock. N Engl J Med 2012;367:1287–96.
30. Thiele H, Zeymer U, Neumann FJ, et al. Intra-aortic balloon counterpulsation in acute myocardial infarction complicated by cardiogenic shock (IABP-SHOCK II): final 12 month results of a randomised, open-label trial. Lancet 2013;382:1638–45.
31. Thiele H, Sick P, Boudriot E, et al. Randomized comparison of intra-aortic balloon support with a percutaneous left ventricular assist device in patients with revascularized acute myocardial infarction complicated by cardiogenic shock. Eur Heart J 2005;26:1276–83.
32. Seyfarth M, Sibbing D, Bauer I, et al. A randomized clinical trial to evaluate the safety and efficacy of a percutaneous left ventricular assist device versus intra-aortic balloon pumping for treatment of cardiogenic shock caused by myocardial infarction. J Am Coll Cardiol 2008;52:1584–8.
33. Ouweneel DM, Eriksen E, Sjauw KD, et al. Impella CP versus intra-aortic balloon pump in acute myocardial infarction complicated by cardiogenic shock: the IMPRESS trial. J Am Coll Cardiol 2016; 69(3):278–87.
34. O'Neill WW, Schreiber T, Wohns DH, et al. The current use of Impella 2.5 in acute myocardial infarction complicated by cardiogenic shock: results from the USpella Registry. J Interv Cardiol 2014; 27:1–11.
35. Anderson MB, Goldstein J, Milano C, et al. Benefits of a novel percutaneous ventricular assist device for right heart failure: the prospective RECOVER RIGHT study of the Impella RP device. J Heart Lung Transplant 2015;34:1549–60.
36. Ross J Jr, Braunwald E. Aortic stenosis. Circulation 1968;38:61–7.
37. Bach DS, Siao D, Girard SE, et al. Evaluation of patients with severe symptomatic aortic stenosis who do not undergo aortic valve replacement: the potential role of subjectively overestimated operative risk. Circ Cardiovasc Qual Outcomes 2009;2:533–9.
38. Cribier A, Eltchaninoff H, Bash A, et al. Percutaneous transcatheter implantation of an aortic valve prosthesis for calcific aortic stenosis: first human case description. Circulation 2002;106:3006–8.
39. Leon MB, Smith CR, Mack M, et al. Transcatheter aortic-valve implantation for aortic stenosis in

patients who cannot undergo surgery. N Engl J Med 2010;363:1597–607.
40. Makkar RR, Fontana GP, Jilaihawi H, et al. Transcatheter aortic-valve replacement for inoperable severe aortic stenosis. N Engl J Med 2012;366: 1696–704.
41. Kapadia SR, Tuzcu EM, Makkar RR, et al. Long-term outcomes of inoperable patients with aortic stenosis randomly assigned to transcatheter aortic valve replacement or standard therapy. Circulation 2014;130:1483–92.
42. Kapadia SR, Leon MB, Makkar RR, et al. 5-year outcomes of transcatheter aortic valve replacement compared with standard treatment for patients with inoperable aortic stenosis (PARTNER 1): a randomised controlled trial. Lancet 2015; 385:2485–91.
43. Popma JJ, Adams DH, Reardon MJ, et al. Transcatheter aortic valve replacement using a self-expanding bioprosthesis in patients with severe aortic stenosis at extreme risk for surgery. J Am Coll Cardiol 2014;63:1972–81.
44. Yakubov SJ, Adams DH, Watson DR, et al. 2-year outcomes after iliofemoral self-expanding transcatheter aortic valve replacement in patients with severe aortic stenosis deemed extreme risk for surgery. J Am Coll Cardiol 2015;66:1327–34.
45. Webb JG, Doshi D, Mack MJ, et al. A randomized evaluation of the SAPIEN XT transcatheter heart valve system in patients with aortic stenosis who are not candidates for surgery. JACC Cardiovasc Interv 2015;8:1797–806.
46. Herrmann HC, Thourani VH, Kodali SK, et al. One-year clinical outcomes with SAPIEN 3 transcatheter aortic valve replacement in high-risk and inoperable patients with severe aortic stenosis. Circulation 2016;134:130–40.
47. Smith CR, Leon MB, Mack MJ, et al. Transcatheter versus surgical aortic-valve replacement in high-risk patients. N Engl J Med 2011;364: 2187–98.
48. Kodali SK, Williams MR, Smith CR, et al. Two-year outcomes after transcatheter or surgical aortic-valve replacement. N Engl J Med 2012;366: 1686–95.
49. Mack MJ, Leon MB, Smith CR, et al. 5-year outcomes of transcatheter aortic valve replacement or surgical aortic valve replacement for high surgical risk patients with aortic stenosis (PARTNER 1): a randomised controlled trial. Lancet 2015;385: 2477–84.
50. Adams DH, Popma JJ, Reardon MJ, et al. Transcatheter aortic-valve replacement with a self-expanding prosthesis. N Engl J Med 2014;370: 1790–8.
51. Reardon MJ, Adams DH, Kleiman NS, et al. 2-year outcomes in patients undergoing surgical or self-expanding transcatheter aortic valve replacement. J Am Coll Cardiol 2015;66:113–21.
52. Manoharan G, Walton AS, Brecker SJ, et al. Treatment of symptomatic severe aortic stenosis with a novel resheathable supra-annular self-expanding transcatheter aortic valve system. JACC Cardiovasc Interv 2015;8:1359–67.
53. Meredith IT, Walters DL, Dumonteil N, et al. 1-year outcomes with the fully repositionable and retrievable lotus transcatheter aortic replacement valve in 120 high-risk surgical patients with severe aortic stenosis: results of the REPRISE II study. JACC Cardiovasc Interv 2016;9:376–84.
54. D'Errigo P, Barbanti M, Ranucci M, et al. Transcatheter aortic valve implantation versus surgical aortic valve replacement for severe aortic stenosis: results from an intermediate risk propensity-matched population of the Italian OBSERVANT study. Int J Cardiol 2013;167:1945–52.
55. Leon MB, Smith CR, Mack MJ, et al. Transcatheter or surgical aortic-valve replacement in intermediate-risk patients. N Engl J Med 2016;374:1609–20.
56. Thourani VH, Kodali S, Makkar RR, et al. Transcatheter aortic valve replacement versus surgical valve replacement in intermediate-risk patients: a propensity score analysis. Lancet 2016;387: 2218–25.
57. Thyregod HG, Steinbruchel DA, Ihlemann N, et al. Transcatheter versus surgical aortic valve replacement in patients with severe aortic valve stenosis: 1-year results from the all-comers NOTION randomized clinical trial. J Am Coll Cardiol 2015;65: 2184–94.
58. Sondergaard L, Steinbruchel DA, Ihlemann N, et al. Two-year outcomes in patients with severe aortic valve stenosis randomized to transcatheter versus surgical aortic valve replacement: the all-comers Nordic Aortic Valve Intervention randomized clinical trial. Circ Cardiovasc Interv 2016;9(6):e003665.
59. NCT02675114 A Prospective, Randomized, Controlled, Multi-center Study to Establish the Safety and Effectiveness of the SAPIEN 3 Transcatheter Heart Valve in Low Risk Patients Requiring Aortic Valve Replacement Who Have Severe, Calcific, Symptomatic Aortic Stenosis. ClinicalTrials.gov. 5-26-2016. 11-23-2016.
60. NCT02701283 Transcatheter Aortic Valve Replacement with the Medtronic Transcatheter Aortic Valve Replacement System in Patients at Low Risk for Surgical Aortic Valve Replacement. ClinicalTrials.gov. 10-26-2016. 11-23-2016.
61. Trichon BH, Felker GM, Shaw LK, et al. Relation of frequency and severity of mitral regurgitation to survival among patients with left ventricular systolic dysfunction and heart failure. Am J Cardiol 2003; 91:538–43.

62. Goel SS, Bajaj N, Aggarwal B, et al. Prevalence and outcomes of unoperated patients with severe symptomatic mitral regurgitation and heart failure: comprehensive analysis to determine the potential role of MitraClip for this unmet need. J Am Coll Cardiol 2014;63:185–6.
63. Feldman T, Kar S, Rinaldi M, et al. Percutaneous mitral repair with the MitraClip system: safety and midterm durability in the initial EVEREST (Endovascular Valve Edge-to-Edge REpair Study) cohort. J Am Coll Cardiol 2009;54:686–94.
64. Franzen O, van der Heyden J, Baldus S, et al. MitraClip® therapy in patients with end-stage systolic heart failure. Eur J Heart Fail 2011;13:569–76.
65. Auricchio A, Schillinger W, Meyer S, et al. Correction of mitral regurgitation in nonresponders to cardiac resynchronization therapy by MitraClip improves symptoms and promotes reverse remodeling. J Am Coll Cardiol 2011;58:2183–9.
66. Taramasso M, Denti P, Buzzatti N, et al. Mitraclip therapy and surgical mitral repair in patients with moderate to severe left ventricular failure causing functional mitral regurgitation: a single-centre experience. Eur J Cardiothorac Surg 2012;42: 920–6.
67. Maisano F, Franzen O, Baldus S, et al. Percutaneous mitral valve interventions in the real world: early and 1-year results from the ACCESS-EU, a prospective, multicenter, nonrandomized post-approval study of the MitraClip therapy in Europe. J Am Coll Cardiol 2013;62:1052–61.
68. Armoiry X, Brochet E, Lefevre T, et al. Initial French experience of percutaneous mitral valve repair with the MitraClip: a multicentre national registry. Arch Cardiovasc Dis 2013;106:287–94.
69. Grasso C, Capodanno D, Scandura S, et al. One- and twelve-month safety and efficacy outcomes of patients undergoing edge-to-edge percutaneous mitral valve repair (from the GRASP Registry). Am J Cardiol 2013;111:1482–7.
70. Toggweiler S, Zuber M, Surder D, et al. Two-year outcomes after percutaneous mitral valve repair with the MitraClip system: durability of the procedure and predictors of outcome. Open Heart 2014;1: e000056.
71. Yeo KK, Yap J, Yamen E, et al. Percutaneous mitral valve repair with the MitraClip: early results from the MitraClip Asia-Pacific Registry (MARS). EuroIntervention 2014;10:620–5.
72. Taramasso M, Maisano F, Latib A, et al. Clinical outcomes of MitraClip for the treatment of functional mitral regurgitation. EuroIntervention 2014;10: 746–52.
73. Glower DD, Kar S, Trento A, et al. Percutaneous mitral valve repair for mitral regurgitation in high-risk patients: results of the EVEREST II study. J Am Coll Cardiol 2014;64:172–81.
74. Nickenig G, Estevez-Loureiro R, Franzen O, et al. Percutaneous mitral valve edge-to-edge repair: in-hospital results and 1-year follow-up of 628 patients of the 2011-2012 Pilot European Sentinel Registry. J Am Coll Cardiol 2014;64:875–84.
75. Lesevic H, Sonne C, Braun D, et al. Acute and midterm outcome after MitraClip therapy in patients with severe mitral regurgitation and left ventricular dysfunction. Am J Cardiol 2015;116: 749–56.
76. Puls M, Lubos E, Boekstegers P, et al. One-year outcomes and predictors of mortality after MitraClip therapy in contemporary clinical practice: results from the German transcatheter mitral valve interventions registry. Eur Heart J 2016;37:703–12.
77. Feldman T, Foster E, Glower DD, et al. Percutaneous repair or surgery for mitral regurgitation. N Engl J Med 2011;364:1395–406.
78. Mauri L, Foster E, Glower DD, et al. 4-year results of a randomized controlled trial of percutaneous repair versus surgery for mitral regurgitation. J Am Coll Cardiol 2013;62:317–28.
79. Feldman T, Kar S, Elmariah S, et al. Randomized comparison of percutaneous repair and surgery for mitral regurgitation: 5-year results of EVEREST II. J Am Coll Cardiol 2015;66:2844–54.
80. Conradi L, Treede H, Rudolph V, et al. Surgical or percutaneous mitral valve repair for secondary mitral regurgitation: comparison of patient characteristics and clinical outcomes. Eur J Cardiothorac Surg 2013;44:490–6.
81. NCT01626079 Cardiovascular Outcomes Assessment of the Mitraclip Percutaneous Therapy for Heart Failure Patients with Functional Mitral Regurgitation. ClinicalTrials.gov. 6-6-2016. 11-23-2016.
82. NCT02444338 A Randomized Study of the MitraClip Device in Heart Failure Patients with Clinically Significant Functional Mitral Regurgitation. ClinicalTrials.gov. 8-30-2016. 11-23-2016.
83. NCT02592889 MitraClip in Non-responders to Cardiac Resynchronization Therapy. ClinicalTrials.gov. 10-29-2015. 11-23-2016.
84. NCT01920698 Multicentre Randomized Study of Percutaneous Mitral Valve Repair MitraClip Device in Patients with Severe Secondary Mitral Regurgitation. ClinicalTrials.gov. 9-21-2015. 11-23-2016.
85. Lipiecki J, Siminiak T, Sievert H, et al. Coronary sinus-based percutaneous annuloplasty as treatment for functional mitral regurgitation: the TITAN II trial. Open Heart 2016;3:e000411.
86. Schofer J, Siminiak T, Haude M, et al. Percutaneous mitral annuloplasty for functional mitral regurgitation: results of the CARILLON Mitral Annuloplasty Device European Union Study. Circulation 2009;120:326–33.
87. Siminiak T, Wu JC, Haude M, et al. Treatment of functional mitral regurgitation by percutaneous

annuloplasty: results of the TITAN Trial. Eur J Heart Fail 2012;14:931–8.
88. NCT02325830 The REDUCE FMR Trial: Safety and Efficacy of the CARILLON Mitral Contour System® in Reducing Functional Mitral Regurgitation (FMR) Associated with Heart Failure. ClinicalTrials.gov. 10-13-2016. 11-25-2016.
89. Rogers JH, Thomas M, Morice MC, et al. Treatment of heart failure with associated functional mitral regurgitation using the ARTO system: initial results of the first-in-human MAVERIC trial (mitral valve repair clinical trial). JACC Cardiovasc Interv 2015; 8:1095–104.
90. Nickenig G, Schueler R, Dager A, et al. Treatment of chronic functional mitral valve regurgitation with a percutaneous annuloplasty system. J Am Coll Cardiol 2016;67:2927–36.
91. NCT01740583 A Feasibility Study of the Mitralign Annuloplasty System for the Treatment of Chronic Functional Mitral Valve Regurgitation. ClinicalTrials.gov. 10-13-2016. 11-25-2016.
92. NCT01899573 A Study of Percutaneous Left Ventricular Reshaping of Mitral Apparatus to Reduce Functional Mitral Regurgitation and Improve LV Function using the Accucinch® System. ClinicalTrials.gov. 10-21-2016. 11-25-2016.
93. NCT02153892 Feasibility of the AccuCinch® System for Left Ventricular Reshaping of the Mitral Apparatus to Reduce Functional Mitral Regurgitation and Improve Left Ventricular Function (LVRECOVER). ClinicalTrials.gov. 10-21-2016. 11-25-2016.
94. Maisano F, Taramasso M, Nickenig G, et al. Cardioband, a transcatheter surgical-like direct mitral valve annuloplasty system: early results of the feasibility trial. Eur Heart J 2016;37:817–25.
95. Nickenig G, Hammerstingl C, Schueler R, et al. Transcatheter mitral annuloplasty in chronic functional mitral regurgitation: 6-month results with the Cardioband percutaneous mitral repair system. JACC Cardiovasc Interv 2016;9:2039–47.
96. NCT02703311 REPAIR - Transcatheter Repair of Mitral Insufficiency with Cardioband System. ClinicalTrials.gov. 11-20-2016. 11-25-2016.
97. Ussia GP, Quadri A, Cammalleri V, et al. Percutaneous transfemoral-transseptal implantation of a second-generation CardiAQ mitral valve bioprosthesis: first procedure description and 30-day follow-up. EuroIntervention 2016;11:1126–31.
98. Cheung A, Webb J, Verheye S, et al. Short-term results of transapical transcatheter mitral valve implantation for mitral regurgitation. J Am Coll Cardiol 2014;64:1814–9.
99. Abdul-Jawad AO, Dumont E, Dagenais F, et al. Initial experience of transcatheter mitral valve replacement with a novel transcatheter mitral valve: procedural and 6 month follow up results. J Am Coll Cardiol 2015;66:1011–9.
100. Quarto C, Davies S, Duncan A, et al. Transcatheter mitral valve implantation: 30-day outcome of first-in-man experience with an apically tethered device. Innovations (Phila) 2016;11:174–8.
101. Topilsky Y, Nkomo VT, Vatury O, et al. Clinical outcome of isolated tricuspid regurgitation. JACC Cardiovasc Imaging 2014;7:1185–94.
102. O'Neill BP, O'Neill WW. Tricuspid valve intervention: new direction and new hope. J Am Coll Cardiol 2016;68:1034–6.
103. Rodes-Cabau J, Hahn RT, Latib A, et al. Transcatheter therapies for treating tricuspid regurgitation. J Am Coll Cardiol 2016;67:1829–45.
104. NCT02098200 Percutaneous Treatment of Tricuspid Valve Regurgitation with the TriCinch System™ (PREVENT). ClinicalTrials.gov. 7-24-2015. 11-27-2016.
105. NCT02339974 Heterotopic Implantation of the Edwards-Sapien XT Transcatheter Valve in the Inferior Vena Cava for the Treatment of Severe Tricuspid Regurgitation (HOVER). ClinicalTrials.gov. 1-6-2016. 11-27-2016.
106. NCT02387697 Treatment of Severe Secondary Tricuspid Regurgitation in Patients With Advance Heart Failure With Caval Vein Implantation of the Edwards Sapien XT Valve (TRICAVAL). ClinicalTrials.gov. 3-12-2015. 11-27-2016.
107. NCT02471807 Early Feasibility Study of the Edwards FORMA Tricuspid Transcatheter Repair System. ClinicalTrials.gov. 11-16-2016. 11-27-2016.
108. NCT02787408 Repair of Tricuspid Valve Regurgitation Using the Edwards Tricuspid Transcatheter Repair System (SPACER). ClinicalTrials.gov. 9-26-2016. 11-27-2016.
109. NCT02574650 Early Feasibility of the Mitralign Percutaneous Tricuspid Valve Annuloplasty System (PTVAS) Also Known as TriAlign™ (SCOUT). ClinicalTrials.gov. 8-17-2016. 11-27-2016.
110. Jategaonkar S, Scholtz W, Schmidt H, et al. Percutaneous closure of atrial septal defects: echocardiographic and functional results in patients older than 60 years. Circ Cardiovasc Interv 2009;2:85–9.
111. Nakagawa K, Akagi T, Taniguchi M, et al. Transcatheter closure of atrial septal defect in a geriatric population. Catheter Cardiovasc Interv 2012;80: 84–90.
112. Thilen M, Christersson C, Dellborg M, et al. Catheter closure of atrial septal defect in the elderly (≥65 years). A worthwhile procedure. Int J Cardiol 2016;218:25–30.
113. Takaya Y, Akagi T, Kijima Y, et al. Long-term outcome after transcatheter closure of atrial septal defect in older patients: impact of age at procedure. JACC Cardiovasc Interv 2015;8:600–6.
114. Sorajja P, Cabalka AK, Hagler DJ, et al. Long-term follow-up of percutaneous repair of paravalvular

prosthetic regurgitation. J Am Coll Cardiol 2011;58: 2218–24.

115. Angulo-Llanos R, Sarnago-Cebada F, Rivera AR, et al. Two-year follow up after surgical versus percutaneous paravalvular leak closure: a non-randomized analysis. Catheter Cardiovasc Interv 2016;88:626–34.
116. Calvert PA, Northridge DB, Malik IS, et al. Percutaneous device closure of paravalvular leak: combined experience from the United Kingdom and Ireland. Circulation 2016;134:934–44.
117. Dharmarajan K, Chaudhry SI. New approaches to reduce readmissions in patients with heart failure. JAMA Intern Med 2016;176:318–20.
118. Adamson PB, Magalski A, Braunschweig F, et al. Ongoing right ventricular hemodynamics in heart failure: clinical value of measurements derived from an implantable monitoring system. J Am Coll Cardiol 2003;41:565–71.
119. Bourge RC, Abraham WT, Adamson PB, et al. Randomized controlled trial of an implantable continuous hemodynamic monitor in patients with advanced heart failure: the COMPASS-HF study. J Am Coll Cardiol 2008;51:1073–9.
120. U.S. Food and Drug Administration. Circulatory System Devices Panel - March 1, 2007. Rockville (MD): US Food and Drug Administration; 2015.
121. Ritzema J, Melton IC, Richards AM, et al. Direct left atrial pressure monitoring in ambulatory heart failure patients: initial experience with a new permanent implantable device. Circulation 2007;116: 2952–9.
122. Ritzema J, Troughton R, Melton I, et al. Physician-directed patient self-management of left atrial pressure in advanced chronic heart failure. Circulation 2010;121:1086–95.
123. Abraham WT, Adamson PB, Costanzo MR, et al. Hemodynamic Monitoring in Advanced Heart Failure: Results from the LAPTOP-HF Trial. J Card Fail 2016;22:940.
124. Abraham WT, Adamson PB, Bourge RC, et al. Wireless pulmonary artery haemodynamic monitoring in chronic heart failure: a randomised controlled trial. Lancet 2011;377:658–66.
125. Adamson PB, Abraham WT, Bourge RC, et al. Wireless pulmonary artery pressure monitoring guides management to reduce decompensation in heart failure with preserved ejection fraction. Circ Heart Fail 2014;7:935–44.
126. Ponikowski P, Voors AA, Anker SD, et al. 2016 ESC guidelines for the diagnosis and treatment of acute and chronic heart failure: the task force for the diagnosis and treatment of acute and chronic heart failure of the European Society of Cardiology (ESC). Developed with the special contribution of the Heart Failure Association (HFA) of the ESC. Eur Heart J 2016;37:2129–200.
127. Hasenfuss G, Hayward C, Burkhoff D, et al. A transcatheter intracardiac shunt device for heart failure with preserved ejection fraction (REDUCE LAP-HF): a multicentre, open-label, single-arm, phase 1 trial. Lancet 2016;387:1298–304.
128. Kaye DM, Hasenfuss G, Neuzil P, et al. One-year outcomes after transcatheter insertion of an interatrial shunt device for the management of heart failure with preserved ejection fraction. Circ Heart Fail 2016;9.
129. Feldman T, Komtebedde J, Burkhoff D, et al. Transcatheter interatrial shunt device for the treatment of heart failure: rationale and design of the randomized trial to REDUCE elevated left atrial pressure in heart failure (REDUCE LAP-HF I). Circ Heart Fail 2016;9:e003025.
130. NCT02511912 Reducing Lung Congestion Symptoms Using the V-wave Shunt in Advanced Heart Failure (RELIEVE-HF). ClinicalTrials.gov. 7-27-2015. 12-3-2016.
131. Jones RH, Velazquez EJ, Michler RE, et al. Coronary bypass surgery with or without surgical ventricular reconstruction. N Engl J Med 2009;360: 1705–17.
132. Buckberg GD, Athanasuleas CL. The STICH trial: misguided conclusions. J Thorac Cardiovasc Surg 2009;138:1060–4.
133. Conte J. An indictment of the STICH trial: "True, true, and unrelated". J Heart Lung Transplant 2010;29:491–6.
134. Mazzaferri EL Jr, Gradinac S, Sagic D, et al. Percutaneous left ventricular partitioning in patients with chronic heart failure and a prior anterior myocardial infarction: results of the PercutAneous Ventricular RestorAtion in Chronic Heart failUre PaTiEnts Trial. Am Heart J 2012;163:812–20.
135. Costa MA, Mazzaferri EL Jr, Sievert H, et al. Percutaneous ventricular restoration using the parachute device in patients with ischemic heart failure: three-year outcomes of the PARACHUTE first-in-human study. Circ Heart Fail 2014;7:752–8.
136. Thomas M, Nienaber CA, Ince H, et al. Percutaneous ventricular restoration (PVR) therapy using the Parachute device in 100 subjects with ischaemic dilated heart failure: one-year primary endpoint results of PARACHUTE III, a European trial. EuroIntervention 2015;11:710–7.
137. Costa MA, Pencina M, Nikolic S, et al. The parachute IV trial design and rationale: percutaneous ventricular restoration using the parachute device in patients with ischemic heart failure and dilated left ventricles. Am Heart J 2013;165: 531–6.
138. Torre-Amione G, Alo K, Estep JD, et al. Spinal cord stimulation is safe and feasible in patients with advanced heart failure: early clinical experience. Eur J Heart Fail 2014;16:788–95.

139. Tse HF, Turner S, Sanders P, et al. Thoracic Spinal Cord Stimulation for Heart Failure as a Restorative Treatment (SCS HEART study): first-in-man experience. Heart Rhythm 2015;12:588–95.
140. Zipes DP, Neuzil P, Theres H, et al. Determining the feasibility of spinal cord neuromodulation for the treatment of chronic systolic heart failure: the DEFEAT-HF study. JACC Heart Fail 2016;4:129–36.
141. De Ferrari GM, Crijns HJ, Borggrefe M, et al. Chronic vagus nerve stimulation: a new and promising therapeutic approach for chronic heart failure. Eur Heart J 2011;32:847–55.
142. Premchand RK, Sharma K, Mittal S, et al. Autonomic regulation therapy via left or right cervical vagus nerve stimulation in patients with chronic heart failure: results of the ANTHEM-HF trial. J Card Fail 2014;20:808–16.
143. Zannad F, De Ferrari GM, Tuinenburg AE, et al. Chronic vagal stimulation for the treatment of low ejection fraction heart failure: results of the Neural Cardiac Therapy for Heart Failure (NECTAR-HF) randomized controlled trial. Eur Heart J 2015;36:425–33.
144. NCT02113033 Vagal Nerve Stimulation: Safeguarding Heart Failure Patients (VANGUARD). ClinicalTrials.gov. 7-16-2015. 12-6-2016.
145. NCT02545582 VITARIA Registry Study. ClinicalTrials.gov. 3-11-2016. 12-6-2016.
146. Gronda E, Seravalle G, Brambilla G, et al. Chronic baroreflex activation effects on sympathetic nerve traffic, baroreflex function, and cardiac haemodynamics in heart failure: a proof-of-concept study. Eur J Heart Fail 2014;16:977–83.
147. Abraham WT, Zile MR, Weaver FA, et al. Baroreflex activation therapy for the treatment of heart failure with a reduced ejection fraction. JACC Heart Fail 2015;3:487–96.
148. NCT00718939 Rheos® Diastolic Heart Failure Trial. ClinicalTrials.gov. 10-19-2016. 12-6-2016.
149. Davies JE, Manisty CH, Petraco R, et al. First-in-man safety evaluation of renal denervation for chronic systolic heart failure: primary outcome from REACH-Pilot study. Int J Cardiol 2013;162:189–92.
150. NCT01639378 Renal Artery Denervation in Chronic Heart Failure Study (REACH). ClinicalTrials.gov. 11-10-2016. 12-6-2016.
151. Verloop WL, Beeftink MM, Nap A, et al. Renal denervation in heart failure with normal left ventricular ejection fraction. Rationale and design of the DIASTOLE (Denervation of the Renal Sympathetic nerves in Heart Failure with Normal LV Ejection Fraction) trial. Eur J Heart Fail 2013;15:1429–37.
152. NCT02085668 Renal Denervation in Patients With Chronic Heart Failure. ClinicalTrials.gov. 3-17-2014. 12-6-2016.
153. NCT02041130 Renal Denervation in Heart Failure Patients With Preserved Ejection Fraction (RESPECT-HF). ClinicalTrials.gov. 1-15-2015. 12-6-2016.
154. NCT01840059 Renal Denervation in Heart Failure With Preserved Ejection Fraction (RDT-PEF). ClinicalTrials.gov. 9-14-2015. 12-6-2016.
155. NCT02471729 Effect at 6 Months of Renal Denervation in Chronic Heart Failure d'Insuffisance Cardiaque (DENRENIC). ClinicalTrials.gov. 10-18-2016. 12-6-2016.
156. NCT02638324 Supportive Treatment of Severe Heart Failure by Renal Denervation (Heart-RND). ClinicalTrials.gov. 12-17-2015. 12-6-2016.
157. Kuo WT, Banerjee A, Kim PS, et al. Pulmonary embolism response to fragmentation, embolectomy, and catheter thrombolysis (PERFECT): Initial results from a prospective multicenter registry. Chest 2015;148:667–73.
158. Bajaj NS, Kalra R, Arora P, et al. Catheter-directed treatment for acute pulmonary embolism: systematic review and single-arm meta-analyses. Int J Cardiol 2016;225:128–39.
159. Kucher N, Boekstegers P, Muller OJ, et al. Randomized, controlled trial of ultrasound-assisted catheter-directed thrombolysis for acute intermediate-risk pulmonary embolism. Circulation 2014;129:479–86.
160. Piazza G, Hohlfelder B, Jaff MR, et al. A prospective, single-arm, multicenter trial of ultrasound-facilitated, catheter-directed, low-dose fibrinolysis for acute massive and submassive pulmonary embolism: the SEATTLE II study. JACC Cardiovasc Interv 2015;8:1382–92.

Surgical Revascularization in Older Adults with Ischemic Cardiomyopathy

Sahil Khera, MD, MPH, Julio A. Panza, MD*

KEYWORDS

• Coronary artery bypass graft • Revascularization • Cardiomyopathy • Left ventricular dysfunction

KEY POINTS

- With the totality of data supporting coronary artery bypass graft (CABG) for mortality benefit, symptomatic angina, and quality of life improvement, the authors subscribe to the concept that CABG should be a class I indication for patients with ischemic cardiomyopathy and severe left ventricular (LV) dysfunction.
- As the population ages and more patients are referred for CABG, however, a careful risk-benefit assessment should be an important part of the consideration regarding revascularization strategies.
- A heart team approach in consultation with a referring cardiologist, interventional cardiologist, and a cardiothoracic surgeon is critical to arrive at the best decision for each patient.
- The underlying substrate, clinical judgment, coronary anatomy, functional status, end-of-life issues, and patient preferences must all be considered as part of the decision-making process.
- Age, alone, should not be a contraindication because there are data to support a reduction in cardiovascular mortality with CABG in older patients.

Coronary artery disease affects a substantial portion of the population and dictates short-term, medium-term, and long-term morbidity and mortality. According to the 2016 American Heart Association heart disease and stroke statistics update, coronary artery disease accounted for 1 in 7 deaths in the United States in 2013 with an American suffering a coronary event every 34 seconds.[1] There has been a paradigm shift in the presentation and mode of death of coronary artery disease in the past 2 decades. The rapid recognition of acute coronary syndromes and increased availability and utilization of percutaneous coronary interventions coupled with excellent secondary preventive pharmacotherapies have led to a shift from sudden cardiac death and early in-hospital mortality to longer survival.[2–5] The longer survival, however, translates into a substantial proportion of the population living with heart failure due to scarred myocardium or myocardium with poor contractile reserve and LV dilatation and remodeling. One in 5 survivors of first myocardial infarction develops heart failure within 5 years of the initial presentation.[6]

Currently, 6 million Americans are living with heart failure and the prevalence is projected to increase by 46% from 2012 to 2030.[1,7] The etiology of heart failure in the United States has shifted in

Division of Cardiology, Department of Medicine, Westchester Medical Center, New York Medical College, 100 Woods Road, Valhalla, NY 10595, USA
* Corresponding author. Division of Cardiology, Westchester Medical Center, 100 Woods Road, Macy Pavilion, Room 102, Valhalla, NY 10595.
E-mail address: Julio.panza@wmchealth.org

Heart Failure Clin 13 (2017) 571–580
http://dx.doi.org/10.1016/j.hfc.2017.02.010
1551-7136/17/

recent years, with 60% to 62% of patients with LV systolic dysfunction diagnosed with coronary artery disease as the likely etiology.[8,9] Heart failure due to ischemic heart disease portends a poorer prognosis compared with systolic dysfunction due to nonischemic etiologies.[10] Aging is associated with an increased risk of coronary artery disease (22.8% of men and 13.9% of women aged 60–79 years and 35.5% of men and 20.8% of women aged 80 years) and an increase in incident heart failure (which doubles with every 10-year increase in men 65–85 years of age and triples for women aged 65–74 and 75–84 years).[1,11,12] Aging is not only a risk factor for coronary artery events and heart failure but also a risk factor for increased morbidity and mortality post–surgical revascularization due to increased frailty, comorbidities, and poorer functional status.[13] Elderly patients with multivessel coronary artery disease and low ejection fraction (EF) with LV dilatation present a challenge to both referring physicians and the operating surgeons.

ISCHEMIC CARDIOMYOPATHY

Although Raftery and colleagues[14] described the causal relationship between coronary artery disease and congestive cardiomyopathy in 1969, it was Burch and coworkers[15] who introduced the term "ischemic cardiomyopathy" a year later. Ischemic cardiomyopathy is defined by LV systolic dysfunction with EF less than or equal to 40% in the setting of coronary artery disease. Despite the inconsistencies and variability in the definitions of ischemic cardiomyopathy in the past, the authors believe that physician judgment in assessing severity of coronary artery disease is paramount.[10,16] In particular, attention should be paid to the extent of coronary artery disease, regional wall motion abnormalities, and exclusion of alternative etiologies of LV systolic dysfunction. The diagnosis of ischemic cardiomyopathy not only provides prognostic information but also helps guide therapy, especially surgical revascularization, which is not a consideration in nonischemic etiologies of dilated cardiomyopathy.

Balancing the potential benefits of surgical revascularization to the risks of increased operative and postoperative mortality in elderly patients with low EF and multiple comorbidities poses unique challenges to caregivers. Availability of multivessel percutaneous coronary interventions, which is a viable option in surgically high or prohibitive risk patients, often offers a lower-risk partial revascularization strategy that may be considered by patients and physicians alike. Hence, deciding the appropriate revascularization strategy in a background of goal-directed medical and device therapies for a particular patient is imperative. In this article, based on contemporary data from the Surgical Treatment for Ischemic Heart Failure (STICH) trial, the authors emphasize the rationale and simplify patient selection for surgical revascularization in elderly patients with ischemic cardiomyopathy.[17]

RATIONALE FOR REVASCULARIZATION

Myocardial scarring and fibrosis after myocyte cell death are central to the development of ischemic cardiomyopathy. Myocardial scarring leads to adverse ventricular remodeling, cavity dilatation, papillary muscle malalignment, and secondary mitral regurgitation. The chronic volume overload sets a vicious cycle by worsening LV geometry, impairing pump function, and accelerating mitral regurgitation. Most of the LV remodeling occurs due to scarring and fibrosis, but chronic hibernating myocardium (adaptive changes secondary to chronic ischemia that lead to loss in contractile proteins and lower oxygen demands of the myocardial tissue) can induce molecular and structural changes, which are reversible with successful revascularization.[18–22] The target for revascularization, however, are these reversible forms of myocardial dysfunction that render the myocardium hypocontractile but viable and are frequently present in patients with ischemic cardiomyopathy.[23] The substrate for ischemic cardiomyopathy is extremely heterogeneous with normal, stunned, hibernating, and scarred myocardium coexisting simultaneously not only in a patient but also in a cross-section of myocardial tissue. Many imaging modalities have been used to prospectively quantify the extent of viable hibernating myocardium and guide patient selection, including using single-photon emission CT (SPECT), dobutamine stress echocardiography, cardiac magnetic resonance, and PET, but there is no single best imaging modality that accurately guides patient selection due to this heterogeneous substrate.[24]

Improvement in global and regional LVEF has been reported after revascularization of viable but hypocontractile myocardium in numerous studies and provides the rationale for offering revascularization on top of maximally tolerated guideline-recommended medical therapy.[25,26] Hibernating myocardium, viability studies, and revascularization have been the areas of intense basic, translation, and clinical research in the field of ischemic cardiomyopathy, but there remain controversies in appropriate patient selection for surgical revascularization of ischemic cardiomyopathy.

CORONARY ARTERY BYPASS GRAFT SURGERY — THE PRE "SURGICAL TREATMENT FOR ISCHEMIC HEART FAILURE TRIAL" ERA

CABG surgery remains the most commonly performed cardiac surgery worldwide.[27,28] Three major trials and subsequent meta-analyses established the long-term mortality benefits of CABG (vs medical therapy alone) in the management of multivessel coronary artery disease. These 3 trials, of historic importance, were the Veterans Administration Cooperative Study (1972–1974), European Coronary Artery Surgery Study (1973–1976), and the Coronary Artery Surgery Study (1975–1979).[29–33]

There are important setbacks in using the results of these trials for the contemporary management of ischemic cardiomyopathy in older patients—none of the trials included patients greater than 65 years of age, female gender was under-represented (<10% in the Coronary Artery Surgery Study and none in the Veterans Administration Cooperative Study or European Coronary Artery Surgery Study), none of them included patients with severe LV dysfunction (EF <36%), the utilization of a background medical therapy considered suboptimal in contemporary medicine (lack of use of aspirin, statins, cardioselective β-blockers, angiotensin-converting enzyme inhibitors, and aldosterone receptor antagonists in the 1970s). Saphenous venous grafts were the conduits of choice in the United States in the 1970s and none of these trials looked specifically at the internal mammary artery conduits, which are associated with a clear survival benefit.[27,34,35]

Despite the reduced generalizability of these 3 trials to patients with ischemic cardiomyopathy, there were signs of survival benefits associated with CABG in patients with ischemic cardiomyopathy from the CASS registry. The registry included 651 patients (excluded from the main trial) with severe LV dysfunction and LVEF less than or equal to 35% (420 medically managed and 231 surgically managed). At 5-year follow-up, survival was the greatest for patients with EF less than 26% when treated surgically (43% survival with medical treatment vs 63% survival with surgery, $P<.05$). Patients with predominantly anginal symptoms benefited the most.[36] Data from Duke University Medical Center's[37] 25-year single-center experience also confirmed the long-term survival benefit of CABG versus medical therapy in patients with New York Heart Association class greater than or equal to II, 1 or more epicardial coronary vessels with a greater than or equal to 75% stenosis, and LVEF less than 40%.

More recently, the Bypass Angioplasty Revascularization Investigation 2 Diabetes (BARI 2D) and Clinical Outcomes Utilizing Revascularization and Aggressive Drug Evaluation (COURAGE) trials showed no clear survival benefits of revascularization (CABG or percutaneous coronary intervention in BARI-2D and percutaneous coronary intervention in COURAGE) compared with the contemporary medical management.[38,39] Again, none of these studies focused on patients with ischemic cardiomyopathy and severely reduced LV function (BARI-2D mean EF 57.2 ± 11.0% and COURAGE excluded EF <30%). As a result of the paucity of information form properly conducted clinical trials, most patients with ischemic cardiomyopathy were managed based solely on physician and patient preferences. The STICH trial was undertaken primarily to address that knowledge gap.[17]

SURGICAL TREATMENT FOR ISCHEMIC HEART FAILURE TRIAL

The STICH trial was a multicenter nonblinded randomized controlled trial sponsored by the National Heart, Lung, and Blood Institute. The trial had 2 major hypotheses: hypothesis 1—role of surgical revascularization in patients with ischemic cardiomyopathy and hypothesis 2 —role of surgical ventricular reconstruction in patients with ischemic cardiomyopathy. This article does not discuss ventricular reconstruction. The hypothesis 1 of the trial compared CABG plus background guideline–directed medical therapy with medical therapy alone in patients with ischemic cardiomyopathy and LVEF less than or equal to 35%.[17] The trial randomized 1212 patients to either CABG plus medical therapy (610 patients) or medical therapy alone (602 patients). Median age of the CABG arm was 60 years and 12% of patients in either arm were women. The design of the trial allowed for up to a 20% rate of crossovers (to mirror a real-world scenario) and 17% of patients in the medical therapy arm underwent CABG because of progressive symptoms, acute decompensation, or family/physician decision after randomization. The medical adherence throughout the trial was excellent (>85% were on β-blocker, statin, or angiotensin-converting enzyme inhibitor/angiotensin receptor blocker at the latest follow-up in either arm). At least 1 arterial graft was used in 91% of patients who underwent CABG compared with 9.9% of patients in the earlier CABG trials.[40] Final follow-up data at median 56 months (range 12–100 months) was available for 99.6% of patients.[17]

The recently published STICH Extension Study provided data on long-term follow-up (median 9.8 years, range 3.5 years–13.4 years) on 97.9% or patients initially enrolled in the STICH trial.[41] All-cause death (primary outcome) was seen in 58.9% of patients in the CABG plus medical therapy arm compared with 66.1% in the medical therapy group on long-term follow-up—a statistically significant 16% decrease in rate of all-cause mortality over 10 years in the CABG group (**Fig. 1**). Ischemic cardiomyopathy has extremely poor prognosis with 62.5% of the entire study cohort dead at a 9.8-year median follow-up despite background goal-directed medical therapy.[41] The STICH Extension Study established the mortality benefits of CABG plus medical therapy over medical therapy in patients with ischemic cardiomyopathy. A STICH substudy also reported better Kansas City Cardiomyopathy Questionnaire scores at 36 months in the CABG plus medical therapy group (vs medical therapy alone group), establishing benefits beyond mortality and a better quality of life with CABG.[42] With the higher short-term risks of surgical revascularization, appropriate patient selection and identifying the subset of patients who will benefit the most is the key.

PATIENT SELECTION —VIABILITY, ISCHEMIA, ANGINA, OR ANATOMY?

Chronic ischemic insults may render the myocardium to a quiescent state of chronic systolic dysfunction with preserved cellular viability (hibernating myocardium) through the loss of contractile proteins. These are adaptive changes to decrease myocardial oxygen demand in the context of decreased supply. As discussed previously, myocardial viability is an area of intense interest in the field of coronary revascularization. Multiple older studies have reported the utilization of viability detection as a means of preoperative stratification and identifying patients who will benefit the most from revascularization.[43–49] The STICH viability substudy reported the effects of myocardial viability (assessed using dobutamine stress echocardiography and SPECT) on outcomes at a 5.1-year follow-up.[50] Patients with demonstrable myocardial viability (irrespective of treatment arm) were more likely to survive at the end of follow-up on univariate analysis (37% vs 51%; odds ratio [OR] 0.64; 95% CI, 0.48–0.86; P = .003). This benefit was no longer statistically significant after multivariable adjustment for significant prognostic variables. Myocardial viability was also associated with reduced cardiovascular mortality. There was no significant interaction, however, between the treatment effect of CABG and the presence or absence of myocardial viability on all-cause mortality or cardiovascular mortality. In other words, the presence of myocardial viability did not accurately identify those patients more likely to benefit from surgical revascularization. Viability testing was optional during the enrollment of patients and only half of the entire cohort underwent the test. In addition, neither MRI nor PET was used for the assessment of myocardial viability in this trial due to the general lack of availability of these modalities in the recruiting sites. These limitations notwithstanding, the utility of routine myocardial viability assessment to identify patients who will derive maximal benefits from surgical revascularization is seriously questioned by these findings.

In a retrospective observation series of more than 13,000 patients who underwent adenosine or exercise stress SPECT myocardial perfusion scintigraphy, patients with extensive ischemia and less scar were more likely to benefit from early revascularization on long term follow-up.[51] The STICH ischemia substudy was designed to test the hypothesis that a similar extends to patients with ischemic cardiomyopathy.[52] From the STICH trial, 399 patients underwent stress testing (197 CABG plus medical therapy arm and 202 medical therapy alone arm); 64% of them had inducible myocardial ischemia during stress testing. Patients with and without ischemia were well balanced in terms of age, multivessel coronary artery disease, LVEF, prior myocardial infarction, and treatment arm. Surprisingly, there were no differences in all-cause mortality, cardiovascular mortality, or death plus cardiovascular hospitalization rate between the 2 subgroups. The study also demonstrated no significant benefits of CABG plus medical therapy over medical therapy alone based on presence of myocardial ischemia. The study suffered from limitations like small sample size, lack of scar quantification, and optional use of ischemia testing during trial randomization but provided useful, albeit negative, prospective data on the current utility of basing patients selection entirely on myocardial ischemia.

Angina is commonly reported by patients with coronary artery disease and denotes viable tissue that is at risk of infarction.[53] Guidelines recommend revascularization in stable ischemic heart disease for patients with persistent anginal symptoms despite maximal medical therapy. Whether this translates to benefits of CABG in patients with ischemic cardiomyopathy or identifying a subset of patients who will benefit from CABG was largely unknown. The STICH angina substudy reported data on all 1212 patients enrolled in the main STICH trial (63.5% with angina, majority

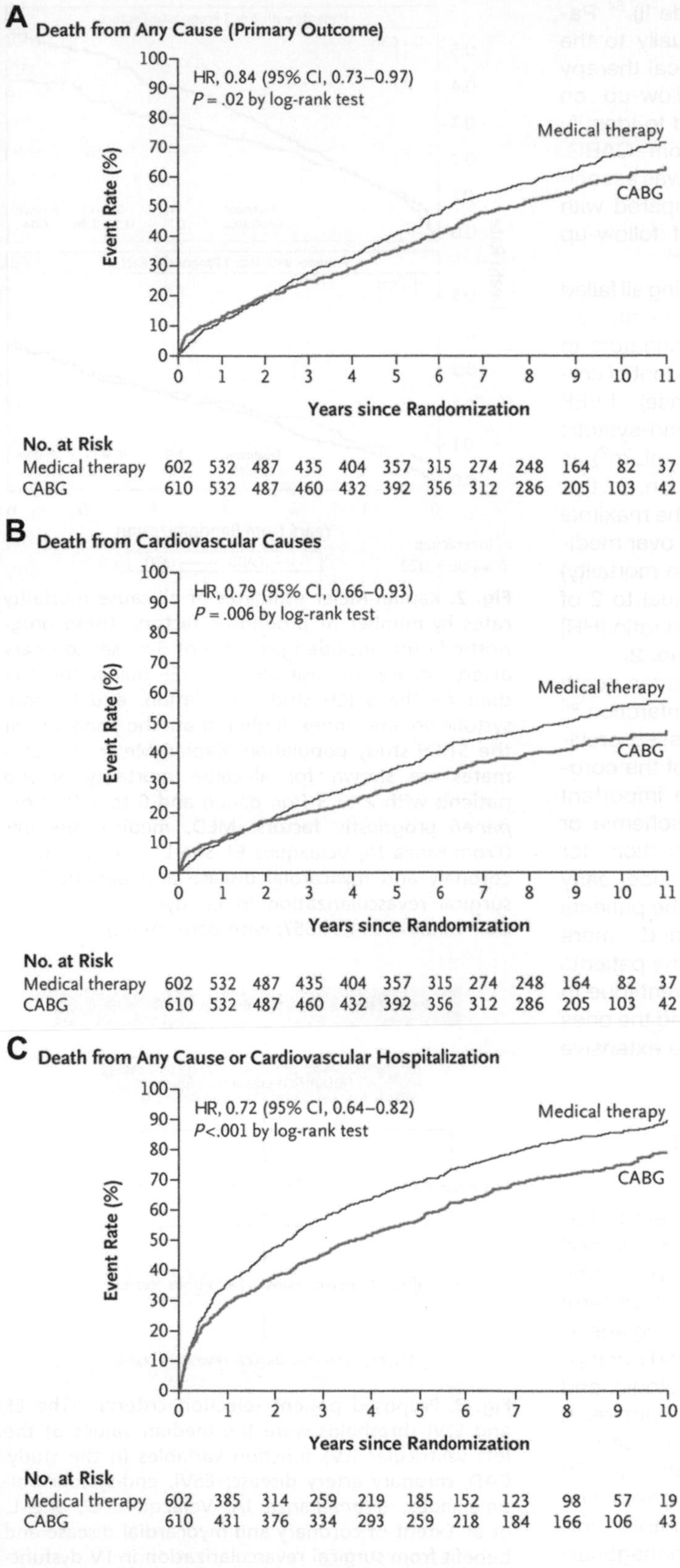

Fig. 1. Kaplan-Meier estimates of the rates of death from any cause (*A*), death from cardiovascular causes (*B*), and death from any cause or hospitalization for cardiovascular causes (*C*). (*From* Velazquez EJ, Lee KL, Jones RH, et al. Coronary-artery bypass surgery in patients with ischemic cardiomyopathy. N Engl J Med 2016;374:1517; with permission.)

Canadian Cardiovascular Society grade II).[54] Patients with angina were assigned equally to the CABG plus medical therapy and medical therapy alone groups. After 56 months' follow-up on 99.6% of patients, angina per se failed to identify patients who benefited the most from CABG. CABG plus medical therapy, however, was associated with improvement in angina compared with medical therapy alone at the end of follow-up (OR 0.70; 95% CI, 0.55–0.90; $P< .01$).[54]

Myocardial viability and ischemia testing all failed to guide patient selection for CABG in ischemic cardiomyopathy. This led the STICH investigators to consider poor anatomic variables like extent of coronary artery disease (3-vessel disease), LVEF (below the median of 27%), and LV end-systolic volume index (above the median of 79 mL/m^2) as potential tools to guide patient selection. In this landmark study, patients who derived the maximal benefits of CABG plus medical therapy over medical therapy alone (in terms of all-cause mortality) were the ones with greater than or equal to 2 of those poor prognostic variables (hazard ratio [HR] 0.71; 95% CI, 0.56–0.89; $P = .004$)[55] (**Fig. 2**).

CABG has been shown to reduce sudden death and death due to recurrent myocardial infarction.[56] The conjunction of the findings, discussed previously, indicates that anatomic extent of the coronary and myocardial disease is more important than physiologic variables, such as ischemia or viability, in appropriate patient selection for CABG in ischemic cardiomyopathy. Hence, early revascularization should be offered to the patients with worse anatomic variables and more advanced disease because those are the patients more likely to have another coronary event (due to the more extensive vascular disease) and the ones less likely to survive it (due to the more extensive myocardial disease) (**Fig. 3**).

CORONARY ARTERY BYPASS GRAFT SURGERY AND AGE

CABG is associated with mortality benefit in patients with ischemic cardiomyopathy as supported by data from the STICH trial and STICH Extension Study. There is greater risk, however, of short-term mortality associated with CABG. Increasing age itself is a risk factor for 30-day mortality and postoperative complications (respiratory, neurologic, and renal) after CABG.[13,57–59] Age, along with renal dysfunction, LV size, atrial fibrillation, and cardiopulmonary bypass time, was a predictor of 30-day mortality in the STICH trial.[60] High-volume surgical centers have reported favorable outcomes for CABG in octogenarian and nonagenarians.[61] A recent analysis of the STICH Extension

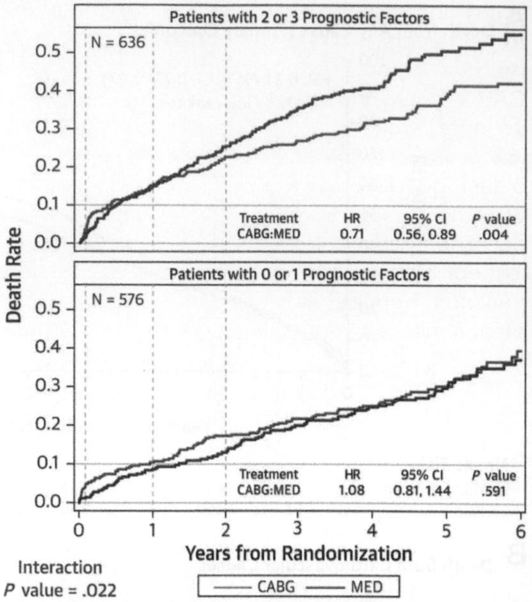

Fig. 2. Kaplan-Meier estimates of all-cause mortality rates by number of prognostic factors. These prognostic factors included presence of 3-vessel coronary artery disease (stenosis >50%), LVEF below the median for the STICH study population, and LV end-systolic volume index higher than the median for the STICH study population. Kaplan-Meier rate estimates are shown for all-cause mortality among patients with 2 to 3 (*top panel*) and 0 to 1 (*bottom panel*) prognostic factors. MED, medical therapy. (*From* Panza JA, Velazquez EJ, She L, et al. Extent of coronary and myocardial disease and benefit from surgical revascularization in LV dysfunction. J Am Coll Cardiol 2014;64:557; with permission.)

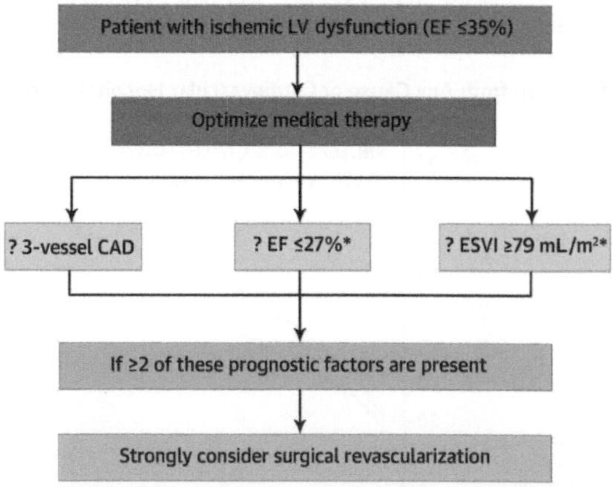

Fig. 3. Proposed patient selection criteria. *The EF and ESVI thresholds were the median values of the left ventricular (LV) function variables in the study. CAD, coronary artery disease; ESVI, end-systolic volume index. (*From* Panza JA, Velazquez EJ, She L, et al. Extent of coronary and myocardial disease and benefit from surgical revascularization in LV dysfunction. J Am Coll Cardiol 2014;64:560; with permission.)

Study according to age quartiles (≤54 years, >54 to ≤60 years, >60 to ≤67 years, and >67 years) reported increased all-cause mortality after CABG in the oldest quartile compared with the youngest quartile at median 9.8 years follow-up (68% vs 48%, $P<.001$).[62] In the youngest and oldest quartile, mean EF was 28%, and there were no differences in number of conduits used, baseline device therapy, or medication use (except higher warfarin and thiazide use in older patients). Perioperative complications (new-onset atrial fibrillation, worsening renal impairment, and inotrope utilization) were higher in the oldest quartile.

More importantly, this article explored the effects of age on the outcomes of CABG. In this analysis, surgical revascularization was associated with a reduction in all-cause mortality in the younger quartile but not in oldest quartile (HR 0.66; 95% CI, 0.49–0.89 in ≤54 years vs HR 0.82; 95% CI, 0.63–1.06 in >67 years). CABG plus medical therapy (vs medical therapy alone), however, reduced cardiovascular mortality consistently across all age quartiles (HR 0.61; 95%

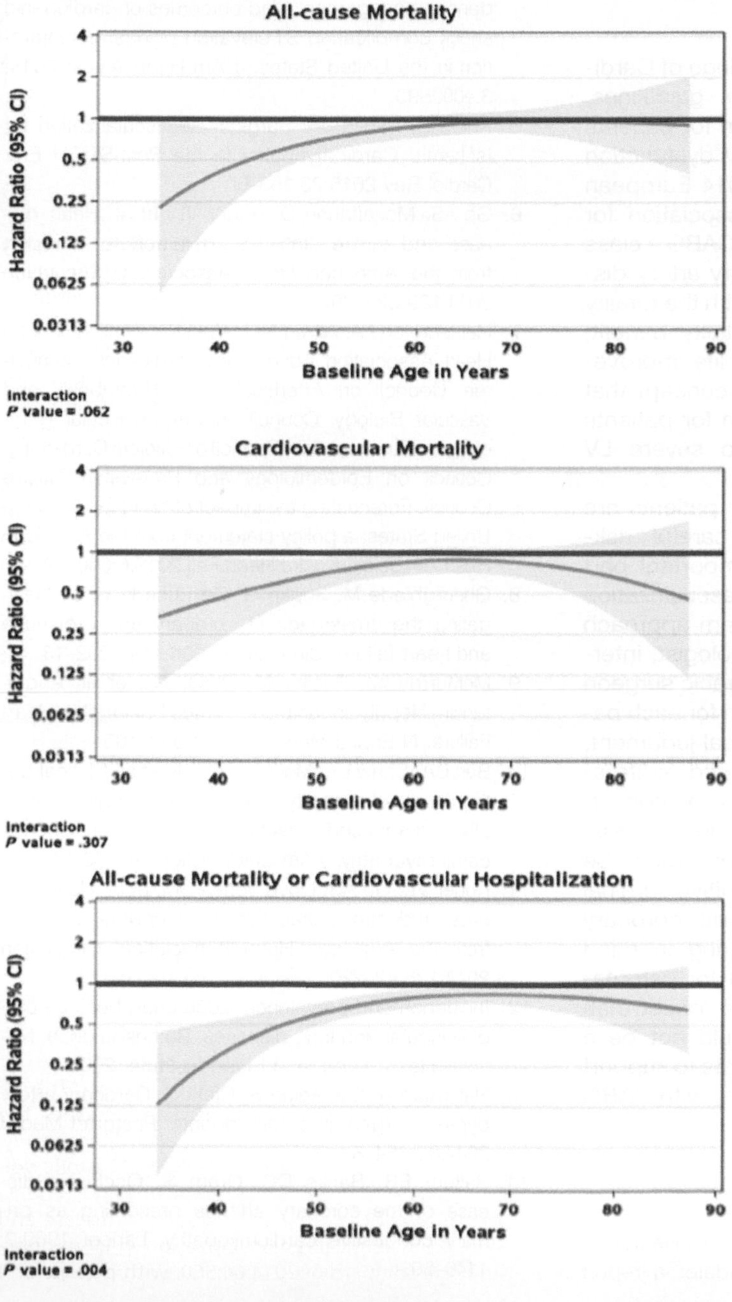

Fig. 4. HR (*solid line*) and 95% CI (*gray area*) for the effect of CABG versus medical therapy across the range of ages. (*From* Petrie MC, Jhund PS, She L, et al. Ten-year outcomes after coronary artery bypass grafting according to age in patients with heart failure and left ventricular systolic dysfunction: an analysis of the extended follow-up of the STICH trial [surgical treatment for ischemic heart failure]. Circulation 2016;134:1321; with permission.)

CI, 0.43–0.85 in ≤54 years vs HR 0.70; 95% CI, 0.50–0.97 in >67 years; $p_{interaction}$ 0.307) (**Fig. 4**).[62] The clinical implication of these findings is that older patients are more likely to die of noncardiovascular causes (compared with the relatively younger cohort) and CABG provided cardiovascular mortality benefits to the older patient population. Hence, CABG should also be offered as valid therapeutic alternative to older patients as long as comorbidities do not seem to impose a counterbalance to the beneficial effect of CABG on cardiovascular mortality.

SUMMARY

According to the older American College of Cardiology/American Heart Association guidelines, CABG is a class IIb recommendation for patients with coronary artery disease and LV dysfunction (EF <35%).[63,64] The more recent 2014 European Society of Cardiology/European Association for Cardio-Thoracic Surgery report give CABG a class I indication for patients with coronary artery disease and severe LV dysfunction.[65] With the totality of data supporting CABG for mortality benefit, symptomatic angina, and quality of life improvement, the authors subscribe to the concept that CABG should be a class I indication for patients with ischemic cardiomyopathy and severe LV dysfunction.

As the population ages and more patients are referred for CABG, however, a careful risk-benefit assessment should be an important part of the consideration regarding revascularization strategies. In this regard, a heart team approach in consultation with a referring cardiologist, interventional cardiologist, and cardiothoracic surgeon is critical to arrive at the best decision for each patient. The underlying substrate, clinical judgment, coronary anatomy, functional status, end-of-life issues, and patient preferences must all be considered as part of the decision-making process. Percutaneous coronary intervention may be offered to patients with high or prohibitive surgical risk and ischemic cardiomyopathy with coronary lesions amenable to stenting, bearing in mind that data regarding mortality benefit for percutaneous coronary intervention are less robust than for CABG. Finally, age, alone, should not be a contraindication because there are data to support a reduction in cardiovascular mortality with CABG in older patients.

REFERENCES

1. Mozaffarian D, Benjamin EJ, Go AS, et al. Heart disease and stroke statistics-2016 update: a report from the American Heart Association. Circulation 2016;133:e38–360.
2. Khera S, Kolte D, Aronow WS, et al. Non-ST-elevation myocardial infarction in the United States: contemporary trends in incidence, utilization of the early invasive strategy, and in-hospital outcomes. J Am Heart Assoc 2014;3:e000995.
3. Khera S, Kolte D, Palaniswamy C, et al. ST-elevation myocardial infarction in the elderly - Temporal Trends in incidence, utilization of percutaneous coronary intervention and outcomes in the United States. Int J Cardiol 2013;168:3683–90.
4. Kolte D, Khera S, Aronow WS, et al. Trends in incidence, management, and outcomes of cardiogenic shock complicating ST-elevation myocardial infarction in the United States. J Am Heart Assoc 2014; 3:e000590.
5. Khera S, Panza JA. Surgical Revascularization for Ischemic Cardiomyopathy in the Post-STICH Era. Cardiol Rev 2015;23:153–60.
6. Go AS, Mozaffarian D, Roger VL, et al. Heart disease and stroke statistics–2014 update: a report from the American Heart Association. Circulation 2014;129:e28–292.
7. Heidenreich PA, Albert NM, Allen LA, et al, American Heart Association Advocacy Coordinating Committee, Council on Arteriosclerosis, Thrombosis and Vascular Biology, Council on Cardiovascular Radiology and Intervention, Council on Clinical Cardiology, Council on Epidemiology and Prevention, Stroke Council. Forecasting the impact of heart failure in the United States: a policy statement from the American Heart Association. Circ Heart Fail 2013;6:606–19.
8. Gheorghiade M, Sopko G, De Luca L, et al. Navigating the crossroads of coronary artery disease and heart failure. Circulation 2006;114:1202–13.
9. McMurray JJ, Packer M, Desai AS, et al. Angiotensin–Neprilysin Inhibition versus Enalapril in Heart Failure. N Engl J Med 2014;371:993–1004.
10. Bart BA, Shaw LK, McCants CB Jr, et al. Clinical determinants of mortality in patients with angiographically diagnosed ischemic or nonischemic cardiomyopathy. J Am Coll Cardiol 1997;30:1002–8.
11. Roger VL, Go AS, Lloyd-Jones DM, et al. Heart disease and stroke statistics–2012 update: a report from the American Heart Association. Circulation 2012;125:e2–220.
12. Incidence and prevalence: 2006 chart book on cardiovascular and lung diseases. Bethesda (MD): National Heart, Lung, and Blood Institute; 2006.
13. Natarajan A, Samadian S, Clark S. Coronary artery bypass surgery in elderly people. Postgrad Med J 2007;83:154–8.
14. Raftery EB, Banks DC, Oram S. Occlusive disease of the coronary arteries presenting as primary congestive cardiomyopathy. Lancet 1969;2: 1146–50.

15. Burch GE, Giles TD, Colcolough HL. Ischemic cardiomyopathy. Am Heart J 1970;79:291–2.
16. Felker GM, Shaw LK, O'Connor CM. A standardized definition of ischemic cardiomyopathy for use in clinical research. J Am Coll Cardiol 2002;39:210–8.
17. Velazquez EJ, Lee KL, Deja MA, et al. Coronary-artery bypass surgery in patients with left ventricular dysfunction. N Engl J Med 2011;364:1607–16.
18. Braunwald E, Rutherford JD. Reversible ischemic left ventricular dysfunction: evidence for the "hibernating myocardium". J Am Coll Cardiol 1986;8:1467–70.
19. Armstrong WF. "Hibernating" myocardium: asleep or part dead? J Am Coll Cardiol 1996;28:530–5.
20. Wijns W, Vatner SF, Camici PG. Hibernating myocardium. N Engl J Med 1998;339:173–81.
21. Briceno N, Schuster A, Lumley M, et al. Ischaemic cardiomyopathy: pathophysiology, assessment and the role of revascularization. Heart 2016;102:397–406.
22. Rahimtoola SH. The hibernating myocardium. Am Heart J 1989;117:211–21.
23. Heusch G, Schulz R. Characterization of hibernating and stunned myocardium. Eur Heart J 1997;18:D102–10.
24. Schuster A, Morton G, Chiribiri A, et al. Imaging in the management of ischemic cardiomyopathy: special focus on magnetic resonance. J Am Coll Cardiol 2012;59:359–70.
25. Bax J, van der Wall EE, Harbinson M. Radionuclide techniques for the assessment of myocardial viability and hibernation. Heart 2004;90(S5):v26–33.
26. Shivalkar B, Maes A, Borgers M, et al. Only hibernating myocardium invariably shows early recovery after coronary revascularization. Circulation 1996;94:308–15.
27. Sedov VM, Nemkov AS. Vasilii Ivanovich Kolesov: pioneer of coronary surgery. Eur J Cardiothorac Surg 2014;45:220–4.
28. Head SJ, Kieser TM, Falk V, et al. Coronary artery bypass grafting: part 1—the evolution over the first 50 years. Eur Heart J 2013;34:2862–72.
29. Murphy ML, Hultgren HN, Detre K, et al. Treatment of chronic stable angina. A preliminary report of survival data of the randomized Veterans Administration cooperative study. N Engl J Med 1977;297:621–7.
30. Takaro T, Hultgren HN, Lipton MJ, et al. The VA cooperative randomized study of surgery for coronary arterial occlusive disease II. Subgroup with significant left main lesions. Circulation 1976;54:III107–17.
31. Coronary-artery bypass surgery in stable angina pectoris: survival at two years. European Coronary Surgery Study Group. Lancet 1979;1:889–93.
32. Long-term results of prospective randomised study of coronary artery bypass surgery in stable angina pectoris. European Coronary Surgery Study Group. Lancet 1982;2:1173–80.
33. Coronary artery surgery study (CASS): a randomized trial of coronary artery bypass surgery. Survival data. Circulation 1983;68:939–50.
34. Loop FD, Lytle BW, Cosgrove DM, et al. Influence of the internal-mammary-artery graft on 10-year survival and other cardiac events. N Engl J Med 1986;314:1–6.
35. Fitzgibbon GM, Kafka HP, Leach AJ, et al. Coronary bypass graft fate and patient outcome: angiographic follow-up of 5,065 grafts related to survival and reoperation in 1,388 patients during 25 years. J Am Coll Cardiol 1996;28:616–26.
36. Alderman EL, Fisher LD, Litwin P, et al. Results of coronary artery surgery in patients with poor left ventricular function (CASS). Circulation 1983;68:785–95.
37. O'Connor CM, Velazquez EJ, Gardner LH, et al. Comparison of coronary artery bypass grafting versus medical therapy on long-term outcome in patients with ischemic cardiomyopathy (a 25-year experience from the duke cardiovascular disease databank). Am J Cardiol 2002;90:101–7.
38. BARI 2D Study Group, Frye RL, August P, Brooks MM, et al. A randomized trial of therapies for type 2 diabetes and coronary artery disease. N Engl J Med 2009;360:2503–15.
39. Boden WE, O'Rourke RA, Teo KK, et al. Optimal medical therapy with or without PCI for stable coronary disease. N Engl J Med 2007;356:1503–16.
40. Yusuf S, Zucker D, Peduzzi P, et al. Effect of coronary artery bypass graft surgery on survival: overview of 10-year results from randomised trials by the coronary artery bypass graft surgery trialists collaboration. Lancet 1994;344:563–70.
41. Velazquez EJ, Lee KL, Jones RH, et al. Coronary-artery bypass surgery in patients with ischemic cardiomyopathy. N Engl J Med 2016;374:1511–20.
42. Mark DB, Knight JD, Velazquez EJ, et al. Quality-of-life outcomes with coronary artery bypass graft surgery in ischemic left ventricular dysfunction: a randomized trial. Ann Intern Med 2014;161:392–9.
43. Pagley PR, Beller GA, Watson DD, et al. Improved outcome after coronary bypass surgery in patients with ischemic cardiomyopathy and residual myocardial viability. Circulation 1997;96:793–800.
44. Cuocolo A, Petretta M, Nicolai E, et al. Successful coronary revascularization improves prognosis in patients with previous myocardial infarction and evidence of viable myocardium at thallium-201 imaging. Eur J Nucl Med 1998;25:60–8.
45. Sicari R, Ripoli A, Picano E, et al. The prognostic value of myocardial viability recognized by low dose dipyridamole echocardiography in patients with chronic ischaemic left ventricular dysfunction. Eur Heart J 2001;22:837–44.

46. Petrasinovic Z, Ostojic M, Beleslin B, et al. Prognostic value of myocardial viability determined by a 201Tl SPECT study in patients with previous myocardial infarction and mild-to-moderate myocardial dysfunction. Nucl Med Commun 2003;24:175–81.
47. Meluzin J, Cerný J, Spinarová L, et al. Prognosis of patients with chronic coronary artery disease and severe left ventricular dysfunction. The importance of myocardial viability. Eur J Heart Fail 2003;5: 85–93.
48. Sawada SG, Dasgupta S, Nguyen J, et al. Effect of revascularization on long-term survival in patients with ischemic left ventricular dysfunction and a wide range of viability. Am J Cardiol 2010;106:187–92.
49. Senior R, Kaul S, Raval U, et al. Impact of revascularization and myocardial viability determined by nitrate-enhanced Tc-99m sestamibi and Tl-201 imaging on mortality and functional outcome in ischemic cardiomyopathy. J Nucl Cardiol 2002;9: 454–62.
50. Bonow RO, Maurer G, Lee KL, et al. Myocardial viability and survival in ischemic left ventricular dysfunction. N Engl J Med 2011;364:1617–25.
51. Hachamovitch R, Rozanski A, Shaw LJ, et al. Impact of ischaemia and scar on the therapeutic benefit derived from myocardial revascularization vs. medical therapy among patients undergoing stress-rest myocardial perfusion scintigraphy. Eur Heart J 2011;32:1012–24.
52. Panza JA, Holly TA, Asch FM, et al. Inducible myocardial ischemia and outcomes in patients with coronary artery disease and left ventricular dysfunction. J Am Coll Cardiol 2013;61:1860–70.
53. Warren J. Remarks on angina pectoris. N Engl J Med Surg 1812;1:1–11.
54. Jolicœur EM, Dunning A, Castelvecchio S, et al. Importance of angina in patients with coronary disease, heart failure, and left ventricular systolic dysfunction: insights from STICH. J Am Coll Cardiol 2015;66:2092–100.
55. Panza JA, Velazquez EJ, She L, et al. Extent of coronary and myocardial disease and benefit from surgical revascularization in LV dysfunction. J Am Coll Cardiol 2014;64:553–61.
56. Carson P, Wertheimer J, Miller A, et al. The STICH trial (Surgical Treatment for Ischemic Heart Failure): mode-of-death results. JACC Heart Fail 2013;1: 400–8.
57. Alexander K, Anstrom K, Muhlbaier L, et al. Outcomes of cardiac surgery in patients age ≥80 years: results from the National Cardiovascular Network. J Am Coll Cardiol 2000;35(3):731–8.
58. Maraschini A, Seccareccia F, D'Errigo P, et al. Role of gender and age on early mortality after coronary artery bypass graft in different hospitals: data from a national administrative database. Interact Cardiovasc Thorac Surg 2010;11:537–42.
59. Rocha ASC, Pitella FJM, Lorenzo AR, et al. Age influences outcomes in 70-year or older patients undergoing isolated coronary artery bypass graft surgery. Rev Bras Cir Cardiovasc 2012;27:45–51.
60. Wrobel K, Stevens SR, Jones RH, et al. Influence of baseline characteristics, operative conduct, and postoperative course on 30-day outcomes of coronary artery bypass grafting among patients with left ventricular dysfunction: results from the surgical treatment for ischemic heart failure (STICH) trial. Circulation 2015;132:720–30.
61. Ghanta RK, Shekar PS, McGurk S, et al. Long-term survival and quality of life justify cardiac surgery in the very elderly patient. Ann Thorac Surg 2011;92: 851–7.
62. Petrie MC, Jhund PS, She L, et al. Ten-year outcomes after coronary artery bypass grafting according to age in patients with heart failure and left ventricular systolic dysfunction: an analysis of the extended follow-up of the STICH trial (surgical treatment for ischemic heart failure). Circulation 2016; 134:1314–24.
63. Hillis LD, Smith PK, Anderson JL, et al. 2011 ACCF/AHA guideline for coronary artery bypass graft surgery: a report of the American College of Cardiology Foundation/American Heart Association Task Force on Practice Guidelines. Circulation 2011;124: e652–735.
64. Fihn SD, Gardin JM, Abrams J, et al. 2012 ACCF/AHA/ACP/AATS/PCNA/SCAI/STS guideline for the diagnosis and management of patients with stable ischemic heart disease: a report of the American College of Cardiology Foundation/American Heart Association Task Force on Practice Guidelines, and the American College of Physicians, American Association for Thoracic Surgery, Preventive Cardiovascular Nurses Association, Society for Cardiovascular Angiography and Interventions, and Society of Thoracic Surgeons. J Am Coll Cardiol 2012;60:e44–164.
65. Windecker S, Kolh P, Alfonso F, et al. 2014 ESC/EACTS Guidelines on myocardial revascularization: the Task Force on Myocardial Revascularization of the European Society of Cardiology (ESC) and the European Association for Cardio-Thoracic Surgery (EACTS)Developed with the special contribution of the European Association of Percutaneous Cardiovascular Interventions (EAPCI). Eur Heart J 2014; 35:2541–619.

Cardiac Resynchronization Therapy in Older Adults with Heart Failure

Phillip H. Lam, MD[a,b], George E. Taffet, MD[c], Ali Ahmed, MD, MPH[a,d,e], Steve Singh, MD[f,*]

KEYWORDS

• Heart failure • Cardiac resynchronization therapy • Older adults • Mortality

KEY POINTS

- Heart failure is a disease of poor prognosis marked by frequent hospitalizations, premature death, and impaired quality of life.
- Cardiac resynchronization therapy (CRT), or biventricular pacing, has led to significant improvement in both survival and symptoms in patients with heart failure and reduced ejection fraction (HFrEF) and evidence of a left bundle branch pattern on electrocardiogram.
- The beneficial effects of CRT, especially in combination with ICD, are not as well documented for the older population as they are for younger individuals with HFrEF, but do not reveal dramatic effects of age on outcomes.
- Placement of CRT, like other pacemakers, is well-tolerated in older patients and complications are infrequent.

CASE PRESENTATION

An 84-year-old man with a past medical history of coronary artery disease and ischemic cardiomyopathy with a recent left ventricular ejection fraction (LVEF) of 20% to 25% as demonstrated by echocardiogram, presents to the cardiology clinic with progressive dyspnea on exertion. Despite being on a medical regimen of lisinopril, carvedilol, spironolactone, and furosemide at stable doses over the past 3 months, the patient is not able to ambulate for more than 2 blocks without having to rest owing to his shortness of breath. An electrocardiogram in clinic reveals a normal sinus rhythm with a left bundle branch block (LBBB) and a QRS interval of 165 msec. He wants to know if there are any additional therapies available to treat his heart failure (HF) and symptoms.

INTRODUCTION

HF is a common chronic disease that carries a poor prognosis. It is a disease marked by frequent hospitalizations and premature death

Conflict of Interest: None.

[a] Center for Health and Aging, Veterans Affairs Medical Center, 50 Irving Street NW, Washington, DC 20422, USA; [b] MedStar Heart and Vascular Institute, Georgetown University/MedStar Washington Hospital Center, 110 Irving Street NW, Washington, DC 20010, USA; [c] Department of Medicine, George Washington University, 2150 Pennsylvania Avenue NW, Suite 8-416, Washington, DC 20037, USA; [d] Department of Medicine, University of Alabama at Birmingham, 933 19th Street South, CH19 201, Birmingham, AL 35294, USA; [e] Department of Geriatrics and Cardiovascular Medicine, Baylor College of Medicine, 1200 Binz Street, Suite 1470, Houston, TX 77004, USA; [f] Department of Cardiology, Veterans Affairs Medical Center, 50 Irving Street NW, Washington, DC 20422, USA
* Corresponding author.
E-mail address: steve.singh@va.gov

Heart Failure Clin 13 (2017) 581–587
http://dx.doi.org/10.1016/j.hfc.2017.02.011
1551-7136/17/

despite optimal medical therapy. It is also associated with a dramatic impairment in quality of life, especially in older patients, when associated with other comorbidities.[1] Despite advances in medical therapy for patients with HF and reduced ejection fraction (HFrEF), defined as an LVEF of 40% or less, mortality and hospitalizations with advanced disease are still increased, and the quality of life continues to be poor in this population.

The advent of cardiac resynchronization therapy (CRT), also known as biventricular pacing, has led to a significant improvement in both survival and symptom management in select patients with HFrEF. This improvement is achieved through a standard atrial and ventricular pacing lead placed in the right atrium and right ventricle with a third lead that is advanced into a lateral or posterolateral branch of the coronary sinus to allow synchronized pacing of both the right and left ventricles (**Fig. 1**). Beneficial changes as seen in randomized clinical trials include not only an increase in survival, but also improved contractile function and ventricular remodeling and a significant improvement in quality of life.[2–7] Despite all of its benefits, data on the role of CRT in older patients has been scarce, because this population is not well-represented in most of the large-scale clinical trials. In this article, we review the role of CRT in the treatment of older patients, defined as patients over the age of 65 years, with HFrEF.

EVOLUTION OF CARDIAC RESYNCHRONIZATION THERAPY

Conduction defects leading to a delay in the onset of right and left ventricular systole occur in about 30% of patients with HFrEF.[8,9] This dyssynchrony can be seen on an electrocardiogram as a QRS interval of greater than or equal to 120 msec with a LBBB morphology. The delay in conduction leads to an impaired ability of the weak heart to eject blood, worsening flow through the mitral valve and leading to progression of HF, and a subsequent impaired quality of life and increased risk of death. The development of atrial-synchronized biventricular pacing that helps to coordinate contraction between these 2 chambers has improved not only cardiac contractility and enhanced quality of life, but also survival as demonstrated by several major randomized clinical trials (**Table 1**).

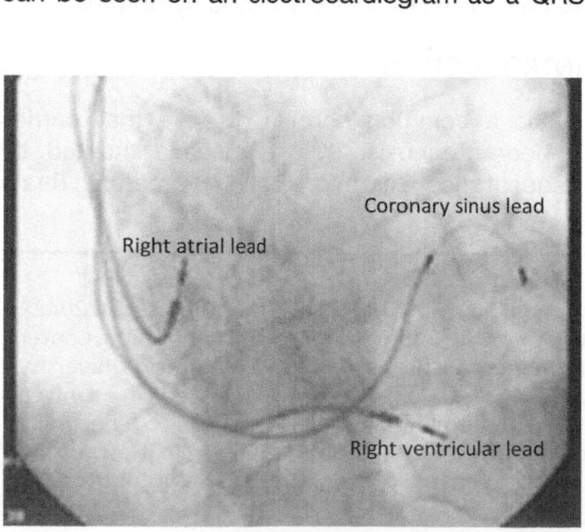

Fig. 1. An anterior-posterior fluoroscopic projection showing all 3 leads involved in cardiac resynchronization therapy.

The MIRACLE (Multicenter Insync Randomized Clinical Evaluation) study was the first double-blind randomized control trial to achieve its primary outcome of improved 6 minute walk test (*P* = .005), quality of life (*P* = .001), and New York Heart Association (NYHA) functional class (*P*<.001) in patients with HFrEF who received CRT plus medical therapy compared with medical therapy alone.[2] In the trial, patients with HF associated with an LVEF of 35% or less and a QRS interval of 130 msec or more were randomized to either receive CRT and medical therapy or medical therapy alone.

The addition of CRT to an implantable cardioverter defibrillator (ICD) was explored in the MIRACLE-ICD (Multicenter Insync ICD Randomized Clinical Evaluation) study, which once again achieved a primary outcome of improved quality of life (*P* = .02) and NYHA functional class (*P* = .007) in patients with systolic HF who received CRT in addition to an ICD for life-threatening arrhythmias.[3]

The COMPANION trial (Comparison of Medical Therapy, Pacing, and Defibrillation in Heart Failure) was the first study to compare CRT-pacing (CRT-P) and CRT-defibrillator (CRT-D) plus medical therapy to optimal pharmacologic therapy alone and included mortality as one of its outcomes. Patients in both the CRT-D and CRT-P groups had a 20% decrease in death or hospitalization compared with the medical therapy group (**Table 2**).[4] Compared with medical therapy alone, the reduction in mortality was noted to be greater in patients receiving CRT-D than those receiving CRT-P at 36% (*P* = .003) and 24% (*P* = .059), respectively.[4]

The CARE-HF trial (Cardiac Resynchronization in Heart Failure) randomized patients with NYHA functional class III or IV HF owing to HFrEF and evidence of cardiac dyssynchronization, defined as a QRS duration of 120 msec or greater, to either receive CRT-P and medical therapy or optimal pharmacologic therapy alone.[5] Patients in the CRT-P had a significant reduction in death from any cause or hospitalization for major cardiovascular events compared with those receiving only

Table 1
Major randomized controlled trials and outcomes in patients with heart failure and reduced ejection fraction receiving CRT

Study	Year	Mean Age of Intervention Group	Number of Patients	Results
MIRACLE	2002	63.9 ± 10.7	453	Improved NYHA functional class, 6-min walk test, and quality of life
MIRACLE-ICD	2003	66.6 ± 11.3	369	Improved NYHA functional class, 6-min walk test, and quality of life
COMPANION	2004	65.0 ± 11.0	1520	Decreased all-cause mortality or all-cause hospitalization
CARE-HF	2005	67 (60–73)	813	Decreased all-cause mortality or cardiovascular hospitalization
MADIT-CRT	2009	65.0 ± 11.0	1820	Decrease all-cause mortality of heart failure hospitalization
RAFT	2010	66.6 ± 9.4	1798	Decreased death from any cause or hospitalization for heart failure

Abbreviations: CRT, cardiac resynchronization therapy; NYHA, New York Heart Association.

medical therapy ($P = .001$; **Table 3**).[5] Secondary outcomes revealed a reduction in death from any cause ($P<.002$) and HF hospitalization ($P<.001$), along with an improvement in quality of life ($P<.001$), and left ventricular ejection function ($P<.001$) in patients who received CRT-P plus optimal medical therapy compared with medical therapy alone.[5] Both the COMPANION and CARE-HF trials helped to established CRT as treatment for patients with HFrEF (NYHA functional class III or IV) and a wide QRS complex. In all these studies, patients like the one in our case presentation were underrepresented.

Although the body of evidence for CRT and its benefits in patients with HFrEF is vast for patients with NYHA functional class III or IV, little was known about its efficacy in patients with mild to moderate HF (NYHA functional class I or II).

Table 2
Percentage free of death or hospitalization in patients enrolled in the COMPANION trial

	0.5 y	1 y	1.5 y	2 y	2.5 y
Pacemaker	58.5	43.7	32.1	23.3	18.5
Pacemaker + defibrillator	58.5	43.7	32.1	23.3	18.5
Medications alone	55	31.4	22	17.9	11.6
Difference favoring devices	3.5	12.3	10.1	5.4	6.9

Data from Bristow MR, Saxon LA, Boehmer J, et al. Cardiac-resynchronization therapy with or without an implantable defibrillator in advanced chronic heart failure. N Engl J Med 2004;350(21):2140–50.

The MADIT-CRT trial (Multicenter Automatic Defibrillator Implantation Trial with Cardiac Resynchronization Therapy), one of the largest randomized CRT trials with a sample size of 1820 patients, randomized patients with HFrEF, NYHA functional class I or II, and QRS duration of 130 msec or greater to receive either CRT-D or ICD alone.[6] Although it achieved its primary outcome of total mortality or HF hospitalizations reduction at 34% in the CRT-D group compared with the ICD group ($P = .001$), it was largely driven by the reduction in HF hospitalizations[6] (**Table 4**).

The RAFT trial (Resynchronization–Defibrillation for Ambulatory Heart Failure) randomized patients with NYHA class II or III HF, LVEF of 30% or less, and a QRS duration of greater than or equal to 120 msec to receive either an ICD alone or ICD plus CRT. The study revealed a significant reduction in death from any cause or hospitalization for HF in the group who received both an ICD and CRT compared with ICD alone ($P<.001$; **Table 5**).[7] Other outcomes, including all-cause mortality, were also lower in the group that received both ICD and CRT ($P = .003$).[7] Taken together, both the MADIT-CRT and RAFT trials provide evidence of the clinical efficacy of CRT in patients with mild-to-moderate HF in addition to patients with moderate-to-severe HF.

The evolution of CRT over the last 15 years has led to the establishment of a national consensus for the placement of CRT in patients with evidence of left ventricular dysfunction and cardiac dyssynchrony. Given the significant improvement in not only survival, but also other parameters such as quality of life in patients with HFrEF, it is currently

Table 3
Percentage free of death or cardiovascular hospitalization in patients enrolled in the CARE-HF trial

	0.5 y	1 y	1.5 y	2 y	2.5 y	3 y	3.5 y
Cardiac resynchronization	83	72	67	62	59	57	54
Medical therapy	79	65	56	49	43	33	30
Difference favoring cardiac resynchronization therapy	4	7	11	13	16	24	24

Data from Cleland JG, Daubert JC, Erdmann E, et al. The effect of cardiac resynchronization on morbidity and mortality in heart failure. N Engl J Med 2005;352(15):1539–49.

a class I indication for the placement of CRT in patients with LVEF of 35% or less, sinus rhythm, left bundle branch block with a QRS duration of 150 msec or greater, and NYHA functional class II, III, or ambulatory IV who are already on goal directed medical therapy as stated in the recent 2012 American College of Cardiology/American Heart Association guidelines.[10] It is also reasonable to consider CRT in patients who have QRS duration of 120 to 149 msec, a class IIa indication.[10]

CLINICAL EFFICACY OF CARDIAC RESYNCHRONIZATION THERAPY IN OLDER PATIENTS

Despite the emergence of CRT for the HFrEF population, to date it remains unclear whether the favorable results from the trials are generalizable to older patients. Few older adults were included during the randomization period. Furthermore, none of the trials have specifically addressed the benefit of CRT in this population. In both the COMPANION and CARE-HF trials, the mean age was about 65 years and the benefit of CRT was seen in patients above the mean age. A subgroup analysis in the COMPANION trial revealed both a reduction in all-cause mortality or all-cause hospitalization and all-cause mortality in patients over the age of 65 years who received CRT-D compared with patients who only received pharmacologic therapy, with an estimated relative risk reduction of 20% to 25% within each group.[4] Subsequent analyses of both the MIRACLE and MIRACLE-ICD trials also revealed a comparable benefit of CRT in older patients to those who were younger.[11] Patients in both studies who were 65 years of age and older had a similar significant improvement in NYHA functional class ($P = .002$) and LVEF ($P = .03$) when compared with patients under the age of 65.[11] The benefits of CRT in the older population extend beyond those with moderate to severe HF. In the MADIT trial, which looked at a population with mild to moderate HF, patients in the age of 60 to 74 years old age group and the greater than 74 years old age group had a similar reduction in combined all-cause mortality or HF readmission when compared with those who were less than the age of 60 ($P<.001$, $P<.001$, and $P = .043$ in each group, respectively).[12]

Equivalent benefits of CRT in older adults were also noted in several observational studies when comparing this population with younger patients. Several studies have noted improvement in both echocardiographic findings of improved LV function and comparable survival benefits when comparing older patients to those who were younger.[13,14] In one study, patients with HFrEF over the age of 70 who received CRT had similar improvement in functional class ($P<.05$), quality of life ($P<.05$), and ejection fraction ($P<.05$) when compared with their less than 70 years old age group counterparts.[13] Older adults receiving CRT not only demonstrated comparable clinical benefits compared with those who were younger, but also displayed similar survival outcomes, with

Table 4
Percentage free of heart failure hospitalization in patients enrolled in the MADIT-HF trial

	0.5 y	1 y	1.5 y	2 y	2.5 y	3 y	3.5 y
CRT + ICD	95.6	92.1	88.4	85.1	82.4	79.9	78.5
ICD only	92.7	88.4	81.7	77.7	74.5	70.7	67.5
Difference favoring ICD + CRT	2.9	3.7	6.7	7.4	7.9	9.2	11

Abbreviations: CRT, cardiac resynchronization therapy; ICD, implantable cardioverter-defibrillator.
Data from Moss AJ, Hall WJ, Cannom DS, et al. Cardiac resynchronization therapy for the prevention of heart-failure events. N Engl J Med 2009;361(14):1329–38.

Table 5
Percentage free of death or heart failure hospitalization in patients enrolled in the RAFT trial

	0.5 y	1 y	1.5 y	2 y	2.5 y	3 y	3.5 y	4 y	4.5 y	5 y
CRT + ICD	93.7	88.6	84.4	81.3	77.5	73.7	69.5	66	60.6	57.8
ICD only	90.8	85.4	80.3	75.6	70.8	66	60.3	55.9	52.4	47.6
Difference favoring ICD + CRT	2.9	3.2	4.1	5.7	6.7	7.7	9.2	10.1	8.2	10.2

Abbreviations: CRT, cardiac resynchronization therapy; ICD, implantable cardioverter-defibrillator.
Data from Tang AS, Wells GA, Talajic M, et al. Cardiac-resynchronization therapy for mild-to-moderate heart failure. N Engl J Med 2010;363(25):2385–95.

one study revealing similar survival at 2-year follow-up when comparing patients over the age of 75 with patients under 75 years of age ($P = .961$).[14,15]

IMPACT OF COMORBIDITIES ON THE EFFICACY OF CARDIAC RESYNCHRONIZATION THERAPY

Geriatricians have concerns that typical multimorbid geriatric patients may be excluded from getting devices such as CRT and ICD. Although the burden of comorbidities such as atrial fibrillation, diabetes mellitus, and chronic kidney disease may preclude some patients from receiving CRT given the concern for the cost of the device placement over its potential benefits, there have been several studies that have shown a clinical benefit of CRT in patients with these comorbidities.[16–18] In one meta-analysis of prospective cohort studies comparing the impact of CRT for patients in atrial fibrillation and sinus rhythm, mortality is similar in both groups at 1-year follow-up ($P = .13$).[16] In a study from Fantoni and colleagues,[17] diabetic HF patients treated with CRT had outcomes not different from their nondiabetic counterparts for death from any cause ($P = .710$), cardiovascular death ($P = .679$), HF death ($P = .806$), and sudden death ($P = .972$). In HF patients with renal dysfunction, a prominent comorbidity in this population, CRT has not only demonstrated an improvement in renal function recovery, but it was shown to also improve patients with severe renal dysfunction. A study of 73 consecutive patients with an average age of greater than 70 receiving either CRT or ICD revealed an improvement in both estimated glomerular filtration rate and functional status in patients who received CRT compared with those who received ICD ($P = .04$ and $P<.001$, respectively).[18] Although age was not studied specifically as a marker of response to CRT in the landmark randomized trials, it is reasonable to apply these findings to an older population based on these subsequent analyses. Therefore, in patients with a good life expectancy, regardless of age, CRT should be considered in patients with HFrEF and existing comorbidities.

COMPLICATIONS OF IMPLANTATION

The complications of CRT are similar to the placement of any standard pacemaker device. These include pneumothorax, bleeding from perforation of vessels or the myocardium, infection, and arrhythmias. Overall, the implantation of any pacemaker device, including CRT, is safe and well-tolerated. The low rate of perioperative complications can also be applied to geriatric patients. Subgroup analyses of both the MIRACLE and MIRACLE-ICD did not reveal an increase of adverse events after CRT implantation in this population.[11] Another study also revealed a similar rate of device-related complication such as the dislodgement of LV leads and pocket erosions in patients younger than and older than 80 years of age.[15] However, these studies are either post hoc analyses or observational studies, which are limitations. To date, there have been no prospective, randomized trials addressing the safety of CRT in the geriatric population.

COST EFFECTIVENESS OF CARDIAC RESYNCHRONIZATION THERAPY

HF is the leading cause for hospital admission and readmission in the United States in patients over the age of 65, which creates a significant health care and financial burden.[19] It has been shown that a readmission for HF not only increases cost and cumulative duration of stay in older patients with HF, it also has clinical implications for patient survival.[20] This has created a significant push from the government to reduce this number, leading to the creation of the Affordable Care Act, which penalizes hospitals with a high rate of hospital readmissions in patients with HF.

CRT has been shown to not only improve survival, but reduce cost and hospitalizations. In the CARE-HF trial, the rate of hospitalization for worsening HF was significantly lower in patients who received CRT compared with those who received only pharmacologic therapy.[5] This observation was also seen in patients with mild to moderate HFrEF as demonstrated in the RAFT trial.[7] A cost analysis of the COMPANION trial was performed over a 2-year period, follow-up hospitalizations were reduced by 29% and 37% in the CRT-P group and CRT-D group, respectively.[21] This translated to a saving of $43,000 per quality-adjusted life-year for CRT-P and $19,600 per quality-adjusted life-year for those who received CRT-D at 7 years.[21] Although this analysis did not make calculations based on patient age, the mean age of the COMPANION trial was 67 years, suggesting that CRT may be a cost-effective method in the prevention of hospitalization in this particular population.

BIVENTRICULAR PACING ALONE IN OLDER ADULTS

As demonstrated in the CARE-HF trial, biventricular pacing alone without an ICD improves survival compared to optimal medical therapy.[4] In addition to the hemodynamic and functional benefits, biventricular pacing may also reduce the number of ventricular arrhythmias, decreasing the need for ICD shocks.[22,23] ICDs have been shown to have a significant impact on a patient's quality of life. The conversion of a malignant arrhythmia can lead to various psychological complications, including anxiety and depression.[24,25] Such findings lead to the debate of whether CRT alone is preferred to CRT plus ICD in patients with HFrEF, and in particular in an older population. The significant reduction in mortality and hospitalizations when CRT is added to ICD compared with ICD alone as demonstrated in the MADIT-HF trial also raises the question of whether ICD alone is beneficial in patient outcomes, particularly in the older adults.[6] Further complicating the decision to implant the type of device, the recent DANISH trial (Danish Study to Assess the Efficacy of ICDs in Patients with Nonischemic Systolic Heart Failure on Mortality),[26] which randomized patients with nonischemic cardiomyopathy and NYHA functional class II through IV symptoms to receive either and ICD plus optimal therapy or optimal medical therapy alone, revealed no survival benefit in the group who received an ICD compared with medical therapy alone ($P = .28$; **Table 6**). In both groups, about 58% of the patients had CRT. Subgroup analyses of the trial revealed a lack of benefit of ICD in patients over the age of 59 years.[26]

Table 6
All-cause mortality rate (%) in patients enrolled in the DANISH trial

	1 y	2 y	3 y	4 y	5 y	6 y
ICD	3.5	5.4	9.9	14.3	18.8	23.4
Control	3.5	8	12.6	18.2	24.5	27.7

Abbreviation: ICD, implantable cardioverter defibrillator.
Data from Kober L, Thune JJ, Nielsen JC, et al. Defibrillator implantation in patients with nonischemic systolic heart failure. N Engl J Med 2016;375(13):1221–30.

Taking into consideration the data that have been presented and discussed, it is reasonable to consider implantation of only CRT in symptomatic older patients with HFrEF and evidence of dyssynchrony on optimal medical therapy without the addition of ICD. However, current guidelines state that an ICD is still indicated in patients with HFrEF, regardless of age, who have a reasonable expectation of survival with an acceptable functional status for at least 1 year.[27] Perhaps a prospective, randomized trial will definitively answer the question of the benefit of CRT in older adults.

SUMMARY: CLINICAL DECISION

Our patient meets the criteria for both an ICD and CRT implantation. His ejection fraction is less than 35% and he has a left bundle branch block with a QRS duration of greater than 150 msec. Because he maintains an active lifestyle, which includes mowing the lawn and spending time outdoors with his family, and he wishes to continue to be able to perform these activities, the decision was made to pursue with a CRT and ICD combination placement.

REFERENCES

1. Antonio N, Elvas L, Goncalves L, et al. Cardiac resynchronization therapy in the elderly: a realistic option for an increasing population? Int J Cardiol 2012; 155(1):49–51.
2. Abraham WT, Fisher WG, Smith AL, et al. Cardiac resynchronization in chronic heart failure. N Engl J Med 2002;346(24):1845–53.
3. Young JB, Abraham WT, Smith AL, et al. Combined cardiac resynchronization and implantable cardioversion defibrillation in advanced chronic heart failure: the MIRACLE ICD Trial. JAMA 2003;289(20): 2685–94.
4. Bristow MR, Saxon LA, Boehmer J, et al. Cardiac-resynchronization therapy with or without an implantable defibrillator in advanced chronic heart failure. N Engl J Med 2004;350(21):2140–50.
5. Cleland JG, Daubert JC, Erdmann E, et al. The effect of cardiac resynchronization on morbidity and

mortality in heart failure. N Engl J Med 2005;352(15):1539–49.

6. Moss AJ, Hall WJ, Cannom DS, et al. Cardiac-resynchronization therapy for the prevention of heart-failure events. N Engl J Med 2009;361(14):1329–38.
7. Tang AS, Wells GA, Talajic M, et al. Cardiac-resynchronization therapy for mild-to-moderate heart failure. N Engl J Med 2010;363(25):2385–95.
8. Farwell D, Patel NR, Hall A, et al. How many people with heart failure are appropriate for biventricular resynchronization? Eur Heart J 2000;21(15):1246–50.
9. Aaronson KD, Schwartz JS, Chen TM, et al. Development and prospective validation of a clinical index to predict survival in ambulatory patients referred for cardiac transplant evaluation. Circulation 1997;95(12):2660–7.
10. 2012 Writing Group Members, Tracy CM, Epstein AE, Darbar D, et al. 2012 ACCF/AHA/HRS focused update of the 2008 guidelines for device-based therapy of cardiac rhythm abnormalities: a report of the American College of Cardiology Foundation/American Heart Association Task Force on Practice Guidelines. J Thorac Cardiovasc Surg 2012;144(6):e127–45.
11. Kron J, Aranda JM, Miles WM, et al. Benefit of cardiac resynchronization in elderly patients: results from the Multicenter Insync Randomized Clinical Evaluation (MIRACLE) and Multicenter Insync ICD Randomized Clinical Evaluation (MIRACLE-ICD) trials. J Interv Card Electrophysiol 2009;25(2):91–6.
12. Thomas S, Moss AJ, Zareba W, et al. Cardiac resynchronization in different age groups: a MADIT-CRT long-term follow-up substudy. J Card Fail 2016;22(2):143–9.
13. Bleeker GB, Schalij MJ, Molhoek SG, et al. Comparison of effectiveness of cardiac resynchronization therapy in patients <70 versus > or =70 years of age. Am J Cardiol 2005;96:420–2.
14. Delnoy PP, Ottervanger JP, Luttikhuis HO, et al. Clinical response of cardiac resynchronization therapy in the elderly. Am Heart J 2008;155(4):746–51.
15. Achilli A, Turreni F, Gasparini M, et al. Efficacy of cardiac resynchronization therapy in very old patients: the Insync/Insync ICD Italian registry. Europace 2007;9(9):732–8.
16. Upadhyay GA, Choudhry NK, Auricchio A, et al. Cardiac resynchronization in patients with atrial fibrillation. a meta-analysis of prospective cohort studies. J Am Coll Cardiol 2008;52(15):1239–46.
17. Fantoni C, Regoli F, Ghanem A, et al. Long-term outcome in diabetic heart failure patients treated with cardiac resynchronization therapy. Eur J Heart Fail 2008;10(3):298–307.
18. Höke U, Khidir MJ, van der Velde ET, et al. Cardiac resynchronization therapy in CKD stage 4 patients. Clin J Am Soc Nephrol 2015;10(10):1740–8.
19. Jencks SF, Williams MV, Coleman EA. Rehospitalizations among patients in the Medicare fee-for-service program. N Engl J Med 2009;360(14):1418–28.
20. Arundel C, Lam P, Khosla R, et al. Association of 30-day all-cause readmission with long-term outcomes in hospitalized older Medicare beneficiaries with heart failure. Am J Med 2016;129(11):1178–84.
21. Feldman AM, De Lissovoy G, Bristow MR, et al. Cost effectiveness of cardiac resynchronization therapy in the Comparison of Medical Therapy, Pacing, and Defibrillation in Heart Failure (COMPANION) trial. J Am Coll Cardiol 2005;46(12):2311–21.
22. Voigt A, Barrington W, Ngwu O, et al. Biventricular pacing reduces ventricular arrhythmic burden and defibrillator therapies in patients with heart failure. Clin Cardiol 2006;29(2):74–7.
23. Higgins SL, Yong P, Sheck D, et al. Biventricular pacing diminishes the need for implantable cardioverter defibrillator therapy. Ventak CHF investigators [see comment]. J Am Coll Cardiol 2000;36(3):824–7.
24. Sears SF, Sowell LV, Kuhl EA, et al. Quality of death: implantable cardioverter defibrillators and proactive care. Pacing Clin Electrophysiol 2006;29(6):637–42.
25. Sears SF, Lewis TS, Kuhl EA, et al. Predictors of quality of life in patients with implantable cardioverter defibrillators. Psychosomatics 2005;46(5):451–7.
26. Køber L, Thune JJ, Nielsen JC, et al. Defibrillator implantation in patients with nonischemic systolic heart failure. N Engl J Med 2016;375(13):1221–30.
27. Epstein AE, DiMarco JP, Ellenbogen KA, et al. ACC/AHA/HRS 2008 guidelines for device-based therapy of cardiac rhythm abnormalities. Hear Rhythm 2008;5(6):934–55.

Treatment of Ventricular Arrhythmias and Use of Implantable Cardioverter-Defibrillators to Improve Survival in Older Adult Patients with Cardiac Disease

Jason T. Jacobson, MD, Sei Iwai, MD,
Wilbert S. Aronow, MD*

KEYWORDS

• Ventricular arrhythmia • ICD • Ablation • Antiarrhythmic drugs • Autonomic modulation

KEY POINTS

- Ventricular arrhythmias in patients with cardiac disease are caused by similar mechanisms regardless of the underlying disease and are treated much the same way regardless of age.
- Antiarrhythmic drugs and catheter ablation are accepted therapies to prevent recurrence but do not prevent sudden cardiac death.
- The implantable cardioverter-defibrillator is the only therapy proved to prevent mortality in patients with ventricular arrhythmias and cardiac disease; however, it is unclear whether this benefit is as robust in the elderly.

INTRODUCTION

The causes and substrates for heart failure (HF) are myriad and are discussed elsewhere in this issue of *Heart Failure Clinics*. The risk of ventricular arrhythmia (VA) depends on the cause and severity of HF and the degree of ventricular dysfunction. Structural heart disease (SHD) can take many forms. Ischemic cardiomyopathy (ICM) occurs in the setting of healed myocardial infarction (MI), leaving behind an area of fibrotic scar. This condition is in contrast with nonischemic cardiomyopathy (NICM), a term that encompasses many different causes, such as viral cardiomyopathy (CMP), cardiac sarcoidosis, and idiopathic dilated cardiomyopathy. Frequently, the exact cause of NICM goes undetermined. Therefore, this group is treated as a whole.

SUBSTRATE AND MECHANISM OF VENTRICULAR ARRHYTHMIAS

The initiation and maintenance of VA in SHD is a complex process that requires an abnormal electrical milieu (substrate), an initiating event (such as ectopic beats), and the modulating factors that influence both (such as autonomic balance). Much is known about the substrate and its role in

This is an updated version of an article that appeared in *Heart Failure Clinics*, Volume 3, Issue 4.

Division of Cardiology, Department of Medicine, Westchester Medical Center, New York Medical College, Macy Pavilion, 100 Woods Road, Valhalla, NY 10595, USA
* Corresponding author. Westchester Medical Center, New York Medical College, Macy Pavilion, Room 141, Valhalla, NY 10595.
E-mail address: wsaronow@aol.com

Heart Failure Clin 13 (2017) 589–605
http://dx.doi.org/10.1016/j.hfc.2017.02.015
1551-7136/17/

arrhythmogenesis. A common end point of many CMPs is the development of ventricular fibrosis and scar. Be it scar from MI, fibrosis from infiltrative CMP such as cardiac sarcoidosis, or fibrofatty replacement in arrhythmogenic right ventricular cardiomyopathy, this process is the common substrate for VA of all causes. Fibrotic pattern varies depending on the cause of SHD. Although MI causes a predominantly subendocardial scar in a vascular distribution, NICM-associated fibrosis can be midmyocardial or epicardial without a correlation to coronary artery territory.[1] Scar deposition is rarely a homogeneous process; usually, surviving myocardial fibers are interspersed in areas of fibrosis.[2] Although these surviving fibers do not participate in systolic function, they are capable of impulse conduction and do so during sinus rhythm.[2–4]

The best-studied process for ventricular tachycardia (VT) is that of monomorphic VT (unchanging QRS morphology and rate) in chronic healed MI. Conduction in infarcted areas is generally slow because of decreased gap junctions at the intercalated disks and also because of more frequent conduction between parallel myocytes, leading to nonlinear, zigzag conduction.[5,6] These areas of surviving myocardium within scar display longer refractory periods and thus encounter transient unidirectional block caused by premature ventricular contractions (PVCs) or changes in heart rate (such as supraventricular tachycardia).[7]

The most important modulating factor behind VA is the sympathetic nervous system. The exact mechanism by which catecholamines influence VA in SHD is not clearly delineated in humans. In addition to enhancement of ectopic activity (caused by both enhanced automaticity and triggered activity) that may initiate sustained VA,[8–10] inhomogeneities in sympathetic innervation of infarcted areas can lead to ectopy as well as changes in potassium channel activity[11] and thus a dispersion of refractory periods.

MEDICAL THERAPY

Antiarrhythmic Drugs

When discussing management of VA in HF, the greatest focus is on sustained arrhythmia and the prevention of sudden cardiac death (SCD). Because no AAD has been reliably shown to prevent SCD, an ICD is indicated in most patients with sustained VA and HF.[12] Several trials have investigated AAD for treatment of complex ventricular ectopy in patients with SHD (mostly post-MI) before the wide adoption of the ICD. Other randomized trials have focused mostly on comparing AAD selection strategies to reduce mortality in patients who have had a sustained VA, rather than strictly preventing VA recurrence. Additional management considerations pertain to preventing recurrent symptomatic VA episodes, especially those that lead to ICD shocks, which have been associated with increased morbidity and mortality.[13] In the ICD era, AAD use in patients with HF has been relegated to prevention of shocks. Because of the increased SCD risk of the class Ic AAD,[14] these agents (flecainide and propafenone) are largely avoided, even in patients with an ICD.

Ventricular ectopy and nonsustained ventricular tachycardia

Based on the observation that frequent ventricular premature beats (VPBs) in post-MI patients are a marker for mortality,[15–18] several trials were undertaken to determine whether treatment with AAD would be protective in this population. The Cardiac Arrhythmia Suppression Trial (CAST) investigated the effects of the class Ic agents flecainide or encainide versus placebo in patients with prior MI, decreased ejection fraction (EF), and at least 6 VPB/h (average) on Holter monitoring at least 6 days after MI.[14] The primary end point of death or resuscitated cardiac arrest was reached in 63 AAD patients versus 26 on placebo ($P = .0001$). Of these, 43 (AAD) and 16 (placebo) were caused by arrhythmia. Most of the nonarrhythmic end points were caused by MI complicated by cardiogenic shock or HF, suggesting that the negative inotropic effects of these drugs exacerbated the ischemic events.[14] Another class Ic AAD, propafenone, was investigated in the Cardiac Arrest Study Hamburg (CASH) trial, compared with amiodarone, metoprolol, and ICD in patients resuscitated from cardiac arrest caused by sustained VA.[19] The propafenone arm of this trial was terminated early because of a 61% higher all-cause mortality compared with the other arms.[20] Because of these findings, the class Ic AAD are largely avoided in patients with coronary artery disease (CAD) and/or SHD.

Amiodarone is a class III AAD that also has class I, II, and IV effects. The Basel Antiarrhythmic Study of Infarct Survival (BASIS) randomized patients before hospital discharge post-MI who also had asymptomatic Lown class 3 or 4b VAs on 24-hour Holter monitor.[21] Three-hundred and twelve patients were randomized to control, empiric amiodarone, or individualized AAD treatment with several class I and III AAD. Compared with the control group, only amiodarone decreased mortality (5% vs 13%; $P<.05$) and sudden death/sustained VT/ventricular fibrillation (VF) (5% vs 17%; $P<.01$). In the Canadian Amiodarone Myocardial

Infarction Arrhythmia Trial (CAMIAT), patients post-MI with at least 10 VPB/h, VT less than 120 beats/min (BPM), or nonsustained VT (NSVT) greater than 120 BPM[22] were randomized to amiodarone or placebo. There was no significant difference between amiodarone and placebo for arrhythmic death alone, cardiac mortality, or all-cause mortality in this trial. The investigators concluded that their study was underpowered to detect a significant decrease in all-cause mortality. At the least, amiodarone was not associated with excess mortality in CAMIAT.

Sustained ventricular tachycardia/fibrillation and aborted sudden death

Although the Electrophysiologic Study Versus Electrocardiographic Monitoring (ESVEM) trial was not designed to specifically evaluate AAD efficacy, it does offer some assessment of recurrence of VA. The primary article evaluated 2 strategies for choosing which AAD to use in patients with documented VT or VF, SCD, or unmonitored syncope. All subjects underwent baseline electrophysiologic study (EPS) with inducible sustained VA and 48 hours of continuous electrocardiogram (ECG) monitoring showing at least 10 VPB/h.[23] Patients were then randomized to AAD selection guided by serial EPS or 24-hour Holter monitoring until an AAD suppressed VA on repeat testing.[23] Seven AAD were tested (sotalol, propafenone, mexiletine, imipramine, pirmenol, procainamide, and quinidine). No significant difference was found in the end points of arrhythmia recurrence or death.[24] Regarding the risk reduction (RR) at 4 years, the end points of arrhythmia recurrence (RR, 0.43; 95% confidence interval [CI], 0.29–0.62; $P<.001$) and death from arrhythmia (RR, 0.50; 95% CI, 0.26–0.96; $P = .04$), sotalol was superior to all the other AAD combined.[25]

Another trial that evaluated different strategies for AAD selection was the Cardiac Arrest in Seattle: Conventional Versus Amiodarone Drug Evaluation (CASCADE) study.[26] Empiric amiodarone was compared in a randomized fashion with conventional EPS or Holter-guided therapy with one of many AAD (procainamide, quinidine, disopyramide, tocainide, mexiletine, encainide, flecainide, propafenone, moricizine).[26,27] The patient population was composed of survivors of cardiac arrest caused by VF who also had VT/VF inducible at EPS and/or at least 10 VPB/h, couplets, or VT on Holter. The conventional therapy group was started on AAD and progressed through the list until a response was seen on repeat testing.[26,27] As the ICD became more readily available and reports of efficacy appeared, as well as a high mortality on interim analysis of CASCADE, the protocol was changed midstudy to include ICD implantation if surgically feasible (early devices required sternotomy and did not have the capability to store electrograms from treated arrhythmias for confirmation of arrhythmia detection).[27] At 2 years, 78% of the amiodarone group and 52% of the conventional therapy group remained free of cardiac death, resuscitated arrest, and sustained VT requiring cardioversion and ICD shocks, decreasing to 41% and 20% at 6 years ($P<.001$).[26] Although this study did show the superiority of empiric amiodarone compared with a conventional AAD choice determined by repeated EPS or Holter monitor, the investigators thought that an ICD should be offered to all study participants later in the study because of the high 1-year incidence of cardiac death and arrhythmic mortality.[27]

Implantable cardioverter-defibrillator shock reduction

Sotalol, a class III potassium channel blocker with β-blocker (BB) activity, was compared with placebo in a randomized, double-blind trial of 302 subjects by Pacifico and colleagues.[28] Patients were stratified by EF (>30%, ≤30%) and all had prior ICD shocks. Sotalol decreased appropriate ICD shocks or death from any cause by 44% compared with placebo (27% vs 42%; $P = -.007$).[28] Delivery of an appropriate first shock was seen in 32% of the placebo group versus 22% of the sotalol group during the 12 month follow-up of the trial.[28]

The Optimal Pharmacological Therapy in Cardioverter-Defibrillator Patients (OPTIC) trial[29] randomized patients receiving ICD shocks for VA to 3 AAD arms: amiodarone (class III) plus BB, sotalol, and BB alone. Four-hundred and twelve patients were randomized: 138 to the BB arm, 140 to the amiodarone arm, and 134 to the sotalol arm. At 1 year, the percentage of patients receiving ICD therapy for VA (antitachycardia pacing [ATP] or shocks) was as follows: amiodarone plus BB, 13%; followed by sotalol, 38.9%; and then BB alone, 45%.[29] Of note, the rate of drug discontinuation was 18.2% for amiodarone and 23.5% for sotalol (vs 5.3% for BB alone) because of side effects,[29] highlighting a significant issue with AAD treatment. In addition, an 11-year follow-up of the Canadian Implantable Defibrillator Study (CIDS) trial showed a 5.5% per year mortality and a 50% discontinuation rate with amiodarone therapy.[30]

One other available class III AAD has been suggested to decrease ICD therapy for VA: dofetilide. In one brief observational report, 50% of patients had a decrease in ICD therapies after starting treatment with dofetilide.[31] In addition, Baquero and colleagues[32] found a significant reduction in monthly VT/VF episodes (1.8 ± 4.5/mo before vs 1.0 ± 3.5/mo on dofetilide; $P = .006$) in 30 patients with ICDs who had failed at least 1 other AAD (63% amiodarone). Azimilide, another class III agent, has been shown to be effective in preventing ICD therapies for recurrent VA in patients with CMP.[33,34] The larger of the 2 trials (633 subjects), the Shock Inhibition Evaluation with Azimilide (SHIELD), randomized patients with secondary prevention ICDs or preexisting ICDs who received a recent shock for VA, to placebo or azimilide in 2 dosages (75 or 125 mg daily) for 1 year. The primary end points were all-cause shocks plus symptomatic tachyarrhythmia terminated by ATP and all-cause shocks. The secondary end point was all appropriate ICD therapies (VA terminated by shocks or ATP), for which a relative RR of 48% (hazard ratio [HR], 0.52; 95% CI, 0.3–0.89; $P = .017$) for 75 mg daily and 62% (HR, 0.38; 95% CI, 0.22–0.65; $P = .0004$) for 125 mg daily was seen at 1 year compared with placebo.[33] As of this writing, azimilide is unavailable in the United States.

Several AAD combinations have been reported with varying success in older nonrandomized studies with small numbers of patients, often only evaluating response during electrophysiology studies. Many have included a class Ic in combination with mexiletine[35](Ib agent) and amiodarone.[36,37] Because of the association with SCD, as stated previously, and proarrhythmia,[37] the Ic agents are generally not used. Mexiletine has also been used in combination with class Ia agents[36,38–40] and amiodarone[41,42] with varying results. Because of side effects and difficulty obtaining the Ia agents, mexiletine is often used in combination with amiodarone because it seems to be clinically effective in refractory VT.[42]

β-Blockers

BBs are considered class II AAD in the Vaughan-Williams classification. In addition to positive effects on mortality, data suggest a decrease in recurrent VA as well. Observational studies in patients with prior SCD and hemodynamically relevant VT have reported a decrease in recurrence.[43–45] Hallstrom and colleagues[43] reported an adjusted relative RR of 38% related to BB therapy in survivors of cardiac arrest. In this same study, a higher mortality was seen with AAD use. In the Antiarrhythmics versus Implantable Defibrillators (AVID) registry,[44] patients on BB but not treated with AAD or ICD showed an approximately 50% reduction in adjusted relative risk of mortality caused by BB therapy. Hreybe and colleagues[45] also showed an increase in time to first ICD shock for VA in patients treated with BB compared with those who were not. In a randomized comparison with sotalol, metoprolol[46] showed a greater survival free of ventricular tachyarrhythmias in patients with implantable defibrillators. This finding is in contrast with the OPTIC trial, which showed greater efficacy for sotalol.[29]

Nonantiarrhythmic Drugs

Although many agents lacking direct ion channel effects have been shown to prevent SCD, few have been shown to prevent the recurrence of VA. It is important to remember that most of these agents may act in preventing the formation/progression of the substrate that leads to VA, thus enacting an indirect antiarrhythmic effect. Agents such as angiotensin-converting enzyme (ACE) inhibitors, angiotensin receptor blockers, aldosterone inhibitors, and 3-hydroxy-3-methyl-glutaryl-coenzyme A reductase inhibitors have not been shown to prevent recurrence of VA.

Fish oil

Polyunsaturated fatty acids (PUFA) commonly found in the oils of certain fishes may have antiarrhythmic effects to prevent recurrences of VA. The data on these compounds are contradictory. Although some studies suggest a benefit,[47–49] others have shown no effect[50] or an increase in VA in patients with ICD,[51] leading to increased therapies. A recent meta-analysis of more than 30,000 patients in 9 trials showed no significant effect on VA.[52] At this time, PUFA cannot be recommended as a viable treatment of VA suppression.

Antianginal agents

The recent addition of ranolazine to the antianginal armamentarium has led to the discovery of antiarrhythmic properties of this drug, following the addition of amiodarone. Ranolazine is a late sodium channel blocker that has antiarrhythmic properties.[53] Although no randomized trials have shown definitive efficacy for VA, case reports and series suggest this compound may have promise.[54–56] These reports have mostly been in patients with recurrent PVCs or ICD therapies for VA, who were also on traditional AAD that were ineffective (usually amiodarone). The addition of ranolazine coincided with an interruption of VT storm or suppression of further ICD therapies.[54–56]

Implantable Cardiac Defibrillator

The utility of the ICD in primary and secondary prevention of SCD in patients at risk is supported by multiple randomized, multicenter trials, establishing this device as the first-line therapy in patients with SHD and VA. Note that although the ICD does prevent SCD, it does not prevent VA. Sustained VA is terminated either with a high-energy shock or, if monomorphic VT of a rate slow enough to respond, with ATP.

Primary prevention trials

Several randomized trials have investigated the utility of the ICD in patients with congestive HF (CHF) at risk for SCD, but have never experienced sustained VA. Primary prevention ICD trials initially focused on patients post-MI with significantly reduced left ventricular EF (LVEF). The Multicenter Automatic Defibrillator Trial (MADIT) randomized 196 patients with prior MI, class I to III CHF, an LVEF less than or equal to 35%, NSVT, and inducible VT on EP study that was not suppressible with procainamide, to an ICD or conventional therapy.[57] Most patients in the conventional therapy arm received amiodarone. The trial was stopped early because it showed a statistically significant, and impressive, 54% reduction in total mortality in the ICD arm at 27 months (16% and 39% in the ICD and conventional therapy groups, respectively). MADIT is notable in that it only enrolled a small number of patients and did not have a control (no arrhythmia therapy) group. In addition, more patients in the ICD group received BBs.

The Multicenter Unsustained Tachycardia Trial (MUSTT) was not designed as an ICD trial, but was intended to test whether EP-guided antiarrhythmic therapy would decrease the risk of SCD.[58] The trial enrolled patients with CAD, LVEF 40% or less, NSVT, HF class I to III, and inducible VT during EP study. NSVT had to occur 4 days or more post-MI or revascularization. Seven-hundred and four inducible patients were randomized to EP-guided therapy (351 patients) or no therapy (353 patients). Of the patients randomized to EP-guided therapy, 29% received antiarrhythmic drugs and 58% received an ICD. Patients only qualified for an ICD if they failed 1 antiarrhythmic agent and remained inducible for VT/VF at repeat EP testing. MUSTT showed a decrease in the combined end point of cardiac arrest or death from arrhythmia at 5 years with EP-guided therapy compared with no antiarrhythmic therapy (25% vs 32%, respectively). Overall mortality was also reduced from 48% to 42% among patients receiving EP-guided therapy. Subgroup analysis revealed that the benefit from EP-guided therapy was entirely caused by the survival benefit of the ICD group. The ICD arm showed a 31% reduction in mortality compared with subjects receiving antiarrhythmic therapy and a 24% mortality reduction compared with those receiving no therapy. Together, MADIT and MUSTT clearly showed the benefit of ICD therapy in patients with a low LVEF, NSVT, and inducible VAs on EP study.

The MADIT-II trial addressed the possibility that patients with CAD and a low LVEF were at sufficiently high risk of SCD, and thus would benefit from an ICD,[59] regardless of inducibility at EPS. In MADIT-II, 1232 patients with prior MI, LVEF less than or equal to 30%, and New York Heart Association (NYHA) class I to III HF were randomly assigned in a 3:2 ratio to receive an ICD or conventional therapy. Patients were excluded if they had an MI within the past month, or if they were revascularized via percutaneous coronary intervention or coronary artery bypass graft (CABG) surgery in the past 3 months. The mean time from MI to enrollment in the trial was 6.5 years. During an average follow-up of 20 months, the mortalities were 19.8% in the conventional therapy group and 14.2% in the ICD group, representing a 31% relative RR for death with ICD therapy. The mortality benefit was caused by a reduction in sudden death (3.8% vs 10.0% in the ICD and conventional therapy arms, respectively). Note that there was a higher rate of hospitalization for HF in the ICD group (20%) than in the conventional therapy group (15%). Potential explanations for this include the ICD preventing arrhythmic death thus leading to more HF, or the effects of right ventricular pacing leading to ventricular dyssynchrony.

These trials were mostly in patients with remote MI. Contrasting evidence was found by the Defibrillation in Acute Myocardial Infarction Trial (DINAMIT) investigators, who assessed the utility of ICD implantation after recent MI.[60] In their study, 674 patients with an MI within 6 to 40 days, LVEF less than or equal to 35%, and impaired cardiac autonomic function (manifest as either depressed heart rate variability or an increased average 24-hour heart rate on Holter monitoring) were randomized to either medical therapy or an ICD. During a mean follow-up of 30 months, there was no difference in overall mortality between the two groups. Although the ICD was effective in reducing death from arrhythmia by 58%, which was a prespecified secondary outcome, this was offset by a 75% increase in nonarrhythmic death in this group. Most of the nonarrhythmic deaths in the ICD group had cardiac causes, suggesting that ICD implantation shifted the mode of death from arrhythmia to HF in this population. Because only 10% of patients were revascularized in the ICD group, recurrent ischemia leading to VT/VF, which normally would have led to cardiac arrest, was prevented by the ICD, but infarction and pump failure was not. However, the trial had a low event rate overall, which may have prevented detection of a difference between the control group and ICD group. It is also possible that the use of impaired autonomic tone as an inclusion criterion may have selected for patients who had a higher propensity to die from HF and not sudden death. Ultimately, the results of DINAMIT suggest that immediate risk stratification of patients post-MI by LVEF and impaired autonomic tone may not be helpful, because the LVEF can recover over time, or scar formation may occur, thus changing the risk of SCD as time progresses.

In addition to DINAMIT, the CABG Patch Trial failed to show the utility of ICD in primary prophylaxis.[61] In CABG Patch, 900 patients scheduled for a CABG with an LVEF less than or equal to 35% and a positive signal-averaged ECG were randomized to CABG and an epicardial ICD or CABG and conventional therapy. There was no reduction in total mortality with the ICD after an average follow-up of 32 months, but the ICD group did have a reduction in arrhythmic death (4% vs 6.9% in the control group). Because most of the deaths were nonarrhythmic, the reduction in arrhythmic death did not affect total mortality. Reasons proposed for the lack of benefit include the beneficial effects of revascularization, including protection against arrhythmia and possible improvement of postoperative LVEF, thereby creating a lower-risk patient population for SCD.

Given the results of MADIT-II, the Sudden Cardiac Death in Heart Failure Trial (SCD-HeFT) (discussed later), MUSTT, as well as DINAMIT and CABG-Patch, current guidelines for patients post-MI with an LVEF less than or equal to 35% with class II to III HF advocate waiting 40 days post-MI before ICD implantation, and waiting 3 months postrevascularization before ICD implantation. Patients post-MI with class I HF must have an LVEF less than or equal to 30% because only MADIT-II specifically included this group of patients. Based on MUSTT, patients with an LVEF less than or equal to 40% and NSVT may undergo EPS and receive an ICD if inducible for VF or sustained VT.[62]

Risk stratification of patients with NICM has proved to be more challenging than in their counterparts with ICM. The Defibrillators in Non-Ischemic Cardiomyopathy Treatment Evaluation (DEFINITE) Trial[63] randomized 458 patients with NICM, LVEF less than 36%, and premature ventricular complexes or NSVT to standard medical therapy or standard medical therapy plus a single-chamber ICD. Of these patients, 86% were on an ACE inhibitor and 85% were on a BB. The ICD group had a significant reduction in arrhythmic death, but a nonsignificant reduction in total mortality. The trial was underpowered because the mortality in the medical therapy arm was lower than the trial design had anticipated, and thus the primary end point may have reached statistical significance if there had been a larger number of study subjects.

SCD-HeFT enrolled 2521 patients with ischemic or nonischemic cardiomyopathy with class II or III HF and an LVEF less than or equal to 35%.[64] Patients were randomized to conventional therapy plus placebo, conventional therapy plus amiodarone, or conventional therapy plus a single-lead ICD. Placebo and amiodarone were administered in double-blind fashion. Amiodarone had no effect on the risk of death (28%) compared with placebo (29%). In contrast, ICD therapy was associated with an absolute decrease in mortality of 7.2% compared with amiodarone and medical therapy with ACE inhibitors and BBs. These results held true for patients with both ischemic and nonischemic cardiomyopathies, a prespecified subgroup analysis.

The results of these primary prevention trials in patients with nonischemic cardiomyopathy led to an indication for ICD implantation in patients with a nonischemic cardiomyopathy, LVEF less than or equal to 35%, and class II or III HF.[62] Importantly in SCD-HeFT, patients had to have a diagnosis of HF for at least 3 months and be on appropriate medical therapy.

The results of the Defibrillator Implantation in Patients with Nonischemic Systolic Heart Failure (DANISH) trial were just published a few months before this writing.[65] This trial was designed to evaluate the added value of the ICD in patients with NICM in the modern era of CHF therapy, including ACE inhibitors or angiotensin receptor blockers, BBs, mineralocorticoid-receptor antagonists, and cardiac resynchronization therapy (CRT) in those eligible. Patients (556) with LVEF less than or equal to 35%, not caused by CAD, and NYHA class II, III, or IV (if CRT planned) were randomized to ICD or standard therapy. An increased N-terminal pro–brain natriuretic peptide (NT-proBNP) level was required as well. After 67.6 months of follow-up, there was a difference in all-cause mortality between those with and without an ICD (21.6% vs 23.4%), although SCD rates were lower in the ICD group (4.3% vs 8.2%; $P = .0005$). However, in subgroup analysis, patients less than 59 years old and those with NT-proBNP less than 1177 pg/ml did experience significant mortality benefit (HR, 0.51 [0.29–0.92] and 0.59 [0.38–0.91]; $P = .02$ for both).[65] It is of interest that the event rate was lower than expected based on prior trials outlined earlier.

Secondary prevention trials

There are 3 randomized trials of ICD for secondary prevention of SCD from VA. Two of these trials, the Canadian Implantable Defibrillator Study (CIDS)[66] and the CASH,[19] showed a nonsignificant decrease in total mortality. CIDS also showed a nonsignificant decrease in arrhythmic death, whereas CASH showed a significant reduction in recurrent SCD. Of note, CIDS also included patients with syncope from VT, VT greater than 150 BPM with presyncope or angina and an EF less than 35%, or unmonitored syncope with subsequent VT longer than 10 seconds or sustained VT induced at electrophysiologic study. Both trials compared the ICD with amiodarone. In addition, CASH included treatment arms consisting of metoprolol and propafenone. Although the metoprolol arm showed similar results to amiodarone, the propafenone arm was discontinued early after showing an unacceptably high mortality.

The AVID randomized more than 1000 subjects to initial treatment with an ICD or treatment with an AAD (amiodarone or sotalol) in patients with VF or VT with syncope, or VT with EF less than 40% and symptoms of hemodynamic compromise.[67] As opposed to CIDS and CASH, AVID showed a clear mortality benefit at 1, 2, and 3 years of follow-up compared with AAD (89.3% vs 82.3%, 81.6% vs 74.7%, and 75.4% vs 64.1% respectively; $P<.02$). These 3 trials were instrumental in establishing the ICD as first-line therapy for hemodynamically significant VA in patients with SHD. However, note that these trials do not address those patients with hemodynamically tolerated VT, or those with SHD and normal/near-normal ventricular function. The data from these studies have been used to support the use of the ICD for these patient populations in the guidelines.[68]

Although the ICD has been a lifesaving therapy for many patients with VA and SHD, it is by no means infallible. Sudden death can still occur at a rate of about 1.3% to 4.5%,[63,69–71] with 16% to 38% caused by refractory VA.[72,73]

Implantable Cardioverter-Defibrillator in the elderly

Although the aforementioned trials included elderly patients, the mean age of subjects was greater than or equal to 65 years in only 2.[58,67] The utility of the ICD in older populations has generated much interest of late because of competing comorbidities that may erase the mortality benefit seen in the pivotal trials. In a meta-analysis of trials of prophylactic amiodarone (6252 patients with prior MI [8 trials] or CHF [5 trials]), the Amiodarone Trialists Meta-Analysis Investigators found that, although both total mortality and SCD rates increased with age, the proportion of SCD decreased from 0.51 before age 50 years to 0.26 after age 80 years, which was not affected by sex, LVEF, or NYHA class.[74]

Several studies have evaluated the benefit of primary prevention ICD in the older population. In a post-hoc analysis of the MADIT-II trial,[75] the investigators found an improved survival with ICD in patients 75 years of age or older (HR, 0.56; 95 CI, 0.29–1.08; $P = .08$) compared with controls of the same age group, which was similar to those less than 75 years of age (HR, 0.63; 0.45–0.88; $P = .01$). Although the HR for the older group did not meet statistical significance, the mortality benefit was similar between the two groups ($P = .75$). The older group had higher blood urea nitrogen levels, more frequent bundle branch block, and a lower use of BBs and statin drugs, but also a lower incidence of diabetes and tobacco use.[75] A meta-analysis of primary prevention trials (ICM and NICM) also failed to show a difference in mortality between younger and older age subgroups, but this analysis was limited by a wide spread in the age cutoff defined in the different trials.[76] Bilchick and colleagues[77] developed a prediction model of mortality up to 4 years after primary prevention ICD implantation and found an increasing HR with advancing age. The HR for age greater than 85 years was 4.03 (3.47–4.68; $P<0,001$). For the final model, an age cutoff of 75 years conferred an HR of 1.70 (1.62–1.80; $P<.0001$) and was combined with NYHA class III CHF, chronic obstructive pulmonary disease, kidney disease, EF less than or equal to 20, and diabetes.[77] A nomogram-derived score in the highest decile conferred a 3-year mortality of 65%,[77] supporting an evaluation of comorbidities when deciding on an ICD. In an analysis of 83,792 Medicare patients (65 years and older), Green and colleagues[78] identified frailty and dementia as additional factors that increase mortality in primary prevention ICD recipients. In addition, the setting of implantation may also affect outcomes. In an analysis of 23,111 elderly (≥66 years) patients who received a primary prevention ICD during a hospital admission for CHF or other comorbidity, mortality and SCD benefits were not seen after adjusting for healthy candidate bias and confounding.[79] Most recently, the DANISH trial was published. As mentioned earlier, this trial studied the added benefit of ICD to contemporary CHF therapy, including CRT. Although the overall trial did not show a mortality benefit, subgroup analysis did show that patients less than 59 years old had a 0.51 HR for mortality (0.29–0.92; $P = .02$), whereas those 68 years of age and older had an HR of 1.19

(0.81–1.73; $P = .38$).[65] Although these studies suggest that the benefit of primary prevention ICD in the elderly is questionable, the overriding message is that overall health seems to matter and that the number and severity of comorbidities needs to be considered.

Regarding patients with secondary prevention ICD, the literature is not as replete. In an analysis of the AVID, CASH, and CIDS trials, Healey and colleagues[80] identified that 252 (13.5%) of 1866 patients were greater than or equal to 75 years old. Despite similar baseline characteristics, the elderly patients did not experience a benefit in mortality (HR, 1.06 [0.69–1.64]; $P = .79$) or arrhythmic death (HR, 0.9 [0.42–1.95]; $P = .79$) at 2.3 years.[80] In a smaller cohort (500) of ICD recipients in Marburg, 40 patients were greater than or equal to 75 years old. Of these, 88% were secondary prevention ICDs, as opposed to 62% in patients less than 75 years old ($P = .002$).[81] In the total cohort, the SCD rate was equally low in both age groups (3% and 2%), but the total mortality was much higher in the older patients (55% vs 21%; $P = .001$) at 5 years.[81] Yung and colleagues[82] analyzed survival in 5399 patients with ICDs in Ontario, 1460 of whom were secondary prevention. The cohort was divided into age groups of 18 to 49, 50 to 59, 60 to 69, 70 to 79, and greater than or equal to 80 years. Mortality increased with age in primary (2.1, 3.0, 5.4, 6.9, and 10.2 per 100 person-years) and secondary (2.2, 3.8, 6.1, 8.7, and 15.5) prevention groups, whereas rates of appropriate shocks were similar across age groups.[82]

No specific randomized trials have evaluated the utility of ICDs in the elderly. The data discussed show variable results depending on the populations, indications, and other comorbidities. There is no current recommended age threshold above which an ICD should be withheld. Suffice it to say, when considering ICD in the elderly, all comorbidities, severity of CHF, and patient goals and wishes should be taken into account with full involvement of the patient in the decision-making process.

SHOCK MORBIDITY AND MORTALITY

ICD therapies can cause significant psychological morbidity. There is a dose-dependent effect of shock frequency on the development of anxiety-related disorders (panic disorder, agoraphobia, and generalized anxiety) and depression.[83,84] Depression can lead to an increase in ICD therapies[85] as well.

In a seeming paradox, recent data have shown an association between ICD shocks and increased mortality. In an analysis of the SCD-HeFT trial, patients who experienced appropriate shocks had a hazard ratio of 5.68 for mortality.[13] It is unclear whether shocks contribute to, or are simply a marker for, risk of death. Patients with a high burden of VA may simply have more advanced disease. It would be expected that those being treated with ATP (discussed later) would have the same mortality if this were so. Data regarding this are conflicting.[86–88] Most recently, an analysis of the Multicenter Automatic Defibrillator Implantation Trial-Reduce Inappropriate Therapy (MADIT-RIT) trial[89] showed that appropriate shocks increased mortality, whereas appropriate ATP did not; however, any inappropriate therapies (shocks or ATP for supraventricular tachyarrhythmias) were also associated with higher mortality.[90] The investigators concluded that this study does provide evidence of the link between ICD shocks for VA and mortality.

SHOCK PREVENTION

Because of the clear morbidity and possible mortality associated with ICD shocks, it is imperative to prevent recurrence. Although AAD can be effective in preventing recurrent shocks for VA, as discussed earlier, evidence-supported ICD programming is crucial in preventing the delivery of shocks that may not be necessary in the first instance.

Modern ICDs are not only capable of delivering shocks to treat VA but can also attempt to terminate VT by overdrive pacing, or ATP. ATP terminates VT by causing conduction block within the VT circuit,[91] without the discomfort and potential morbidity of ICD shocks. Although originally applied only to slower VT because of the fear of inefficacy, syncope, and acceleration to VF when used for VT greater than 200 BPM, subsequent studies largely dispelled these concerns.[92,93] With this revelation, many trials have evaluated overall programming protocols to reduce the incidence of ICD shocks. These trials have used ATP as well as delaying the delivery of therapies in the hopes that VA may prove to be nonsustained and terminate spontaneously without any detriment to the patient. In addition, therapies for slower VT have been minimized in the belief that they pose little risk for sudden death.

The aforementioned MADIT-RIT trial compared 3 ICD programming protocols in a primary prevention population: a standard protocol that would treat VT of 170 to 200 BPM within 2.5 seconds and greater than 200 BPM after 1 second; a delayed-therapy protocol that would treat VT 170 to 200 BPM after 60 seconds of tachycardia, 200 to 249 BPM after 12 seconds, and greater than

250 BPM after 2.5 seconds; and a high-rate protocol that would treat only VA greater than 200 BPM after 2.5 seconds.[89] This trial showed a significant reduction in mortality, appropriate therapies (mostly ATP), and inappropriate therapies in both the delayed therapy and high-rate protocols compared with the standard programming, thus proving that more conservative ICD programming is preferable in primary prevention ICD recipients.[89]

The Effect of Long-Detection Interval Versus Standard Detection Interval for Implantable Cardioverter-Defibrillators on Antitachycardia Pacing and Shock Delivery (ADVANCE III) trial[94] also evaluated delaying therapy delivery, but in both primary and secondary prevention ICD recipients. For primary prevention patients, VA greater than 188 BPM was treated, whereas in the secondary prevention group, VA detection was based on the patients' clinical tachycardia.[94] This trial also showed a decrease in both appropriate and inappropriate ICD therapies with prolonged detection time, but without any difference in mortality for the overall population[94] and in a subgroup analysis of the secondary prevention patients.[95]

ABLATION

Catheter ablation (CA) for the treatment of VA has evolved significantly over the past few decades, greatly aided by better understanding of the arrhythmogenic substrate, as well as technological advances in computer mapping systems and delivery of ablation energy. Initially only an option in the minority of patients with hemodynamically stable VT, CA can now be offered to most patients with VT and VF in the setting of SHD.

Ablation of monomorphic VT in the setting of remote MI is the paradigm on which all VT ablation in SHD is based. The critical isthmus of the VT circuit (discussed earlier) is located within scar using electrode-tipped catheters and rendered electrically inert with ablation energy (most frequently radiofrequency electrical energy). This technique is based on the early experience of surgical subendocardial resection of infarcted myocardium pioneered at the University of Pennsylvania.[96,97] CA offers a minimally invasive approach with less morbidity and has largely supplanted surgical resection.

Contemporary VT ablation uses modern tools to enhance both the mapping and ablation processes. Computer mapping systems are able to follow catheter movements in three-dimensional space and collect data points that denote location and electrical parameters such as activation timing and tissue voltage.[98] These electroanatomic mapping systems allow the reproduction of the endocardial and/or epicardial surface in the computer space, which can be used to guide catheter manipulation with minimal fluoroscopy.[99] Locations with signals of interest can be tagged on the reconstructed geometry and revisited for ablation later in the procedure. Signals showing low voltage consistent with scar/fibrosis, especially those that display multicomponent fractionation, can be involved in VT circuits.[3,4,100]

Mapping can be performed during sinus rhythm and VT. A voltage map is often constructed during sinus rhythm to locate areas of scar.[101] A mapping catheter is moved throughout the ventricle and placed in contact with the myocardium over many cardiac cycles. A three-dimensional geometry of the chamber is created on the mapping system. Confluent areas of low voltage are color coded and fractionated signals and late potentials (occurring after the end of the QRS complex) are tagged on the map to be revisited after VT is induced. If the VT is hemodynamically tolerated, the circuit can be mapped by annotating the activation timing at sites throughout the chamber in reference to the QRS complex and performing pacing maneuvers to prove that the site is a part of the circuit.[102–104] The critical isthmus displays activation during diastole (between QRS complexes), because this low-voltage activity in the scar cannot be seen on the surface ECG. Once this critical isthmus is defined, ablation can terminate the VT and prevent recurrence.[104,105] In addition, patients who show frequent PVC may benefit from their ablation by better targeting reentrant VT and allowing some improvement in LV function.[106–108]

However, most VT (approximately 90%[109]) are not hemodynamically tolerated long enough for traditional mapping. Modern techniques for VT mapping and ablation focus on modification of the scar (substrate modification) guided by induced VT that is quickly terminated. The potential critical isthmus of an observed VT can be located by pacing inside the scar area (pace mapping) during a stable rhythm (sinus or right ventricular paced rhythm). If the resultant paced QRS matches the VT QRS, the site is likely at or near the isthmus, and is ablated.[101,110] During most VT ablation procedures, a combination of mapping during VT that is tolerated, and pace mapping those that are not, is used to maximize outcomes. Note that multiple VT can often be induced during a single procedure and that outcomes are best if all are targeted.[111,112] Observational studies of this approach in patients with ICM[112] and patients with both ICM and NICM[101] experiencing frequent ICD shocks for VT showed a significant reduction in episodes after ablation in at least two-thirds of patients.

The most current ablation techniques consist of extensive ablation targeting all signals that display evidence of slow conduction in the hope of interrupting all possible VT circuits. The complete elimination of all these sites, both endocardially and epicardially, shows promise and predicts long-term success independently of noninducibility of VT at the end of a procedure.[113,114]

Few randomized trials of VT ablation in patients with SHD have been published. Two such studies enrolled only patients with ICM and documented VA. The Prophylactic Catheter Ablation for the Prevention of Defibrillator Therapy (SMASH-VT) trial randomized 128 patients with a recent implantation of ICD for VA or who had a recent ICD therapy for VA after a recent implant, to ablation (substrate modification) or standard medical therapy (patients on class I or III AAD were excluded). There was a significant decrease in ICD therapies between the standard medical therapy and ablation groups (33% vs 12%; $P = .007$).[115]

The Catheter Ablation of Stable Ventricular Tachycardia Before Defibrillator Implantation in Patients with Coronary Heart Disease (VTACH) trial randomized 107 patients with hemodynamically tolerated monomorphic VT to ablation before ICD implantation or ICD and standard medical therapy (without AAD).[116] The ablation approach included traditional mapping of the stable VT and substrate modification as needed for other induced VT. The intention-to-treat analysis showed that the ablation group had a longer ICD therapy-free interval (18.6 vs 5.9 months) and greater VA-free survival at 2 years (47% vs 29%), with the greatest benefit seen in patients with EF greater than 30%.[116] A follow-up on treatment analysis (13% of the ablation group did not undergo the procedure, 19% of the control group were ablated) did show a greater effect of ablation compared with the intention-to-treat analysis: relative RR of VA, 49% versus 39%; and relative RR in cardiac hospitalization, 52% versus 45%.[117]

Until recently, no randomized trials comparing ablation and AAD had been published. The Ventricular Tachycardia Ablation Versus Escalation of Antiarrhythmic Drugs (VANISH) trial was designed to compare escalation of AAD therapy with VT ablation in patients with ICM and recurrent VT despite ongoing treatment with an AAD.[118] All patients had a previously implanted ICD and had an episode of VT (either below the detection rate of the ICD or ICD-terminated episodes) during treatment with amiodarone or another class I or III AAD, within the previous 6 months. Patients were randomized (1:1) to either ablation or intensification of AAD therapy. For patients initially treated with another AAD, this was discontinued and amiodarone was started. For patients initially treated with amiodarone less than 300 mg daily, additional drug loading was followed by maintenance of 300 mg daily. Those patients who were taking at least 300 mg of amiodarone daily had mexiletine, 200 mg thrice daily, added to their regimens. The primary end point was a composite of death or VT storm (at least 3 episodes in a 24-hour period) or appropriate ICD shocks.[118]

Of 132 patients randomized to ablation, 129 underwent the procedure (2 died, 1 withdrew consent). All patients in the escalated-therapy group (127) received the assigned treatment. The primary outcome rate was lower in the ablation group (HR, 0.72; 95% CI, 0.53–0.98; $P = .04$), which was mostly caused by decreases in VT storm and appropriate ICD shocks.[118] Of interest, in subgroup analysis, in those patients who were on amiodarone before the start of the study, outcomes were superior in the ablation group (HR, 0.55; 95% CI, 0.38–0.80; $P = .001$). Of note, no mortality benefit was seen for ablation, even on subgroup analysis,[118] although the study was not powered for this end point alone. Although VANISH does not directly answer the question of superiority of ablation compared with AAD as first-line therapy, it does compliment the data from OPTIC suggesting that amiodarone is superior to sotalol (the only other AAD used at baseline in the escalated-therapy arm) for prevention of recurrent VA in this patient population. In addition, it aids in the decision for ablation, suggesting that patients who are naive to amiodarone may benefit from this drug (if not averse/susceptible to its toxicities), whereas those already on amiodarone would be less likely to benefit from increasing the dose or adding mexiletine.[118]

No randomized trials of ablation for VT in NICM have been published to date. The initial series suggest similar efficacy, but recent data suggest lower success than for VT in ICM.[119] The substrate for VT in these patients is less frequently endocardial and may be midmyocardial or even epicardial in location.[1] The advent of a percutaneous subxiphoid approach to accessing the pericardial space for VT ablation has allowed the ablation of many VT that were previously unaccessible.[120,121] The ability to identify and ablate midmyocardial circuits remains a challenge. In refractory cases, selective intracoronary alcohol ablation can be effective, but needs to be used cautiously.[122] It is hoped that new ablation technologies able to deliver deeper lesions will address this issue in the near future.[123,124]

Once considered an arrhythmia not amenable to ablation, techniques to address VF have been pioneered over the past few years. As SMASH-VT suggests, ablation of VT has the additional effect of decreasing ICD therapies for VF as well,[115] likely explained by the fact that many VF episodes begin as VT, but also likely because of the extensive substrate ablation. Specifically, surviving Purkinje fibers located in areas of scar can induce VF in both ICM and NICM via ectopic beats.[125,126] These areas can be identified as displaying early signals that precede the QRS during sinus rhythm and during ectopic beats. Ablation of these areas can prevent further VF episodes, even if the exact site of ectopic beat origination is not identified.[125,126]

Despite the extensive body of literature on ablation and the expanding application to multiple VA substrates and areas of origin, a definitive mortality benefit has not been proved. In addition, randomized comparisons as a first-line therapy with AAD or ICD have not been published. For these reasons, at this writing, ablation of VA in SHD is largely adjunctive to the ICD in patients who fail, do not tolerate, or do not wish to take AAD.

AUTONOMIC MODULATION

Based on the known benefits of beta-adrenergic blockade previously discussed, and the success of left cardiac sympathetic denervation for patients with long QT syndrome,[127] invasive approaches to autonomic modulation have generated increasing interest for the treatment of VA in SHD. The stellate ganglia provide direct sympathetic innervation to the heart. Several case reports and series have investigated the surgical destruction of the lower third to half of the stellate ganglia for arrhythmia control.[128,129] In 41 patients refractory to AAD and ablation for VA, Vaseghi and colleagues[129] found bilateral stellate ganglia destruction more effective than left-sided ganglion destruction alone (ICD shock–free survival, 48% vs 30%; $P = .04$).

The development of renal artery denervation for the treatment of hypertension[130,131] has generated much interest in the effects on arrhythmia prevention. The renal afferent signals are processed in the central nervous system and affect sympathetic outflow and circulating catecholamine levels. There is also evidence that they directly interact with the stellate ganglia.[132] Several case reports and series have displayed potential benefit in patients wit SHD with refractory VA.[133–135] These data must be tempered by the uncertain efficacy of renal denervation for the treatment of hypertension.[136] In addition, direct spinal cord stimulation, which can help prevent angina by suppressing sympathetic effects on the heart, has been used in 2 patients with refractory VA with good effect.[137] These invasive approaches to cardiac sympathetic blockade offer unique insights into arrhythmogenesis and offer potential future therapies, but have yet to be proved in large-scale trials.

SUMMARY

The treatment of VA in patients with SHD has evolved over the decades from a primarily medical approach to one dominated by technology and invasive interventions. Although the ICD has offered extended life to many patients, recurrent VA are still the cause of significant morbidity. In addition, the elderly may not derive as much benefit as the major ICD trials suggest, depending on comorbidities. A complex, multimodality approach by expert clinicians is necessary for successful management of these patients. Future technologic advances will allow the effective treatment of more patients.

REFERENCES

1. Jackson E, Bellenger N, Seddon M, et al. Ischaemic and non-ischaemic cardiomyopathies–cardiac MRI appearances with delayed enhancement. Clin Radiol 2007;62(5):395–403.
2. de Bakker JM, van Capelle FJ, Janse MJ, et al. Reentry as a cause of ventricular tachycardia in patients with chronic ischemic heart disease: electrophysiologic and anatomic correlation. Circulation 1988;77(3):589–606.
3. Kienzle MG, Miller J, Falcone RA, et al. Intraoperative endocardial mapping during sinus rhythm: relationship to site of origin of ventricular tachycardia. Circulation 1984;70(6):957–65.
4. Cassidy DM, Vassallo JA, Buxton AE, et al. The value of catheter mapping during sinus rhythm to localize site of origin of ventricular tachycardia. Circulation 1984;69(6):1103–10.
5. de Bakker JM, Coronel R, Tasseron S, et al. Ventricular tachycardia in the infarcted, Langendorff-perfused human heart: role of the arrangement of surviving cardiac fibers. J Am Coll Cardiol 1990;15(7):1594–607.
6. Peters NS, Green CR, Poole-Wilson PA, et al. Reduced content of connexin43 gap junctions in ventricular myocardium from hypertrophied and ischemic human hearts. Circulation 1993;88(3):864–75.
7. Rosman J, Hanon S, Shapiro M, et al. Triggers of sustained monomorphic ventricular tachycardia differ among patients with varying etiologies of left ventricular dysfunction. Ann Noninvasive Electrocardiol 2006;11(2):113–7.

8. Huelsing DJ, Spitzer KW, Pollard AE. Spontaneous activity induced in rabbit Purkinje myocytes during coupling to a depolarized model cell. Cardiovasc Res 2003;59(3):620–7.
9. Spitzer KW, Pollard AE, Yang L, et al. Cell-to-cell electrical interactions during early and late repolarization. J Cardiovasc Electrophysiol 2006;17(Suppl 1):S8–14.
10. Philips B, Madhavan S, James C, et al. High prevalence of catecholamine-facilitated focal ventricular tachycardia in patients with arrhythmogenic right ventricular dysplasia/cardiomyopathy. Circ Arrhythm Electrophysiol 2013;6(1):160–6.
11. Kapa S, Venkatachalam KL, Asirvatham SJ. The autonomic nervous system in cardiac electrophysiology: an elegant interaction and emerging concepts. Cardiol Rev 2010;18(6):275–84.
12. Russo AM, Stainback RF, Bailey SR, et al. ACCF/HRS/AHA/ASE/HFSA/SCAI/SCCT/SCMR 2013 appropriate use criteria for implantable cardioverter-defibrillators and cardiac resynchronization therapy: a report of the American College of Cardiology Foundation Appropriate Use Criteria Task Force, Heart Rhythm Society, American Heart Association, American Society of Echocardiography, Heart Failure Society of America, Society for Cardiovascular Angiography and Interventions, Society of Cardiovascular Computed Tomography, and Society for Cardiovascular Magnetic Resonance. J Am Coll Cardiol 2013;61(12):1318–68.
13. Poole JE, Johnson GW, Hellkamp AS, et al. Prognostic importance of defibrillator shocks in patients with heart failure. N Engl J Med 2008;359(10):1009–17.
14. Echt DS, Liebson PR, Mitchell LB, et al. Mortality and morbidity in patients receiving encainide, flecainide, or placebo. The Cardiac Arrhythmia Suppression Trial. N Engl J Med 1991;324(12):781–8.
15. Ruberman W, Weinblatt E, Goldberg JD, et al. Ventricular premature beats and mortality after myocardial infarction. N Engl J Med 1977;297(14):750–7.
16. Bigger JT Jr, Fleiss JL, Kleiger R, et al. The relationships among ventricular arrhythmias, left ventricular dysfunction, and mortality in the 2 years after myocardial infarction. Circulation 1984;69(2):250–8.
17. Mukharji J, Rude RE, Poole WK, et al. Risk factors for sudden death after acute myocardial infarction: two-year follow-up. Am J Cardiol 1984;54(1):31–6.
18. Moss AJ, Davis HT, DeCamilla J, et al. Ventricular ectopic beats and their relation to sudden and nonsudden cardiac death after myocardial infarction. Circulation 1979;60(5):998–1003.
19. Kuck KH, Cappato R, Siebels J, et al. Randomized comparison of antiarrhythmic drug therapy with implantable defibrillators in patients resuscitated from cardiac arrest: the Cardiac Arrest Study Hamburg (CASH). Circulation 2000;102(7):748–54.
20. Siebels J, Cappato R, Ruppel R, et al. Preliminary results of the Cardiac Arrest Study Hamburg (CASH). Cash Investigators. Am J Cardiol 1993;72(16):109F–13F.
21. Burkart F, Pfisterer M, Kiowski W, et al. Effect of antiarrhythmic therapy on mortality in survivors of myocardial infarction with asymptomatic complex ventricular arrhythmias: Basel Antiarrhythmic Study of Infarct Survival (BASIS). J Am Coll Cardiol 1990;16(7):1711–8.
22. Cairns JA, Connolly SJ, Roberts R, et al. Randomised trial of outcome after myocardial infarction in patients with frequent or repetitive ventricular premature depolarisations: CAMIAT. Canadian Amiodarone Myocardial Infarction Arrhythmia Trial Investigators. Lancet 1997;349(9053):675–82.
23. The ESVEM trial. Electrophysiologic study versus electrocardiographic monitoring for selection of antiarrhythmic therapy of ventricular tachyarrhythmias. The ESVEM Investigators. Circulation 1989;79(6):1354–60.
24. Mason JW. A comparison of electrophysiologic testing with Holter monitoring to predict antiarrhythmic-drug efficacy for ventricular tachyarrhythmias. Electrophysiologic Study Versus Electrocardiographic Monitoring Investigators. N Engl J Med 1993;329(7):445–51.
25. Mason JW. A comparison of seven antiarrhythmic drugs in patients with ventricular tachyarrhythmias. Electrophysiologic Study Versus Electrocardiographic Monitoring Investigators. N Engl J Med 1993;329(7):452–8.
26. Randomized antiarrhythmic drug therapy in survivors of cardiac arrest (the CASCADE Study). The CASCADE Investigators. Am J Cardiol 1993;72(3):280–7.
27. Cardiac Arrest in Seattle: Conventional Versus Amiodarone Drug Evaluation (the CASCADE study). Am J Cardiol 1991;67(7):578–84.
28. Pacifico A, Hohnloser SH, Williams JH, et al. Prevention of implantable-defibrillator shocks by treatment with sotalol. d,l-Sotalol Implantable Cardioverter-Defibrillator Study Group. N Engl J Med 1999;340(24):1855–62.
29. Connolly SJ, Dorian P, Roberts RS, et al. Comparison of beta-blockers, amiodarone plus beta-blockers, or sotalol for prevention of shocks from implantable cardioverter defibrillators: the OPTIC Study: a randomized trial. JAMA 2006;295(2):165–71.
30. Bokhari F, Newman D, Greene M, et al. Long-term comparison of the implantable cardioverter defibrillator versus amiodarone: eleven-year follow-up of a subset of patients in the Canadian Implantable Defibrillator Study (CIDS). Circulation 2004;110(2):112–6.

31. Pinter A, Akhtari S, O'Connell T, et al. Efficacy and safety of dofetilide in the treatment of frequent ventricular tachyarrhythmias after amiodarone intolerance or failure. J Am Coll Cardiol 2011;57(3):380–1.
32. Baquero GA, Banchs JE, Depalma S, et al. Dofetilide reduces the frequency of ventricular arrhythmias and implantable cardioverter defibrillator therapies. J Cardiovasc Electrophysiol 2012; 23(3):296–301.
33. Dorian P, Borggrefe M, Al-Khalidi HR, et al. Placebo-controlled, randomized clinical trial of azimilide for prevention of ventricular tachyarrhythmias in patients with an implantable cardioverter defibrillator. Circulation 2004;110(24):3646–54.
34. Singer I, Al-Khalidi H, Niazi I, et al. Azimilide decreases recurrent ventricular tachyarrhythmias in patients with implantable cardioverter defibrillators. J Am Coll Cardiol 2004;43(1):39–43.
35. Mendes L, Podrid PJ, Fuchs T, et al. Role of combination drug therapy with a class IC antiarrhythmic agent and mexiletine for ventricular tachycardia. J Am Coll Cardiol 1991;17(6):1396–402.
36. Foster MT, Peters RW, Froman D, et al. Electrophysiologic effects and predictors of success of combination therapy with class Ia and Ib antiarrhythmic drugs for sustained ventricular arrhythmias. Am J Cardiol 1996;78(1):47–50.
37. Jung W, Mletzko R, Manz M, et al. Efficacy and safety of combination therapy with amiodarone and type I agents for treatment of inducible ventricular tachycardia. Pacing Clin Electrophysiol 1993; 16(4 Pt 1):778–88.
38. Whitford EG, McGovern B, Schoenfeld MH, et al. Long-term efficacy of mexiletine alone and in combination with class Ia antiarrhythmic drugs for refractory ventricular arrhythmias. Am Heart J 1988; 115(2):360–6.
39. Duff HJ, Roden D, Primm RK, et al. Mexiletine in the treatment of resistant ventricular arrhythmias: enhancement of efficacy and reduction of dose-related side effects by combination with quinidine. Circulation 1983;67(5):1124–8.
40. Widerhorn J, Sager PT, Rahimtoola SH, et al. The role of combination therapy with mexiletine and procainamide in patients with inducible sustained ventricular tachycardia refractory to intravenous procainamide. Pacing Clin Electrophysiol 1991; 14(3):420–6.
41. Toivonen L, Kadish A, Morady F. A prospective comparison of class IA, B, and C antiarrhythmic agents in combination with amiodarone in patients with inducible, sustained ventricular tachycardia. Circulation 1991;84(1):101–8.
42. Waleffe A, Mary-Rabine L, Legrand V, et al. Combined mexiletine and amiodarone treatment of refractory recurrent ventricular tachycardia. Am Heart J 1980;100(6 Pt 1):788–93.
43. Hallstrom AP, Cobb LA, Yu BH, et al. An antiarrhythmic drug experience in 941 patients resuscitated from an initial cardiac arrest between 1970 and 1985. Am J Cardiol 1991;68(10):1025–31.
44. Exner DV, Reiffel JA, Epstein AE, et al. Beta-blocker use and survival in patients with ventricular fibrillation or symptomatic ventricular tachycardia: the Antiarrhythmics Versus Implantable Defibrillators (AVID) trial. J Am Coll Cardiol 1999;34(2):325–33.
45. Hreybe H, Bedi M, Ezzeddine R, et al. Indications for internal cardioverter defibrillator implantation predict time to first shock and the modulating effect of beta-blockers. Am Heart J 2005;150(5):1064.
46. Seidl K, Hauer B, Schwick NG, et al. Comparison of metoprolol and sotalol in preventing ventricular tachyarrhythmias after the implantation of a cardioverter/defibrillator. Am J Cardiol 1998;82(6): 744–8.
47. Finzi AA, Latini R, Barlera S, et al. Effects of n-3 polyunsaturated fatty acids on malignant ventricular arrhythmias in patients with chronic heart failure and implantable cardioverter-defibrillators: a substudy of the Gruppo Italiano per lo Studio della Sopravvivenza nell'Insufficienza Cardiaca (GISSI-HF) trial. Am Heart J 2011;161(2):338–43.e1.
48. Madsen T, Christensen JH, Thogersen AM, et al. Intravenous infusion of n-3 polyunsaturated fatty acids and inducibility of ventricular tachycardia in patients with implantable cardioverter defibrillator. Europace 2010;12(7):941–6.
49. Metcalf RG, Sanders P, James MJ, et al. Effect of dietary n-3 polyunsaturated fatty acids on the inducibility of ventricular tachycardia in patients with ischemic cardiomyopathy. Am J Cardiol 2008;101(6):758–61.
50. Brouwer IA, Zock PL, Camm AJ, et al. Effect of fish oil on ventricular tachyarrhythmia and death in patients with implantable cardioverter defibrillators: the Study on Omega-3 Fatty Acids and Ventricular Arrhythmia (SOFA) randomized trial. JAMA 2006; 295(22):2613–9.
51. Raitt MH, Connor WE, Morris C, et al. Fish oil supplementation and risk of ventricular tachycardia and ventricular fibrillation in patients with implantable defibrillators: a randomized controlled trial. JAMA 2005;293(23):2884–91.
52. Khoueiry G, Abi Rafeh N, Sullivan E, et al. Do omega-3 polyunsaturated fatty acids reduce risk of sudden cardiac death and ventricular arrhythmias? A meta-analysis of randomized trials. Heart Lung 2013;42(4):251–6.
53. Verrier RL, Pagotto VP, Kanas AF, et al. Low doses of ranolazine and dronedarone in combination exert potent protection against atrial fibrillation and vulnerability to ventricular arrhythmias during acute myocardial ischemia. Heart Rhythm 2013; 10(1):121–7.

54. Bunch TJ, Mahapatra S, Murdock D, et al. Ranolazine reduces ventricular tachycardia burden and ICD shocks in patients with drug-refractory ICD shocks. Pacing Clin Electrophysiol 2011;34(12):1600–6.
55. Vizzardi E, D'Aloia A, Salghetti F, et al. Efficacy of ranolazine in a patient with idiopathic dilated cardiomyopathy and electrical storm. Drug Discov Ther 2013;7(1):43–5.
56. Yeung E, Krantz MJ, Schuller JL, et al. Ranolazine for the suppression of ventricular arrhythmia: a case series. Ann Noninvasive Electrocardiol 2014; 19(4):345–50.
57. Moss AJ, Hall WJ, Cannom DS, et al. Improved survival with an implanted defibrillator in patients with coronary disease at high risk for ventricular arrhythmia. Multicenter Automatic Defibrillator Implantation Trial Investigators. N Engl J Med 1996; 335(26):1933–40.
58. Buxton AE, Lee KL, Fisher JD, et al. A randomized study of the prevention of sudden death in patients with coronary artery disease. Multicenter Unsustained Tachycardia Trial Investigators. N Engl J Med 1999;341(25):1882–90.
59. Moss AJ, Zareba W, Hall WJ, et al. Prophylactic implantation of a defibrillator in patients with myocardial infarction and reduced ejection fraction. N Engl J Med 2002;346(12):877–83.
60. Hohnloser SH, Kuck KH, Dorian P, et al. Prophylactic use of an implantable cardioverter-defibrillator after acute myocardial infarction. N Engl J Med 2004;351(24):2481–8.
61. Bigger JT Jr. Prophylactic use of implanted cardiac defibrillators in patients at high risk for ventricular arrhythmias after coronary-artery bypass graft surgery. Coronary Artery Bypass Graft (CABG) Patch Trial Investigators. N Engl J Med 1997;337(22): 1569–75.
62. Epstein AE, DiMarco JP, Ellenbogen KA, et al. ACC/AHA/HRS 2008 Guidelines for device-based therapy of cardiac rhythm abnormalities: a report of the American College of Cardiology/American Heart Association Task Force on Practice Guidelines (Writing Committee to Revise the ACC/AHA/NASPE 2002 Guideline Update for Implantation of Cardiac Pacemakers and Antiarrhythmia Devices): developed in collaboration with the American Association for Thoracic Surgery and Society of Thoracic Surgeons. Circulation 2008;117(21): e350–408.
63. Kadish A, Dyer A, Daubert JP, et al. Prophylactic defibrillator implantation in patients with nonischemic dilated cardiomyopathy. N Engl J Med 2004; 350(21):2151–8.
64. Bardy GH, Lee KL, Mark DB, et al. Amiodarone or an implantable cardioverter-defibrillator for congestive heart failure. N Engl J Med 2005; 352(3):225–37.
65. Kober L, Thune JJ, Nielsen JC, et al. Defibrillator implantation in patients with nonischemic systolic heart failure. N Engl J Med 2016;375(13):1221–30.
66. Connolly SJ, Gent M, Roberts RS, et al. Canadian Implantable Defibrillator Study (CIDS): a randomized trial of the implantable cardioverter defibrillator against amiodarone. Circulation 2000; 101(11):1297–302.
67. A comparison of antiarrhythmic-drug therapy with implantable defibrillators in patients resuscitated from near-fatal ventricular arrhythmias. The Antiarrhythmics Versus Implantable Defibrillators (AVID) Investigators. N Engl J Med 1997;337(22):1576–83.
68. Epstein AE, DiMarco JP, Ellenbogen KA, et al. 2012 ACCF/AHA/HRS focused update incorporated into the ACCF/AHA/HRS 2008 guidelines for device-based therapy of cardiac rhythm abnormalities: a report of the American College of Cardiology Foundation/American Heart Association Task Force on Practice Guidelines and the Heart Rhythm Society. J Am Coll Cardiol 2013;61(3):e6–75.
69. Carson P, Anand I, O'Connor C, et al. Mode of death in advanced heart failure: the comparison of medical, pacing, and defibrillation therapies in heart failure (COMPANION) trial. J Am Coll Cardiol 2005;46(12):2329–34.
70. Greenberg H, Case RB, Moss AJ, et al. Analysis of mortality events in the multicenter automatic defibrillator implantation trial (MADIT-II). J Am Coll Cardiol 2004;43(8):1459–65.
71. Packer DL, Prutkin JM, Hellkamp AS, et al. Impact of implantable cardioverter-defibrillator, amiodarone, and placebo on the mode of death in stable patients with heart failure: analysis from the Sudden Cardiac Death in Heart Failure Trial. Circulation 2009;120(22):2170–6.
72. Mitchell LB, Pineda EA, Titus JL, et al. Sudden death in patients with implantable cardioverter defibrillators: the importance of post-shock electromechanical dissociation. J Am Coll Cardiol 2002; 39(8):1323–8.
73. Duray GZ, Schmitt J, Richter S, et al. Arrhythmic death in implantable cardioverter defibrillator patients: a long-term study over a 10 year implantation period. Europace 2009;11(11):1462–8.
74. Krahn AD, Connolly SJ, Roberts RS, et al. Diminishing proportional risk of sudden death with advancing age: implications for prevention of sudden death. Am Heart J 2004;147(5):837–40.
75. Huang DT, Sesselberg HW, McNitt S, et al. Improved survival associated with prophylactic implantable defibrillators in elderly patients with prior myocardial infarction and depressed ventricular function: a MADIT-II substudy. J Cardiovasc Electrophysiol 2007;18(8):833–8.
76. Farley A, Persson R, Garlitski AC, et al. Effectiveness of implantable cardioverter defibrillators for

primary prevention of sudden cardiac death in subgroups a systematic review. Ann Intern Med 2014;160(2):111–21.
77. Bilchick KC, Stukenborg GJ, Kamath S, et al. Prediction of mortality in clinical practice for medicare patients undergoing defibrillator implantation for primary prevention of sudden cardiac death. J Am Coll Cardiol 2012;60(17):1647–55.
78. Green AR, Leff B, Wang Y, et al. Geriatric conditions in patients undergoing defibrillator implantation for prevention of sudden cardiac death: prevalence and impact on mortality. Circ Cardiovasc Qual Outcomes 2016;9(1):23–30.
79. Chen CY, Stevenson LW, Stewart GC, et al. Real world effectiveness of primary implantable cardioverter defibrillators implanted during hospital admissions for exacerbation of heart failure or other acute co-morbidities: cohort study of older patients with heart failure. BMJ 2015;351:h3529.
80. Healey JS, Hallstrom AP, Kuck KH, et al. Role of the implantable defibrillator among elderly patients with a history of life-threatening ventricular arrhythmias. Eur Heart J 2007;28(14):1746–9.
81. Grimm W, Stula A, Sharkova J, et al. Outcomes of elderly recipients of implantable cardioverter defibrillators. Pacing Clin Electrophysiol 2007; 30(Suppl 1):S134–8.
82. Yung D, Birnie D, Dorian P, et al. Survival after implantable cardioverter-defibrillator implantation in the elderly. Circulation 2013;127(24):2383–92.
83. Godemann F, Butter C, Lampe F, et al. Panic disorders and agoraphobia: side effects of treatment with an implantable cardioverter/defibrillator. Clin Cardiol 2004;27(6):321–6.
84. Goodman M, Hess B. Could implantable cardioverter defibrillators provide a human model supporting the learned helplessness theory of depression? Gen Hosp Psychiatry 1999;21(5):382–5.
85. Whang W, Albert CM, Sears SF Jr, et al. Depression as a predictor for appropriate shocks among patients with implantable cardioverter-defibrillators: results from the Triggers of Ventricular Arrhythmias (TOVA) study. J Am Coll Cardiol 2005;45(7): 1090–5.
86. Bencardino G, Di Monaco A, Rio T, et al. The association between ICD interventions and mortality is independent of their modality: clinical implications. J Cardiovasc Electrophysiol 2014;25(12):1363–7.
87. Larsen GK, Evans J, Lambert WE, et al. Shocks burden and increased mortality in implantable cardioverter-defibrillator patients. Heart Rhythm 2011;8(12):1881–6.
88. Sweeney MO, Sherfesee L, DeGroot PJ, et al. Differences in effects of electrical therapy type for ventricular arrhythmias on mortality in implantable cardioverter-defibrillator patients. Heart Rhythm 2010;7(3):353–60.
89. Moss AJ, Schuger C, Beck CA, et al. Reduction in inappropriate therapy and mortality through ICD programming. N Engl J Med 2012;367(24):2275–83.
90. Ruwald AC, Schuger C, Moss AJ, et al. Mortality reduction in relation to implantable cardioverter defibrillator programming in the Multicenter Automatic Defibrillator Implantation Trial-Reduce Inappropriate Therapy (MADIT-RIT). Circ Arrhythm Electrophysiol 2014;7(5):785–92.
91. Josephson M. Clinical cardiac electrophysiology. Philadelphia: Lippincott Williams and Wilkins; 2008.
92. Wathen MS, Sweeney MO, DeGroot PJ, et al. Shock reduction using antitachycardia pacing for spontaneous rapid ventricular tachycardia in patients with coronary artery disease. Circulation 2001;104(7):796–801.
93. Wathen MS, DeGroot PJ, Sweeney MO, et al. Prospective randomized multicenter trial of empirical antitachycardia pacing versus shocks for spontaneous rapid ventricular tachycardia in patients with implantable cardioverter-defibrillators: Pacing Fast Ventricular Tachycardia Reduces Shock Therapies (PainFREE Rx II) trial results. Circulation 2004;110(17):2591–6.
94. Gasparini M, Proclemer A, Klersy C, et al. Effect of long-detection interval vs standard-detection interval for implantable cardioverter-defibrillators on antitachycardia pacing and shock delivery: the ADVANCE III randomized clinical trial. JAMA 2013;309(18):1903–11.
95. Kloppe A, Proclemer A, Arenal A, et al. Efficacy of long detection interval implantable cardioverter-defibrillator settings in secondary prevention population: data from the Avoid Delivering Therapies for Nonsustained Arrhythmias in ICD Patients III (ADVANCE III) trial. Circulation 2014;130(4):308–14.
96. Josephson ME, Harken AH, Horowitz LN. Endocardial excision: a new surgical technique for the treatment of recurrent ventricular tachycardia. Circulation 1979; 60(7):1430–9.
97. Miller JM, Kienzle MG, Harken AH, et al. Subendocardial resection for ventricular tachycardia: predictors of surgical success. Circulation 1984;70(4):624–31.
98. Gepstein L, Hayam G, Ben-Haim SA. A novel method for nonfluoroscopic catheter-based electroanatomical mapping of the heart. In vitro and in vivo accuracy results. Circulation 1997;95(6):1611–22.
99. Nademanee K, Kosar EM. A nonfluoroscopic catheter-based mapping technique to ablate focal ventricular tachycardia. Pacing Clin Electrophysiol 1998;21(7):1442–7.
100. Cassidy DM, Vassallo JA, Miller JM, et al. Endocardial catheter mapping in patients in sinus rhythm: relationship to underlying heart disease and ventricular arrhythmias. Circulation 1986;73(4):645–52.
101. Marchlinski FE, Callans DJ, Gottlieb CD, et al. Linear ablation lesions for control of unmappable

ventricular tachycardia in patients with ischemic and nonischemic cardiomyopathy. Circulation 2000;101(11):1288–96.

102. Ellison KE, Friedman PL, Ganz LI, et al. Entrainment mapping and radiofrequency catheter ablation of ventricular. J Am Coll Cardiol 1998;32(3):724–8.
103. Stevenson WG, Khan H, Sager P, et al. Identification of reentry circuit sites during catheter mapping and radiofrequency ablation of ventricular tachycardia late after myocardial infarction. Circulation 1993;88(4 Pt 1):1647–70.
104. El-Shalakany A, Hadjis T, Papageorgiou P, et al. Entrainment/mapping criteria for the prediction of termination of ventricular tachycardia by single radiofrequency lesion in patients with coronary artery disease. Circulation 1999;99(17):2283–9.
105. Morady F, Harvey M, Kalbfleisch SJ, et al. Radiofrequency catheter ablation of ventricular tachycardia in patients with coronary artery disease. Circulation 1993;87(2):363–72.
106. Bogun F, Crawford T, Chalfoun N, et al. Relationship of frequent postinfarction premature ventricular complexes to the reentry circuit of scar-related ventricular tachycardia. Heart Rhythm 2008;5(3): 367–74.
107. El Kadri M, Yokokawa M, Labounty T, et al. Effect of ablation of frequent premature ventricular complexes on left ventricular function in patients with nonischemic cardiomyopathy. Heart Rhythm 2015;12(4):706–13.
108. Sarrazin JF, Labounty T, Kuhne M, et al. Impact of radiofrequency ablation of frequent post-infarction premature ventricular complexes on left ventricular ejection fraction. Heart Rhythm 2009;6(11):1543–9.
109. Kim YH, Sosa-Suarez G, Trouton TG, et al. Treatment of ventricular tachycardia by transcatheter radiofrequency ablation in patients with ischemic heart disease. Circulation 1994;89(3):1094–102.
110. Soejima K, Suzuki M, Maisel WH, et al. Catheter ablation in patients with multiple and unstable ventricular tachycardias after myocardial infarction: short ablation lines guided by reentry circuit isthmuses and sinus rhythm mapping. Circulation 2001;104(6):664–9.
111. Rothman SA, Hsia HH, Cossu SF, et al. Radiofrequency catheter ablation of postinfarction ventricular tachycardia: long-term success and the significance of inducible nonclinical arrhythmias. Circulation 1997;96(10):3499–508.
112. Stevenson WG, Wilber DJ, Natale A, et al. Irrigated radiofrequency catheter ablation guided by electroanatomic mapping for recurrent ventricular tachycardia after myocardial infarction: the multicenter Thermocool Ventricular Tachycardia Ablation Trial. Circulation 2008;118(25):2773–82.
113. Jaïs P, Maury P, Khairy P, et al. Elimination of local abnormal ventricular activities: a new end point for substrate modification in patients with scar-related ventricular tachycardia. Circulation 2012;125(18): 2184–96.
114. Di Biase L, Santangeli P, Burkhardt DJ, et al. Endo-epicardial homogenization of the scar versus limited substrate ablation for the treatment of electrical storms in patients with ischemic cardiomyopathy. J Am Coll Cardiol 2012;60(2):132–41.
115. Reddy VY, Reynolds MR, Neuzil P, et al. Prophylactic catheter ablation for the prevention of defibrillator therapy. N Engl J Med 2007;357(26):2657–65.
116. Kuck KH, Schaumann A, Eckardt L, et al. Catheter Ablation of Stable Ventricular Tachycardia Before Defibrillator Implantation in Patients with Coronary Heart Disease (VTACH): a multicentre randomised controlled trial. Lancet 2010;375(9708):31–40.
117. Delacretaz E, Brenner R, Schaumann A, et al. Catheter Ablation of Stable Ventricular Tachycardia Before Defibrillator Implantation in Patients with Coronary Heart Disease (VTACH): an on-treatment analysis. J Cardiovasc Electrophysiol 2013;24(5):525–9.
118. Sapp JL, Wells GA, Parkash R, et al. Ventricular tachycardia ablation versus escalation of antiarrhythmic drugs. N Engl J Med 2016;375(2):111–21.
119. Dinov B, Fiedler L, Schönbauer R, et al. Outcomes in catheter ablation of ventricular tachycardia in dilated nonischemic cardiomyopathy compared with ischemic cardiomyopathy: results from the Prospective Heart Centre of Leipzig VT (HELP-VT) Study. Circulation 2014;129(7):728–36.
120. Sosa E, Scanavacca M, d'Avila A, et al. A new technique to perform epicardial mapping in the electrophysiology laboratory. J Cardiovasc Electrophysiol 1996;7(6):531–6.
121. Sosa E, Scanavacca M, D'Avila A, et al. Endocardial and epicardial ablation guided by nonsurgical transthoracic epicardial mapping to treat recurrent ventricular tachycardia. J Cardiovasc Electrophysiol 1998;9(3):229–39.
122. Tokuda M, Sobieszczyk P, Eisenhauer AC, et al. Transcoronary ethanol ablation for recurrent ventricular tachycardia after failed catheter ablation: an update. Circ Arrhythm Electrophysiol 2011;4(6):889–96.
123. Sapp JL, Beeckler C, Pike R, et al. Initial human feasibility of infusion needle catheter ablation for refractory ventricular tachycardia. Circulation 2013;128(21):2289–95.
124. Gizurarson S, Spears D, Sivagangabalan G, et al. Bipolar ablation for deep intra-myocardial circuits: human ex vivo development and in vivo experience. Europace 2014;16(11):1684–8.
125. Sinha AM, Schmidt M, Marschang H, et al. Role of left ventricular scar and Purkinje-like potentials during mapping and ablation of ventricular fibrillation in dilated cardiomyopathy. Pacing Clin Electrophysiol 2009;32(3):286–90.

126. Marrouche NF, Verma A, Wazni O, et al. Mode of initiation and ablation of ventricular fibrillation storms in patients with ischemic cardiomyopathy. J Am Coll Cardiol 2004;43(9):1715–20.
127. Schwartz PJ, Locati EH, Moss AJ, et al. Left cardiac sympathetic denervation in the therapy of congenital long QT syndrome. A worldwide report. Circulation 1991;84(2):503–11.
128. Hayase J, Patel J, Narayan SM, et al. Percutaneous stellate ganglion block suppressing VT and VF in a patient refractory to VT ablation. J Cardiovasc Electrophysiol 2013;24(8):926–8.
129. Vaseghi M, Gima J, Kanaan C, et al. Cardiac sympathetic denervation in patients with refractory ventricular arrhythmias or electrical storm: intermediate and long-term follow-up. Heart Rhythm 2014;11(3):360–6.
130. Krum H, Schlaich M, Whitbourn R, et al. Catheter-based renal sympathetic denervation for resistant hypertension: a multicentre safety and proof-of-principle cohort study. Lancet 2009;373(9671):1275–81.
131. Symplicity HTN-1 Investigators. Catheter-based renal sympathetic denervation for resistant hypertension: durability of blood pressure reduction out to 24 months. Hypertension 2011;57(5):911–7.
132. Huang B, Yu L, Scherlag BJ, et al. Left renal nerves stimulation facilitates ischemia-induced ventricular arrhythmia by increasing nerve activity of left stellate ganglion. J Cardiovasc Electrophysiol 2014;25(11):1249–56.
133. Ukena C, Bauer A, Mahfoud F, et al. Renal sympathetic denervation for treatment of electrical storm: first-in-man experience. Clin Res Cardiol 2012;101(1):63–7.
134. Hoffmann BA, Steven D, Willems S, et al. Renal sympathetic denervation as an adjunct to catheter ablation for the treatment of ventricular electrical storm in the setting of acute myocardial infarction. J Cardiovasc Electrophysiol 2013;24(10):1175–8.
135. Remo BF, Preminger M, Bradfield J, et al. Safety and efficacy of renal denervation as a novel treatment of ventricular tachycardia storm in patients with cardiomyopathy. Heart Rhythm 2014;11(4):541–6.
136. Bhatt DL, Kandzari DE, O'Neill WW, et al. A controlled trial of renal denervation for resistant hypertension. N Engl J Med 2014;370(15):1393–401.
137. Grimaldi R, de Luca A, Kornet L, et al. Can spinal cord stimulation reduce ventricular arrhythmias? Heart Rhythm 2012;9(11):1884–7.

Exercise Therapy for Older Heart Failure Patients

Jerome L. Fleg, MD

KEYWORDS

- Heart failure syndrome • Aerobic training • Resistance training • Exercise therapy
- Aerobic capacity

KEY POINTS

- Both the aging process and heart failure (HF) syndrome are characterized by a dramatic reduction of aerobic capacity caused by a combination of cardiac and peripheral factors. Significant decreases in muscle mass and strength are also common to both conditions.
- Although a growing literature has documented that aerobic exercise training (ET) elicits improvement in peak oxygen consumption (V_{O_2}), submaximal exercise measures, and quality of life in younger HF patients, few HF training studies have included meaningful numbers of older individuals, especially those greater than 80 years of age and older women with HF with reduced ejection fraction (HFrEF). Nevertheless, the modest data available suggest similar benefits in older as in younger HF patients as well as excellent safety.
- Resistance training may provide additional benefit in older patients with HF, especially those with substantial muscle wasting.
- Whether ET can reduce mortality, hospitalizations, and overall health care costs in patients with HFpEF must await the outcome of adequately powered multicenter trials in this large subset of the HF population.

REDUCED AEROBIC CAPACITY: A CENTRAL FEATURE OF NORMATIVE AGING AND HEART FAILURE

Reduction in aerobic capacity, best quantified by peak V_{O_2}, is a central feature of both normative aging and chronic HF. Numerous observational studies over the past half-century have documented declines in peak V_{O_2} of approximately 50% across the adult age span in apparently healthy populations (**Fig. 1**).[1–4] In men, peak V_{O_2} decreases from approximately 45 mL/kg/min in a healthy 25 year old to approximately 25 mL/kg/min in a 75 year old (see **Fig. 1**). Comparable numbers in women are approximately 20% lower because of their smaller proportion of muscle mass and lower hemoglobin levels. A healthy 80-year-old woman typically has a peak V_{O_2} of 15 mL/kg/min to 20 mL/kg/min, a range characteristic of mild HF. Even lower peak V_{O_2} is common in older adults with significant comorbidities, such as pulmonary disease, coronary or peripheral arterial disease, arthritis, and orthopedic or neurologic disorders, that further impair aerobic capacity. Furthermore, recent data suggest that longitudinal age-associated declines in peak V_{O_2} in healthy volunteers accelerate with age, exceeding 20% per decade in the 8th and 9th decades (see **Fig. 1**).[5]

Peak V_{O_2} is the product of cardiac output and arteriovenous oxygen (AVO_2) difference.

In healthy Baltimore Longitudinal Study of Aging volunteers, declines in peak HR and AVO_2

This is an updated version of an article that appeared in *Heart Failure Clinics*, Volume 3, Issue 4.
Division of Cardiovascular Diseases, National Heart, Lung, and Blood Institute, 6701 Rockledge Drive, Room 8154, Bethesda, MD 20892-7936, USA
E-mail address: flegj@nhlbi.nih.gov

Heart Failure Clin 13 (2017) 607–617
http://dx.doi.org/10.1016/j.hfc.2017.02.012
1551-7136/17/Published by Elsevier Inc.

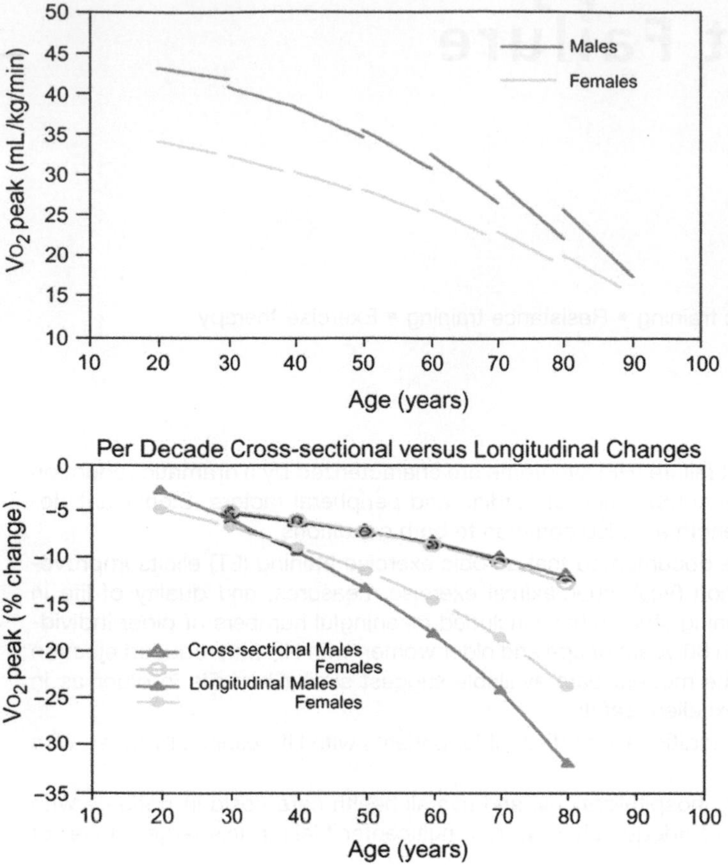

Fig. 1. Cross-sectional and longitudinal changes in peak V_{O_2} per weight in kilograms in healthy adults by age decade and gender. (*Top panel*) The per-decade longitudinal change in peak V_{O_2} for age decades from the 20s through the 70s, predicted from a mixed-effects regression model. Peak V_{O_2} declines more steeply with successive age decades, especially in men. (*Bottom panel*) Per-decade percent cross-sectional and longitudinal changes in peak V_{O_2} by age decade and gender, derived from the mixed-effects model. From the 50s onward, longitudinal declines in peak V_{O_2} substantially exceed cross-sectional declines. (*From* Fleg JL, Morrell CH, Bos AG, et al. Accelerated longitudinal decline of aerobic capacity in healthy older adults. Circulation 2005;12:677; with permission.)

difference make similar contributions to the decline in peak V_{O_2} with aging.[6] In contrast, exercise stroke volume (SV) is not age related among individuals screened for the absence of coronary heart disease by clinical criteria and exercise thallium scintigraphy. In these individuals, enhanced use of the Frank-Starling mechanism augments left ventricular end-diastolic volume (LVEDV), compensating for modest blunting of systolic emptying with age.[7] Plasma catecholamines are increased with age at peak exercise.[8] This exercise hemodynamic profile of normal aging resembles that of β-adrenergic blockade of a young adult.[9]

HF, like aging, is characterized by a major reduction in peak V_{O_2}, which provides powerful prognostic information regarding risk for hospitalization, mortality, and need for ventricular assist devices or cardiac transplantation.[10–12] The impairment in peak V_{O_2} in these patients is attributable to both cardiac and peripheral factors. In patients with systolic HF, also known as HFrEF, peak HR and SV are reduced approximately 20% and 45%, respectively, compared with normal individuals.[13,14] Peripheral factors contributing to reduced AVO_2 difference, thence, peak V_{O_2}, include reduced muscle mass, decreased mitochondrial density in exercising muscle, and peripheral vasoconstriction because of intrinsic abnormalities of smooth muscle vasodilation and neurohormonal factors.[15,16] A similar constellation of peripheral abnormalities contributes to the age-associated decrease in AVO_2 difference at peak exercise (**Table 1**).[17] In patients with HF and preserved systolic function (HFpEF), peak V_{O_2} is reduced to nearly the same degree as in patients who have systolic HF.[18] The reduction in peak exercise SV in these individuals is explained primarily by a lower LVEDV.[19]

DO OLDER PEOPLE WITHOUT HEART FAILURE RESPOND TO AEROBIC TRAINING LIKE YOUNGER ADULTS?

Although early studies suggested that aerobic capacity could not be augmented by exercise training (ET) in healthy older adults, multiple subsequent investigations have documented 10% to 25% increases in peak V_{O_2} in previously sedentary adults through the ninth decade, comparable to

Table 1
Physiologic similarities between normative aging and heart failure

	Aging[a]	Heart Failure
Peak V_{O_2}	↓↓	↓↓↓
Maximal SV	— or ↓	↓↓
Maximal heart rate	↓↓	↓
Maximal AVO_2 difference	↓↓	↓↓
Skeletal muscle mass	↓↓	↓↓
Mitochondrial oxidative enzymes	↓	↓↓↓

[a] Between the third and ninth decades.
From Fleg JL. Can exercise conditioning be effective in older heart failure patients? Heart Failure Rev 2002;7(1):101; with permission.

those seen in young adults.[20–23] In a meta-analysis of 41 trials in 2102 individuals aged 60 and older, aerobic training elicited a 16.3% mean increase in peak V_{O_2}.[24] These improvements in peak V_{O_2} are mediated by enhanced AVO_2 difference and augmented SV secondary to a larger LVEDV; maximal HR is unaffected by ET in healthy older adults.

Aerobic ET has also shown convincing benefits in older patients with coronary heart disease. In clinical studies of patients participating in traditional cardiac rehabilitation programs after a coronary event, individuals older than 70 years have derived relative improvements in exercise capacity similar to those in younger patients.[25–27] For example, Ades and colleagues[26] reported a 16% increase in peak V_{O_2} in 60 patients aged 65 years ± 5 years who underwent 3 months of training beginning 8 weeks after myocardial infarction or coronary revascularization. The increased peak V_{O_2} was entirely attributable to a widened AVO2 difference, similar to the training response in younger coronary patients.

EXERCISE THERAPY IN PATIENTS WITH HEART FAILURE: STATE OF THE EVIDENCE

It may be useful to review the effects of ET in the general HF population before focusing specifically on its role in older HF patients. Multiple studies over the past decade have demonstrated that aerobic ET is effective and safe in patients with HF. Among such patients who were receiving diuretics, converting enzyme inhibitors, and digitalis at baseline, randomized trials have demonstrated increases in peak V_{O_2} of 12% to 33%.[28,29] Patients on β-blockers seem to derive similar training-induced improvements in aerobic capacity.[30] Increased AVO_2 difference is the primary contributor to the training-induced augmentation of peak V_{O_2} in HF patients, with modest increases in cardiac output also observed in some studies.[31] Parallel improvement in ventilatory or lactate threshold is generally observed as well as lower HR and lactate levels at fixed submaximal workloads. These physiologic changes translate into improved exercise tolerance with fewer symptoms, both highly relevant clinical outcomes. Despite early concerns that aerobic training might exacerbate adverse left ventricular (LV) remodeling, especially in coronary patients with preexisting wall motion abnormalities,[32] numerous subsequent investigations have shown no deleterious effects on LV structure or resting function after training.

Augmentation of peripheral blood flow and improved skeletal muscle morphology and function mediate much of the benefit from aerobic ET in HF patients. Increases in peak leg blood flow and oxygen delivery and reduced leg vascular resistance have been observed.[33] Training also augments the blunted endothelium-mediated flow-dependent vasodilation seen in patients who have HFrEF.[34,35] Several studies have shown less muscle acidosis and phosphocreatine depletion and accelerated resynthesis of adenosine triphosphate during recovery from localized limb exercise post-training.[36–38] Increases of approximately 20% in mitochondrial volume density and 41% in cytochrome C oxidase–positive mitochondria were seen after 6 months of aerobic training; these increases correlated with improvements in exercise capacity.[39]

Aerobic training also elicits favorable changes in autonomic function and neurohormonal profile in HF. The characteristic elevations of resting plasma levels of vasopressin, atrial natriuretic peptides, angiotensin, and aldosterone are reduced after training.[40] Decreased norepinephrine spillover is accompanied by a parallel reduction in low-frequency heart rate variability and reciprocal increases in high-frequency peaks, consistent with augmented vagal tone.[41]

Although earlier studies of ET in HF were not adequately powered to detect an effect on clinical events or survival, Belardinelli and colleagues[42] observed reduced rates of hospital admissions and cardiac mortality in patients randomized to 14 months of supervised aerobic training compared with controls. Some of the reduction in events by training in this primarily ischemic sample may have been mediated by improved myocardial perfusion, observed in 75% of trained patients but only 2% of controls. The multicenter

2331 patient Heart Failure: A Controlled Trial Investigating Outcomes of Exercise Training (HF-ACTION) was designed specifically to determine if aerobic ET could reduce all-cause hospitalization and mortality in patients with HFrEF.[43] Adults with stable HFrEF who were receiving optimal medical and device therapy were randomized to 36 sessions of supervised ET followed by home training on a treadmill or cycle ergometer for an additional 2 or more years or to usual care. A modest but significant 11% decrease in the primary endpoint was found on an prespecified analysis that adjusted for prognostic baseline covariates.[43] Similar findings were seen in the subset of 435 patients greater than or equal to 70 years as in younger patients. A major limitation of this study was that only 30% of participants achieved the target weekly goals for exercise min/wk during the home exercise phase, resulting in only a modest increase of 0.6 mL/kg/min in peak V_{O_2} in the group randomized to ET.

AEROBIC EXERCISE TRAINING IN OLDER HEART FAILURE PATIENTS: CLINICAL TRIAL EVIDENCE IN HEART FAILURE WITH REDUCED EJECTION FRACTION

Despite the demonstrated favorable effects of aerobic ET in HF, most such trials have enrolled predominantly younger patients, similar to the age bias observed in nonexercise HF trials.[44] Given the advanced age typical of HF patients in the general community, it is imperative to examine the literature of HF training studies specific to older patients. A review of 29 such trials in 2004 revealed only 4 studies with a mean age greater than 65 years[45]; 11 of these 29 trials included only men, and another 11 enrolled fewer than 25% women. Several more recent trials have provided additional data, however, on training effects in older HF patients, including higher proportions of women.

Results have been generally favorable in those ET trials that have included meaningful numbers of older HF patients (**Table 2**). Willenheimer and coworkers[46] randomized 54 patients of mean age 64 years to 4 months of supervised cycle ergometry or a control group; an improved quality of life but no significant changes in peak V_{O_2} or the dyspnea-fatigue index were found in those who trained. In 67 men with New York Heart Association (NYHA) class 2 or class 3 HF and left ventricular ejection fraction (LVEF) less than 40% who underwent 12 weeks of aerobic training, Wielenga and colleagues[47] observed similar increases in peak V_{O_2} and exercise duration in patients younger versus those older than 65 years; however, the change in peak V_{O_2} was not statistically significant in either group. In a study of 33 older HF patients, Gottlieb and coworkers[48] observed that 6 of 17 patients randomized to a 6-month aerobic training program did not tolerate ET; in the remaining 11 patients, both peak V_{O_2} and 6-minute walk distance (6MWD) increased significantly, but neither daily energy expenditure nor perceived quality of life improved. In 22 HF patients aged 75 years old to 90 years old, a 12-week program of once-weekly exercise sessions resulted in an 11% increase in 6MWD, but no significant improvement was found in quality of life as assessed by the Minnesota Living with Heart Failure Questionnaire (MLHFQ).[49]

Four larger trials of aerobic ET have targeted the older HFrEF population. McKelvie and coworkers[50] randomized 181 NYHA class 2 to class 3 HF patients of mean age 65 years (19% women) with LVEF less than 40% to 3 months of supervised aerobic and resistance training followed by 9 months of home training or to a control group. Most patients received diuretics, converting enzyme inhibitors, and digitalis, and approximately 20% received β-blockers. Peak V_{O_2} in the training group increased 10% after 3 months and 14% after 12 months, whereas minimal changes occurred in controls. Modest increases in 6MWD were observed at 3 and 12 months in both groups, without significant intergroup differences. No significant changes from baseline in radionuclide cardiac function or quality of life occurred in either group.

Austin and colleagues[51] randomized 200 patients, 60 years old to 89 years old (mean 72 years, 34% women), with NYHA class 2 to class 3 HF and LVEF less than 40% to 24 weeks of ET or standard care. Training consisted of an 8-week twice weekly hospital-based cardiac rehabilitation program followed by 16 weeks of supervised community-based exercise sessions for 1 hour weekly. Throughout the 24-week program, patients performed aerobic training and low-resistance/high-repetition strength training and were encouraged to exercise an additional 3 times per week at home. Significant improvement occurred in health-related quality of life, NYHA class (from 2.4 to 2.0) and 6MWD (from 276 m to 320 m) in exercisers, whereas no changes occurred in controls; peak V_{O_2} was not measured. Furthermore, fewer patients in the exercise group (11%) than standard care patients (20%) were hospitalized by week 24 although mortality was similarly low in both groups. The low 12% dropout rate indicates that such a training program is feasible in most older patients with HF.

Table 2
Randomized controlled trials of exercise therapy in older patients with heart failure and reduced ejection fraction

Authors	n	Mean Age	Women (%)	Duration	Mode	Benefits
Austin et al,[51] 2005	200	72	34	24 wk	Aerobic resistance	↑6MWD 16% ↓NYHA class; 16% ↑QOL
Antonicelli et al,[52] 2016[a]	138	77	43	6 mo	Cycle	↑6MWD 33%, ↑QOL, ↓BNP
Witham et al,[53] 2012	107	80	35	24 wk	Walk/resistance	No Δ 6MWD or QOL
Gottlieb et al,[48] 1999	33	65	12	6 mo	Cycle/treadmill	↑Peak Vo_2 – 13% ↑6MWD – 11% No Δ – QOL
McKelvie et al,[50] 2002	181	65	19	12 mo	Cycle/resistance	No Δ 6MWD ↑Peak Vo_2 – 14%
Owen and Croucher,[49] 2000	22	81	25	12 wk	Aerobic/resistance	No Δ – QOL ↑6MWD – 11%
Pu et al,[71] 2001	16	77	100	10 wk	Resistance	No Δ – QOL ↑Strength – 43% ↑6MWD – 13%
Selig et al,[70] 2004	39	65	15	3 mo	Resistance	No Δ – Peak Vo_2 ↑Peak Vo_2 – 11% ↑FBF 20% ↑HRV
Wielenga et al,[47] 1998	67	64	None	12 wk	Walk/cycle	No Δ peak Vo_2
Willenheimer et al,[46] 1998	54	64	28	16 wk	Cycle	↑QOL No Δ – peak Vo_2

Abbreviations: Δ, change; FBF, forearm blood flow; HRV, heart rate variability; QOL, quality of life.
[a] 37% of the 373 patients had LVEF less than 40%.

In the largest trial of ET in older HF patients, Antonicelli and colleagues[52] randomized 343 individuals greater than 70 year old (mean 77 years, 43% women) with either HFrEF (37%) or HFpEF (63%) to 3 months of supervised ET 3 times/wk on a cycle ergometer, followed by 3 additional months of home-telemonitored training or to usual care. The ET group showed substantial improvement in 6MWD (from 299 m to 394 m), quality of life using the MLHFQ, and reduction in N terminal pro–brain natriuretic peptide level whereas no significant improvement in these variables occurred in usual care patients. In addition, all-cause hospitalization occurred in 37% of the latter group but only 15% of the ET group. No syncope, sustained arrhythmia, or falls occurred during the exercise sessions. The changes after ET in HFrEF versus HFpEF patients were not reported.

In contrast to the prior 3 trials, Witham and colleagues[53] reported no improvement in 6MWD or MLHFQ and no decrease in health care costs in 107 patients with HFrEF greater than or equal to 70 year old (mean 80 years, 35% women) after 8 weeks of twice weekly supervised ET followed by 16 weeks of home training. No significant difference in adverse events or hospitalization rate was found between the groups.

A meta-analysis of 7 ET trials comprising 530 HFrEF patients greater than or equal to 70 years (including 4 of the trials reviewed previously but not the large Antonicelli and colleagues[52] trial) concluded that both 6MWD and general quality of life improved significantly after ET whereas no significant effects on peak V_{O_2}, disease-specific quality of life, or hospitalizations were seen.[54] Peak V_{O_2} was measured, however, in only 3 of the smaller studies, and a nonsignificant reduction in hospitalizations from 28.5% in controls to 19.4% in the ET group was observed.

CLINICAL TRIAL EVIDENCE IN OLDER PATIENTS WITH HEART FAILURE WITH PRESERVED EJECTION FRACTION

Given that HFpEF is now recognized as the predominant form of HF in older adults, it is important to examine the evidence related to ET in this common condition. Over the past few years, several ET training trials have targeted these patients. Kitzman and coworkers[55] randomized 53 patients with HFpEF (mean age 70 years, 75% women) to 16 weeks of supervised aerobic ET or to attention control. Peak V_{O_2} increased from 13.8 mL/kg/min to 16.1 mL/kg/min in ET patients whereas there was no significant change in controls. Parallel increases were found in 6MWD and ventilatory anaerobic threshold and in the physical quality of life score in the ET group. A group of 64 HFpEF patients (mean age 65 years, 56% women) were randomized to 3 months (32 sessions) of combined endurance/resistance training or usual care. Peak V_{O_2} increased from 16.1% mL/kg/min to 18.7% mL/kg/min in the ET group and was accompanied by a decrease in LV volumes and diastolic E/e′ ratio and physical function quality of life whereas these were unchanged in controls.[56] A meta-analysis of 6 randomized controlled trials involving 276 patients (mean age 67 years, 69% women) demonstrated a mean 2.72 mL/kg/min in peak V_{O_2} and a 4-point improvement in MLHFQ score compared with controls (**Fig. 2**), but no change was seen in LV systolic or diastolic function.[57]

The mechanism for improvement in peak V_{O_2} from aerobic ET in patients with HFpEF was investigated by Haykowsky and colleagues.[58] After 4 months of ET, peak HR increased from 131 beats/min to 139 beats/min, but no significant change occurred in LVEDV, SV, or cardiac output; 84% of the increase in peak V_{O_2} was mediated by an increase in AV_{O_2} difference. A further analysis from this laboratory found no improvement in either brachial artery flow-mediated dilation or carotid artery distensibility, suggesting that other mechanisms, such as increased skeletal muscle perfusion or oxygen utilization, mediate training-induced increases in peak V_{O_2}.[59] An interesting 20-week trial compared ET to caloric restriction or the combination in 100 obese patients with HFpEF (mean age 67 years, 81% women).[60] Peak V_{O_2} increased similarly in the ET (1.2 mL/kg/min) and diet (1.3 mL/kg/min) groups, and the increase was additive in the group receiving both interventions (2.5 mL/kg/min).The MLHFQ score did not improve significantly, however, in any group.

RESISTANCE TRAINING STUDIES IN OLDER PATIENTS WITH HEART FAILURE

Although most ET trials in HF patients have focused on aerobic exercise to enhance the reduced aerobic capacity, another prominent characteristic of the HF syndrome is skeletal muscle atrophy.[61–63] Muscle atrophy is most pronounced in highly oxidative, fatigue-resistant type I fibers, causing a shift toward glycolytic, more fatigue-prone type II fibers.[62] Normative aging also is accompanied by significant loss of muscle mass,[64,65] which accelerates after the sixth decade and is a major contributor to disability in the elderly. Older patients who have HF are therefore at especially high risk for skeletal muscle wasting.

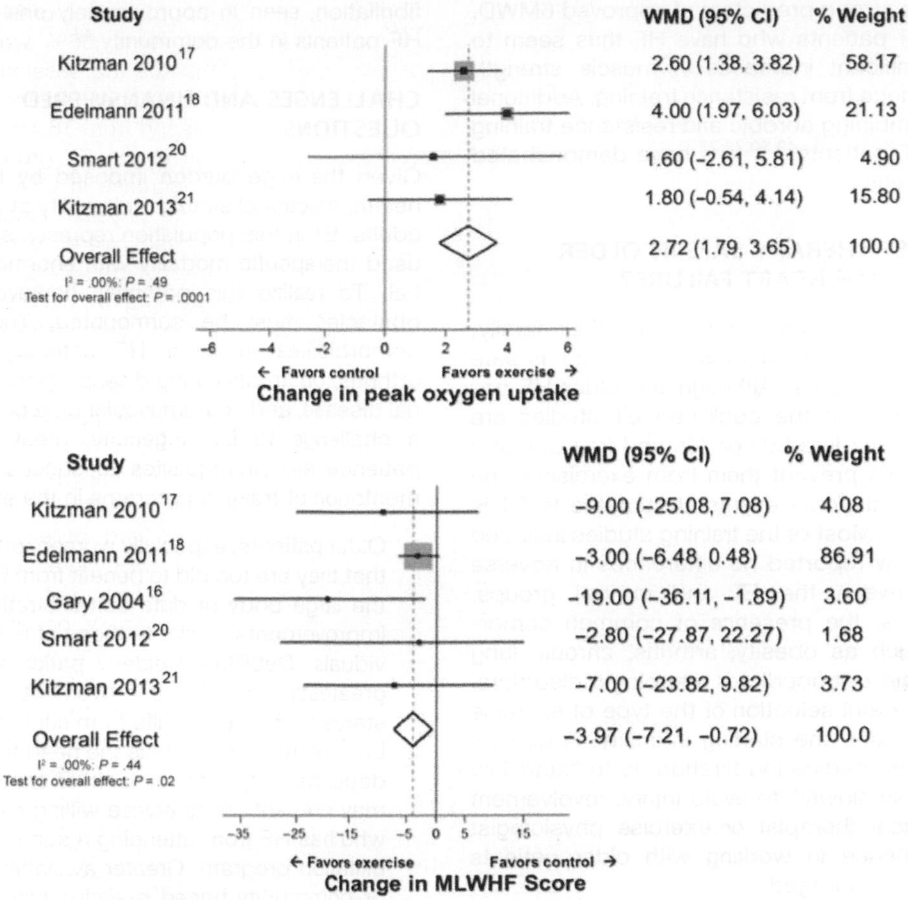

Fig. 2. Forest plot showing effect of ET on cardiorespiratory fitness, measured as peak oxygen uptake (mL/kg/min) and quality of life, estimated using MLWHF score, in participants with HFpEF. WMD, weighted mean difference. (*From* Pandey A, Parashar A, Kumbhani DJ, et al. ET in patients with heart failure and preserved ejection fraction. Meta-analysis of randomized controlled trials. Circ Heart Fail 2015;8:37; with permission.)

High-intensity resistance training has produced dramatic increases in strength and sizable increases in muscle mass in frail elderly nursing home residents in their 80s and 90s who did not have overt HF.[66,67] These improvements were accompanied by increases in gait speed; in some patients, the need for walkers or canes was eliminated. Since these landmark studies, a growing literature has documented beneficial effects of resistance training in patients with HF.

Cider and colleagues[68] observed increased ventilator anaerobic threshold but no improvement in peak V_{O_2}, muscle strength, or quality of life in 24 NYHA class 2 to class 3 HF patients (mean age 63 years, 33% women) randomized to 5 months of circuit weight training twice per week. In another study of 24 HF patients aged 63 years ± 9 years (46% women), Tyni-Lenne and colleagues[69] documented increases in peak V_{O_2}, 6MWD, and quality of life and reduced resting and submaximal plasma norepinephrine in those randomized to 8 weeks of resistance exercises. After 3 months of resistance training, Selig and coworkers[70] observed an increase in peak V_{O_2}, skeletal muscle strength, forearm blood flow, and heart rate variability in a randomized trial of resistance training in 39 class 2 to clas 3 patients aged 65 years ± 11 years (15% women) who had HF.

The relative youth and minimal numbers of women in the studies, discussed previously, of resistance training in HF patients were addressed by Pu and colleagues[71] in a study of 16 women with HF of mean age 77 years randomized to progressive resistance training for 10 weeks. At baseline these women had approximately 40% lower muscle strength than those of similar age who had other chronic diseases. Training was well tolerated and resulted in a 43% increase in strength and 13% increase in 6MWD but no increase in peak V_{O_2}. Increases in type I muscle fiber area (mean 10%) and citrate synthase activity

(35%) were strong predictors of improved 6MWD. Thus, older patients who have HF thus seem to derive significant increases in muscle strength and endurance from resistance training. Additional studies combining aerobic and resistance training in older HF patients[49,50,72,73] have demonstrated similar benefits.

IS EXERCISE THERAPY SAFE IN OLDER PATIENTS WITH HEART FAILURE?

An important concern for patients, their family, and health care providers is whether ET is safe in older HF patients. Although the older HF patients included in the published ET studies are typically in their late 60s or 70s and free of major disorders that prevent them from exercising, the low rates of adverse events attributable to ET is encouraging. Most of the training studies included in this review reported no differences in adverse events between the ET and control groups. Nevertheless, the presence of common comorbidities, such as obesity, arthritis, chronic lung disease, and orthopedic or neurologic disorders, mandate careful selection of the type of exercise intervention and the starting intensity. A general rule, as with medication titration, is to "start low and increase slowly" to avoid injury. Involvement of a physical therapist or exercise physiologist with experience in working with older patients should be encouraged.

LIMITATIONS OF EXISTING TRAINING STUDIES IN OLDER HEART FAILURE PATIENTS

Despite the accumulating evidence that ET is beneficial in older patients with HF, several important limitations of existing studies must be recognized. As discussed previously, few of the studies to date have enrolled a sizable number of patients older than 75 years, the group most representative of HF patients in the general community.[74,75] Similarly, although older women are well represented in ET trials of HFpEF patients, they have been severely underrepresented in existing HFrEF training trials. These deficiencies in recruitment of older HFrEF patients, especially women, also are encountered in standard cardiac rehabilitation programs, representing both a failure of clinicians to refer such patients and logistic difficulties encountered by older patients in attending these programs.[27] The latter issue can be addressed successfully by home-based training, which elicits improvements in exercise capacity parallel to those seen in supervised programs. A further limitation of existing studies is the severe under-representation of patients who have atrial fibrillation, seen in approximately one-quarter of HF patients in the community.[43]

CHALLENGES AND UNANSWERED QUESTIONS

Given the huge burden imposed by HF on the health, functional status, and quality of life in older adults, ET in this population represents an underused therapeutic modality with enormous potential. To realize this potential, however, several obstacles must be surmounted. The multiple comorbidities in older HF patients, including arthritis, obstructive lung disease, peripheral arterial disease, and neuromuscular disorders, provide a challenge to ET. Ingenuity, great care, and patience are prerequisites to successful implementation of training programs in the elderly.

1. Older patients, especially women, often believe that they are too old to benefit from ET, despite the large body of data demonstrating relative improvements similar to those of younger individuals. Debilitated elderly patients have the greatest potential for improvement in functional status and quality of life from such training.
2. Logistic factors, such as the need to care for a dependent spouse or lack of transportation, may prevent an otherwise willing older patient who has HF from attending a supervised rehabilitation program. Greater availability of home or community-based exercise programs may overcome such obstacles and may be more cost effective than traditional hospital-based training.
3. The greatest barrier to recruiting more elderly patients with HF into ET programs may lie within the medical community itself. Physicians and other health care providers must be educated in the benefits of ET in this age group so that they refer such patients to these programs.

Critical questions regarding the benefit of ET in the elderly remain to be answered. Perhaps the most important of these is whether such training prolongs survival or reduces morbidity in older patients who have HF, in particular the large subset with HFpEF. The large HF-ACTION, limited to patients with HFrEF, suggested that aerobic ET could elicit a modest reduction in the combined endpoint of all-cause mortality and hospitalizations as well as similar reduction in cardiovascular endpoints.[43] These positive results, although modest in effect size, resulted in Medicare extending its coverage of cardiac rehabilitation programs to include patients who have HFrEF. A parallel study of similar size is needed to investigate whether patients with HFpEF, who were excluded from HF-ACTION, will benefit from ET. Another important issue is to determine whether a combination of resistance and aerobic training provides greater benefit than aerobic training alone on cardiovascular endpoints, functional measures, and quality of life.

SUMMARY

Both the aging process and HF syndrome are characterized by a dramatic reduction of aerobic capacity caused by a combination of cardiac and peripheral factors. Significant decreases in muscle mass and strength are also common to both conditions. Although a growing literature has documented that aerobic ET elicits improvement in peak Vo_2, submaximal exercise measures, and quality of life in younger HF patients, few HF training studies have included meaningful numbers of older individuals, especially those greater than 80 years of age and older women with HFrEF. Nevertheless, the modest data available suggest similar benefits in older as in younger HF patients as well as excellent safety. Resistance training may provide additional benefit in older patients with HF, especially those with substantial muscle wasting. Whether ET can reduce mortality, hospitalizations, and overall health care costs in patients with HFpEF must await the outcome of adequately powered multicenter trials in this large subset of the HF population.

REFERENCES

1. Buskirk ER, Hodgson JL. Age and aerobic power: the rate of change in men and women. Fed Proc 1987;46:1824–9.
2. Jackson AS, Beard EF, Wier LT, et al. Changes in aerobic power of men ages 25–70 years. Med Sci Sports Exerc 1995;27:113–20.
3. Fleg JL, Lakatta EF. Role of muscle loss in the age-associated reduction in VO2 max. J Appl Physiol (1985) 1988;65:1147–51.
4. Ogawa T, Spina R, Martin WH III, et al. Effects of aging, sex, and physical training on cardiovascular response to dynamic upright exercise. Circulation 1992;86:404–503.
5. Fleg JL, Morrell CH, Bos AG, et al. Accelerated longitudinal decline of aerobic capacity in healthy older adults. Circulation 2005;112:674–82.
6. Fleg JL, O'Connor FC, Becker LC, et al. Cardiac versus peripheral contributions to the age-associated decline in aerobic capacity. J Am Coll Cardiol 1997;29:269A.
7. Fleg JL, O'Connor F, Gerstenblith G, et al. Impact of age on the cardiovascular response to dynamic upright exercise in healthy men and women. J Appl Physiol 1995;78:890–900.
8. Fleg JL, Tzankoff SP, Lakatta EG. Age-related augmentation of plasma catecholamines during dynamic exercise in healthy men. J Appl Physiol 1985; 59:1033–9.
9. Fleg JL, Schulman S, O'Connor F, et al. Effects of acute β-adrenergic receptor blockade on age-associated changes in cardiovascular performance during dynamic exercise. Circulation 1994; 90:2333–41.
10. Stelken AM, Younis LT, Jennison SH, et al. Prognostic value of cardiopulmonary exercise testing using percent achieved of predicted peak oxygen uptake for patients with ischemic and dilated cardiomyopathy. J Am Coll Cardiol 1996;27:345–52.
11. Francis DP, Shamin W, Davies LC, et al. Cardiopulmonary exercise testing for prognosis in chronic heart failure: continuous and independent prognostic value from VE/VCO2 slope and peak VO2. Eur Heart J 2000;21:154–61.
12. Mancini DM, Eisen H, Kussmaul W, et al. Value of peak exercise oxygen consumption for optimal timing of cardiac transplantation in ambulatory patients with heart failure. Circulation 1991;83:778–86.
13. Higginbotham MB, Morris KG, Conn EH, et al. Determinants of variable exercise performance among patients with severe left ventricular dysfunction. Am J Cardiol 1983;51:52–60.
14. Colucci WS, Ribeiro JP, Rocco MB, et al. Impaired chronotropic response to exercise in patients with congestive heart failure. Role of post-synaptic beta-adrenergic desensitization. Circulation 1989; 80:314–23.
15. Sullivan MJ, Hawthorne MH. Exercise intolerance in patients with chronic heart failure. Prog Cardiovasc Dis 1995;38:1–22.
16. Pina IL, Apstein CS, Balady GJ, et al. Exercise and heart failure: a statement from the American Heart Association Committee on Exercise, Rehabilitation and Prevention. Circulation 2003;107:1210–25.
17. Fleg JL. Can exercise conditioning be effective in older heart failure patients? Heart Fail Rev 2002;7: 99–103.
18. Kitzman DW, Little WC, Brubaker PH, et al. Pathophysiologic characterization of isolated diastolic heart failure in comparison to systolic heart failure. JAMA 2002;288:2144–50.
19. Haykowsky MJ, Brubaker PH, John JM, et al. Determinants of exercise intolerance in elderly heart failure patients with preserved ejection fraction. J Am Coll Cardiol 2011;58:265–74.
20. Badenhop DJ, Cleary PA, Schoal SF, et al. Physiological adjustments to higher- and lower-intensity exercise in elders. Med Sci Sports Exerc 1983;15:496–502.
21. Seals DR, Hagberg JM, Hurley BF, et al. Endurance training in older men and women. I. Cardiovascular response to exercise. J Appl Physiol Respir Environ Exerc Physiol 1984;57:1024–9.

22. Hagberg JM, Graves JF, Limacher M, et al. Cardiovascular response of 70- to 79-year old men to ET. J Appl Physiol 1989;66:2589–94.
23. Schulman SP, Fleg JL, Goldberg AP, et al. Continuum of cardiovascular performance across a broad range of fitness levels in healthy older men. Circulation 1996;94:359–67.
24. Huang G, Gibson CA, Tran ZV, et al. Controlled endurance ET and VO2max changes in older adults: a meta-analysis. Prev Cardiol 2005;8:217–25.
25. Lavie CJ, Milani RV, Littman AB. Benefits of cardiac rehabilitation and ET in secondary coronary prevention in the elderly. J Am Coll Cardiol 1993;22:678–83.
26. Ades PA, Waldmann ML, Meyer WL, et al. Skeletal muscle and cardiovascular adaptations to exercise conditioning in older coronary patients. Circulation 1996;94:323–30.
27. Ades PA. Cardiac rehabilitation in older coronary patients. J Am Geriatr Soc 1999;47:98–105.
28. Afzal A, Brawner CA, Keteyian SJ. ET in heart failure. Prog Cardiovasc Dis 1998;41:175–90.
29. Piepoli MT, Flather M, Coats AJ. Overview of studies of ET in chronic heart failure: the need for a prospective randomized multicentre European trial. Eur Heart J 1998;19:830–41.
30. Curnier D, Galinier M, Pathak A, et al. Rehabilitation of patients with congestive heart failure with or without β-blockade therapy. J Card Fail 2001;7:241–8.
31. Hambrecht R, Gielen S, Linke A, et al. Effects of ET on left ventricular function and peripheral resistance in patients with chronic heart failure. JAMA 2000;283:3095–101.
32. Jugdutt BI, Michorowski BL, Kappagoda CT. ET after anterior Q wave myocardial in- farction: importance of regional left ventricular function and topography. J Am Coll Cardiol 1988;12:362–72.
33. Sullivan MJ, Higginbotham MB, Cobb FR. ET in patients with severe left ventricular dys- function: hemodynamic and metabolic effects. Circulation 1988;78:506–15.
34. Hambrecht R, Fiehn E, Weigl C, et al. Regular physical exercise corrects endothelial dysfunction and im- proves exercise capacity in patients with chronic heart failure. Circulation 1998;98:2709–15.
35. Katz SD, Yuen J, Bijou R. Training improves endothelium–dependent vasodilation in resistance vessels of patients with heart failure. J Appl Physiol 1997;82:1488–92.
36. Minotti JR, Johnson EC, Hudson TC, et al. Skeletal muscle response to ET in congestive heart failure. J Clin Invest 1990;86:751–8.
37. Adamopoulos S, Coats AJ, Brunotte F. Physical training improves skeletal muscle metabolism in patients with heart failure. J Am Coll Cardiol 1993;21:1101–6.
38. Stratton JR, Dunn SF, Adamopoulos S, et al. Training partially reverses skeletal muscle metabolic abnormalities during exercise in heart failure. J Appl Physiol 1994;76:1575–82.
39. Hambrecht R, Niebauer J, Fiehn E, et al. Physical training in patients with stable chronic heart failure. Effects on cardiorespiratory fitness and ultrastructural abnormalities of leg muscles. J Am Coll Cardiol 1995;25:1239–45.
40. Braith RW, Welsch MA, Feigenbaum MS, et al. Neuroendocrine activation in heart failure is modified by endurance exercise. J Am Coll Cardiol 1999;34:1170–5.
41. Coats AJ, Adamopoulos S, Radaelli A. Controlled trial of physical training in chronic heart failure. Exercise performance, hemodynamics, ventilation, and autonomic function. Circulation 1992;85:2119–31.
42. Belardinelli R, Georgiou D, Cianci G, et al. Randomized, controlled trial of long-term moderate ET in chronic heart failure: effects on functional capacity, quality of life, and clinical out- come. Circulation 1999;99:1173–82.
43. O'Connor CM, Whellan DJ, Lee KL, et al. Efficacy and safety of ET in patients with chronic heart failure. HF-ACTION randomized controlled trial. JAMA 2009;301:1439–50.
44. Heiat A, Gross CP, Krumholz HM. Representation of the elderly, women, and minorities in heart failure clinical trials. Arch Intern Med 2002;162:1682–8.
45. Rees K, Taylor RS, Singh S, et al. Exercise based rehabilitation for heart failure. Cochrane Database Syst Rev 2004;(3):CD003331.
46. Willenheimer R, Erhardt L, Cline C, et al. ET in heart failure improves quality of life and exercise capacity. Eur Heart J 1998;19:774–81.
47. Wielenga RP, Huisveld IA, Bol E, et al. ET in elderly patients with chronic heart failure. Coron Artery Dis 1998;9:765–70.
48. Gottlieb SS, Fisher ML, Freudenberger R, et al. Effect of ET on peak performance and quality of life in congestive heart failure patients. J Card Fail 1999;3:188–94.
49. Owen A, Croucher L. Effect of an exercise programme for elderly patients with heart failure. Eur J Heart Fail 2000;2:65–70.
50. McKelvie RS, Teo KK, Roberts R, et al. Effects of ET in patients with heart failure: the Exercise Rehabilitation Trial (EXERT). Am Heart J 2002;144:23–30.
51. Austin J, Williams R, Ross L, et al. Randomised controlled trial of cardiac rehabilitation in elderly patients with heart failure. Eur J Heart Fail 2005;7:411–7.
52. Antonicelli R, Spazzafumo L, Scalvini S, et al. Exercise: a "new drug" for elderly patients with chronic heart failure. Aging 2016;8:860–9.
53. Witham MD, Fulton RL, Greig CA, et al. Efficacy and cost of an exercise program for functionally impaired

older patients with heart failure: a randomized controlled trial. Circ Heart Fail 2012;5:209–16.
54. Chen YM, Li Y. Safety and efficacy of ET in elderly heart failure patients: a systematic review and meta-analysis. Int J Clin Pract 2013;67:1192–8.
55. Kitzman DW, Brubaker PH, Morgan TM, et al. ET in older patients with heart failure and preserved ejection fraction: a randomized, controlled, single-blind trial. Circ Heart Fail 2010;3:659–67.
56. Edelmann F, Gelbrich G, Dungen HD, et al. ET improves exercise capacity and diastolic function in patients with heart failure with preserved ejection fraction. Results of the Ex-DHF (ET in Diastolic Heart Failure) pilot study. J Am Coll Cardiol 2011; 58:1780–91.
57. Pandey A, Parashar A, Kumbhani DJ, et al. ET in patients with heart failure and preserved ejection fraction. Meta-analysis of randomized controlled trials. Circ Heart Fail 2015;8:33–40.
58. Haykowsky MJ, Brubaker PH, Stewart KP, et al. Effect of endurance training on the determinants of peak oxygen consumption in elderly patients with stable compensated heart failure and preserved ejection fraction. J Am Coll Cardiol 2012;60:120–8.
59. Kitzman DW, Brubaker PH, Herrington DM, et al. Effect of endurance ET on endothelial function and arterial stiffness in older patients with heart failure and preserved ejection fraction: a randomized, controlled, single-blind trial. J Am Coll Cardiol 2013;62:584–92.
60. Kitzman DW, Brubaker P, Morgan T, et al. Effect of caloric restriction or aerobic ET on peak oxygen consumption and quality of life in obese older patients with heart failure with preserved ejection fraction. A randomized clinical trial. JAMA 2016;315:36–46.
61. Mancini DM, Walter G, Reichek N, et al. Contribution of skeletal muscle atrophy to exercise intolerance and altered muscle metabolism in heart failure. Circulation 1992;85:1364–73.
62. Drexler H, Reide V, Munzel T, et al. Alteration of skeletal muscle in chronic heart failure. Circulation 1992; 85:1751–9.
63. Toth MJ, Gottlieb SS, Fisher ML, et al. Skeletal muscle atrophy and peak oxygen consumption in heart failure. Am J Cardiol 1997;79:1267–9.
64. Kallman DA, Plato CC, Tobin JD. The role of muscle loss in the age-related decline of grip strength: cross-sectional and longitudinal perspectives. J Gerontol 1990;45:M82–8.
65. Faulkner JA, Brooks SV, Zerba E. Muscle atrophy and weakness with aging: contraction-induced in jury as an underlying mechanism. J Gerontol 1995; 50A:124–9.
66. Fiataroni MA, Marks EC, Ryan ND, et al. High intensity strength training in nonagenarians: effects on skeletal muscle. JAMA 1990;263:3029–34.
67. Fiataroni MA, O'Neill EF, Ryan ND, et al. ET and nutritional supplementation for physical frailty in very elderly people. N Engl J Med 1994;330:1769–75.
68. Cider A, Tygessen H, Hedberg M, et al. Peripheral muscle training in patients with clinical signs of heart failure. Scand J Rehabil Med 1997;2:121–7.
69. Tyni-Lenne R, Dencker K, Gordon A, et al. Comprehensive local muscle training increases aer- obic working capacity and quality of life and de- creases neurohormonal activation in patients with chronic heart failure. Eur J Heart Fail 2001;3:47–52.
70. Selig SE, Carey MF, Menzies DG, et al. Moderate- intensity resistance training in patients with chronic heart failure improves strength, endurance, heart rate variability, and forearm blood flow. J Card Fail 2004;10:21–30.
71. Pu CT, Johnson MT, Foreman DE, et al. Randomized trial of progressive resistance training to coun- teract the myopathy of chronic heart failure. J Appl Physiol 2001;90:2341–50.
72. Maiorani A, O'Driscoll G, Cheetham C, et al. Combined aerobic and resistance ET im- proves functional capacity and strength in CHF. J Appl Physiol 2000;88:1565–70.
73. Senden PJ, Sabelis LW, Zonderland ML, et al. The effect of physical training on workload, upper leg muscle function and muscle areas in patients with chronic heart failure. Int J Cardiol 2005;100: 293–300.
74. Kitzman DW, Gardin JM, Gottdiener JS, et al, for the Cardiovascular Health Study Research Group. Importance of heart failure with preserved systolic function in patients > or = 65 years of age. Am J Cardiol 2001;87:413–9.
75. Owan TE, Hodge DO, Herges RM, et al. Trends in prevalence and outcome of heart failure with preserved ejection fraction. N Engl J Med 2006;355: 251–9.

Left Ventricular Assist Device in Older Adults

Chris Caraang, MD, Gregg M. Lanier, MD, Alan Gass, MD, Wilbert S. Aronow, MD, Chhaya Aggarwal Gupta, MD*

KEYWORDS

• Heart failure • Left ventricular assist device • Elderly patients

KEY POINTS

- Because of a limited donor pool for cardiac transplantation, use of a left ventricular assist device (LVAD) has been established as a life-prolonging treatment of patients with advanced heart failure who are ineligible for heart transplantation.
- Selecting the proper patient for an LVAD involves assessment of indications, risk factors, scores for overall outcomes, assessment for right ventricular failure, and optimal timing of implantation.
- LVAD complications remain an Achilles heel of LVAD implants with a 5% to 10% perioperative mortality and complications of bleeding, thrombosis, stroke, infection, right ventricular failure, and device failure.

INTRODUCTION

The population older than 65 years has experienced rapid growth, with census data showing an increase from 34.2 million in 2004 to 44.2 million in 2014. This is projected to more than double to 98 million by 2060.[1] The overall prevalence of heart failure (HF) in the United States and Europe is between 1% and 12% with the number of Medicare beneficiaries (≥65 years) with congestive HF (CHF) being estimated to be at the upper end of the scale at 9% to 12%.[2] The number of patients in New York Heart Association (NYHA) class IV and stage D HF is difficult to estimate, as data are scarce, but Olmstead County data estimate a prevalence of 0.2% in patients age 65 to 74, and 1.4% in those older than 75.[3] Applying a conservative estimate of 0.2% to the overall population older than 65 years, there are 88,400 affected individuals, which exceeds the overall left ventricular assist devices (LVADs) implanted so far of 13,286 between June 2006 and December 2014 reported to the US Interagency Registry for Mechanically Assisted Circulatory Support (INTERMACS).[4]

Identification of patients with stage D HF is important not only because of the limited resources on hand, but because the disease is generally progressive, mortality is high, and treatment options are limited. Treatments include home inotropy, mechanical circulatory support, cardiac transplantation, and palliative care/hospice.

Palliative inotropy may improve symptoms of HF, but has not been shown to prolong life. Orthotopic heart transplantation (OHT) has remained the gold standard for stage D HF. However, because of a limited donor pool, LVAD has been established as a life-prolonging treatment of patients with advanced HF and who are ineligible for heart transplantation.

The National Heart, Lung, and Blood Institute (NHLBI) initiated the artificial heart program in 1964 with the first temporary implantation in 1969 to support a patient awaiting a donor heart.[5] It has evolved to include pulsatile-flow LVADs as

Division of Heart Failure and Heart Transplantation, Department of Medicine, Westchester Medical Center, New York Medical College, Valhalla, NY 10595, USA
* Corresponding author. Cardiology Division, Westchester Medical Center, Macy Pavilion, Room 112, Valhalla, NY 10595.
E-mail address: Chhaya.aggarwal@wmchealth.org

Heart Failure Clin 13 (2017) 619–632
http://dx.doi.org/10.1016/j.hfc.2017.02.013
1551-7136/17/

bridge to transplant (BTT) and as destination therapy (DT) in 2002. And with the subsequent approval of the continuous-flow LVAD (CF-LVAD) HeartMate II (HMII) as a BTT in 2008, the implantation of LVADs has rapidly risen to the point at which annual LVAD implantations exceeded the annual heart transplantations in 2012 (**Fig. 1**), coincidently the year the third-generation LVAD, HVAD (HeartWare International, Inc, Framingham, MA) was approved by the Food and Drug Administration (FDA).[6]

Life expectancy at birth in the general population is 78.8 years, which has been unchanged since 2012.[7] Age is an important factor in heart transplant patient selection. The Randomized Evaluation of Mechanical Assistance for the Treatment of Congestive Heart Failure (REMATCH)[8] trial in 2001 deemed patients older than 65 years as nontransplantable and studied them for LVAD DT. Recent studies show an age at transplantation of 70 being associated with lower survival,[9] whereas age of 72 is listed as a relative contraindication to heart transplantation.[10]

Careful patient selection for a ventricular assist device (VAD) is therefore critical. Only a few studies have evaluated age as a factor in the implantation of the second-generation LVADs. Small studies have shown no significant difference when evaluating the outcome in elderly individuals against their younger cohort.[11–13] This is contrary to other studies that show age related to higher risks in elderly individuals.[6,14,15] Although sample sizes are small, this discrepancy underscores the challenges in investigating elderly patients best suited for an LVAD. This article focuses on patient selection and timing of LVAD implantation in the elderly patient, to optimize the benefits over the risks and improve quality and quantity of life with the application of this new technology for advanced HF.

OUTCOME WITH HOME INOTROPY

In patients with HF with reduced ejection fraction stage D on home inotropes, the results are dismal. In the REMATCH trial, stage D patients on inotropes experienced a 75% mortality at 1 year and virtually no survival at 2 years. The Non-Transplant Eligible Patients who are Inotrope Dependent (INTrEPID) trial[16] showed an 11% 1-year survival. Similarly, the COSI trial[17] demonstrated a 6% 1-year survival (**Fig. 2**). However, in a study by Hashim and colleagues[18] published in 2015 involving 97 Class IV patients on inotropes, guideline-directed medical therapy with 82% of patients on cardiac resynchronization therapy (CRT)–implantable cardioverter defibrillator, the actuarial 1-year survival was reported as 47.6% (38.4% 2-year survival).[19]

HISTORY OF LEFT VENTRICULAR ASSIST DEVICES

The artificial heart program was developed by the NHLBI in 1964 as a heart replacement therapy,[6] which led the first cardiac assist device being successfully implanted in 1966 at the Texas Heart Institute. The HeartMate 1000 IP pneumatic implantable LVAD was then developed and first used by Texas Heart Institute in 1986.[20] Further technological development lead to FDA approval of HeartMate as a BTT in 1994. This BTT strategy was not borne out of evidence-based data, but out of necessity due to lack of available hearts. The updated version, the HeartMate XVE was subsequently approved in 1998 for BTT and as DT in 2002. However, because of the device's size and lack of reliability with malfunction or failure approaching nearly 73% after 2 years,[21] the second-generation LVAD systems, continuous axial-flow pumps, were developed.

The HMII, a second-generation LVAD, is the most widely implanted LVAD to date.[22] It is smaller, with only one moving part, the rotor, suspended in the blood flow path by ruby bearings. It resulted in lower rates of mechanical failure and other complications. The HeartMate II received BTT FDA approval in 2008. It subsequently received DT FDA approval in 2010 based on the trial published by Slaughter and colleagues,[23] in 2009. This trial

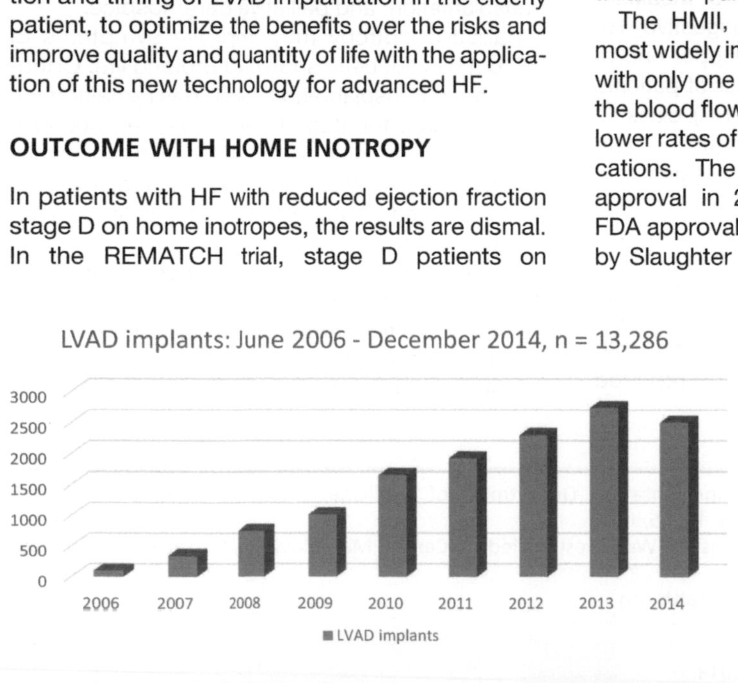

Fig. 1. Implants increasing over time, except for a dip in the total in 2014. (*Data from* Kirklin JK, Naftel DC, Pagani FD, et al. Seventh INTERMACS annual report: 15,000 patients and counting. J Heart Lung Transplant 2015;34(12):1495–504.)

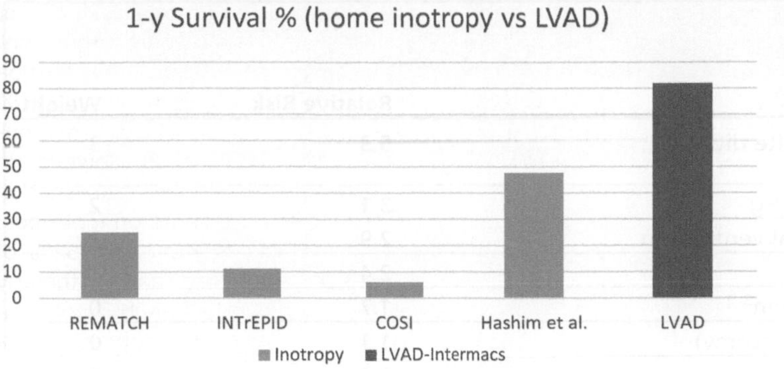

Fig. 2. The 1-year survival of patients on home inotropy compared with CF-LVAD.

compared the HeartMate XVE to the HeartMate II in patients who were not considered transplant eligible. The study found an improvement in survival (1-year and 2-year survival for patients with HeartMate II were 68% and 58%, respectively, compared with 55% and 24% with the HeartMate XVE). There was also substantial improvement in functional capacity and quality of life.

The third-generation, and smaller, implantable LVAD design by HeartWare HVAD eliminated the bearings, and instead, suspended the impeller with magnetic or hydrodynamic suspension systems. This device was studied in a multicenter prospective, nonrandomized trial in the United States between 2008 and 2010 (ADVANCE trial). Noninferiority was shown, with its 6-and 12-month survival at 94.0% and 90.6%, respectively, in the HeartWare group, and 90.2% and 85.7% in the comparison group. It received FDA approval for BTT in 2012.[22]

RISK PREDICTORS OF LEFT VENTRICULAR ASSIST DEVICE MORBIDITY AND MORTALITY

Because the most important factor for overall clinical assessment and improving patient outcomes is careful patient selection, we review the most common risk models. Scores indicating high risk may impact negatively on the decision to place an LVAD. That is, if the patient is such a high risk that he or she is unlikely to survive even with an LVAD, this would be considered a futile implant. Additionally, some risk models predict postoperative mortality, mostly from right ventricular (RV) failure.

Risk Factor Selection Scale

One of the earliest risk models was proposed by Mehmet Oz and colleagues[24] in 1995, called the Risk Factor Selection Scale to determine a patient's suitability for LVAD implantation. It was derived from a cohort of 56 patients who received an LVAD as BTT at Columbia Presbyterian Hospital/The Cleveland Clinic Foundation Centers. It included 7 criteria (total score of 10); a higher score was correlated with worse outcome. An intermediate-risk score, such as 4 to 7, indicated that the implantation may need to be delayed until a favorable clinical status can be achieved (**Table 1**).

Risk Factor Summation Scale

The risk-scoring predictors by Oz and colleagues[24] were then revised by Rao and colleagues[25] to improve its risk discrimination. It used a cohort of 130 consecutive patients with BTT VE HeartMate I LVAD.[25] It found that prior thoracotomy no longer predicted death, and instead, post-pericardiotomy shock, prior LVAD, and right ventricular assist device (RVAD) did. A score of greater than 5 was associated with a perioperative mortality risk of 45% (instead of 12% if the score was $\leq$5, *P*<.001) (**Table 2**).

The Apache II score, developed by Knaus and colleagues[26] was derived from a multi-institutional cohort of 5815 critically ill patients and not from LVAD-related patients. It consisted of 13 preoperative variables, including temperature, mean arterial pressure, heart rate, respiratory rate, partial pressure of arterial oxygen, or alveolar-arterial oxygen gradient if Fio_2 is $\geq$50%, arterial pH, serum sodium, potassium, creatinine, hematocrit, white blood cell count, Glasgow Coma Score, and age.

The Lietz-Miller Destination Therapy Risk Score (DTRS)[27] was developed in a cohort of 222 patients with the XVE HeartMate I LVAD. It includes 9 variables in determining risk factors for 90-day in-hospital mortality (**Table 3**).

Interagency Registry for Mechanically Assisted Circulatory Support Score

INTERMACS places LVAD patients into 7 levels of clinical acuity: 1 ("critical cardiogenic shock"),

Table 1
Risk factor selection scale

Variable	Relative Risk	Weight
Urinary output <30 mL/12 h despite diuretic administration	5.3	3
Central venous pressure >16 mm Hg	3.1	2
Need for preoperative mechanical ventilation	2.9	2
Prothrombin time >16 s	2.4	1
White blood cell count >15,000/mm^3	1.7	0
Recent reoperation (median sternotomy)	1.1	0
Temperature >101.5°F	0.0	0

Data from Oz MC, Goldstein DJ, Pepino P, et al. Screening scale predicts patients successfully receiving long-term implantable left ventricular assist devices. Circulation 1995;92(9):169–73.

2 ("progressive decline despite inotropes"), 3 ("stable but inotrope-dependent"), 4 ("recurrent advanced HF"), 5 ("exertion intolerant"), 6 ("exertion limited"), and 7 ("advanced NYHA III").[28] It predicts complications and mortality after mechanical circulatory support (MCS) implantation.[29] It classifies patients according to hemodynamic status and predicts outcomes in those undergoing MCS implantation. It predicts the prognosis after surgery, hence can be used to select candidates for urgent surgery.

Seattle Heart Failure Risk Score

The Seattle Heart Failure Model (SHFM), reported in 2006, is a multimarker (21-variable) risk assessment model derived during the Prospective Randomized Amlodipine Survival Evaluation (PRAISE)[30] study that involved 1125 patients with NYHA class IIIB or IV. It has been validated in several studies involving nearly 10,000 patients. It also was tested in the REMATCH trial cohort, which showed that it was predictive of outcomes in both the medical (P = .014) and LVAD groups (P = .051) with a 1-year mortality of 30% versus 28% (predicted vs actual) in the medical and 49% versus 52% in the LVAD group.[31] The SHFM also can be used to identify patients who would benefit from LVAD therapy.[32] The SHFM was then updated to include inotropes, intra-aortic balloon pump (IABP), ultrafiltration, mechanical ventilation, and addition of an LVAD. The SHFM has an online calculator that can be accessed at http://SeattleHeartFailureModel.org, where users can view the effect of variables being added or removed, such as HF medications and devices, including the addition of an LVAD.

A study looked at how well these 5 models do in a single-center experience. The APACHE II and SHFM were best able to discriminate high and low risk, hazard ratio, but the SHFM provided good discrimination of short-term deaths.[33] The DTRS was derived from a cohort of pulsatile LVADs, and only a few of the devices used in the INTERMACS study were CF-LVAD. Although the APACHE II and SHFM better predicted patients who were high risk and low risk at 1 year, no score achieved significance in predicting 30-day or 90-day mortality, although SHFM came close (P = .08 and P = .09, respectively).[33] Also, the

Table 2
Revised risk factor summation score

Variable	Sample Size	Relative Risk	Weight
Ventilated	66	5.3	4
Postcardiotomy	38	3.3	2
Pre-LVAD	26	3.3	2
Central venous pressure >16 mm Hg	83	2.1	1
Prothrombin time >16 s	72	2.1	1

Data from Rao V, Oz MC, Flannery MA, et al. Revised screening scale to predict survival after insertion of a left ventricular assist device. J Thorac Cardiovasc Surg 2003;125(4):855–62.

Table 3
Calculation of Destination Therapy Risk Score (DTRS)

Calculation of the DTRS Score	Points
Platelet count ≤148 k/μL	7
Serum albumin ≤3.3 g/dL	5
Presence of vasodilator therapy	4
International normalized ratio >1.1	4
Mean pulmonary artery pressure ≤25 mm Hg	3
Hematocrit ≤34%	2
Blood urea nitrogen >51 U/dL	2
Not on intravenous inotropes	2
Aspartate aminotransferase >45 U/mL	2

Risk Score	Strata of Risk	90-Day Death %
>19	Very high	81
17–19	High	44
9–16	Medium	12
0–8	Low	2

INTERMACS scoring system fell short in the multivariable analysis, given its lack of objective component variables. The SHFM, when compared with DTRS and Risk Factor Summation Scale score, best predicted postimplantation mortality and was able to stratify CF-LVADs into low-risk and high-risk groups.[33]

HeartMate II Risk Score

HeartMate II Risk Score (HMRS) is also an easy-to-calculate score at bedside. It is a predictive tool for post-VAD survival (regardless of BTT or DT indication). The variables include age, serum albumin, creatinine, international normalized ratio (INR), and implant center experience.[15] The score can be used as a starting point for discussion with the patient and family, and to identify variables that can be optimized preoperatively; for example, serum albumin and kidney function. The formula: $0.0274 \times \text{Age} - 0.723 \times \text{Albumin (g/dL)} + 0.74 \times \text{Creatinine (mg/dL)} + 1.136 \times \text{PT-INR} + 0.807 \times$ (0 or 1, considering center volume higher than 15).[15] Stratification includes: low (<1.58) and medium (≥1.58 to ≤2.48). The risk score found good discrimination of risk at 90 days, as well as 1 year and 2 years.

POSTIMPLANTATION RIGHT VENTRICULAR FAILURE

Most morbidity and mortality post-LVAD is related to RV failure. LVADs are a great technology to assist a failing LV, but do nothing to support the RV. LVAD implantation results in an increase in venous return to the RV that may overwhelm RV function, cause a right-to-left interventricular septal shift, and increase tricuspid regurgitation. The risk for death is 44% with RV failure requiring an RVAD (vs 21% when no RVAD is required) after an LVAD.[34] Parameters that have been identified that reflect poor preoperative RV performance include high central venous pressure (CVP), high CVP to pulmonary capillary wedge pressure ratio, low cardiac index, low RV stroke work index (RVSWI), and high pulmonary vascular resistance (PVR).[35]

Several predictors, including the Michigan, Penn, and Utah scores were retrospectively evaluated in 69 patients. The Michigan score resulted in the highest discrimination although only modest results.[36]

1. The Michigan score, also called Right Ventricular Failure Risk Score (RVFRS)[37] was derived from retrospectively analyzed preoperative data of 197 patients who underwent an LVAD implantation. From this, clinical, echocardiographic, laboratory, and hemodynamic predictors of RV failure were developed, including preoperative parenteral inotropic requirement, severe RV dysfunction, RVSWI less than 450 mm Hg*mL/m^2, pulmonary artery systolic pressure less than 50 mm Hg. The receiver operating characteristic curve of the RVFRS showed it was a more discriminative predictor than right atrial systolic pressure, pulmonary artery systolic pressure, transpulmonary gradient (TPG), PVR, severe RV systolic dysfunction, and RVSWI alone with a *P*<.05. The score assigns points to vasopressor requirement, aspartate aminotransferase (AST) ≥80, bilirubin ≥2.0, and creatinine ≥2.3. This resulted in a specificity of 88%, negative predictive value (for predicting absence of RV failure) of 80%, and positive predictive value (correctly predicting RV failure) of 80%. Risk strata is summarized in **Table 4**.
2. Fitzpatrick and colleagues[38] identified 6 independent high-risk predictors with weighted coefficients, and constructed them into a risk score. A systolic blood pressure ≤96 mm Hg (score 13), Cardiac Index ≤2.2 L/min/m^2 (score 18), RVSWI ≤0.25 mm Hg L/m^2 (score 18), creatinine ≥1.9 mg/dL (score 17), severe preoperative RV dysfunction (16), and prior cardiac surgery (score 16) as independent risk factors for right HF. A multiplier of 1 is given for each criterion met, for a total possible score of 98. A score ≥50 successfully predicted the need for a biventricular assist device (BiVAD) with greater than 80% sensitivity and specificity.

Table 4
Right ventricular failure risk score and right ventricular failure by score strata

Calculation of Right Ventricular Failure Risk Score	Points
Vasopressor requirement	4
Aspartate aminotransferase ≥80 IU/L	2
Bilirubin ≥2.0 mg/dL	2.5
Creatinine ≥2.3 mg/dL	3
Risk Score (Sum of Points)	**Strata of Risk**
≤3.0	Low
4.0–5.0	Intermediate
≥5.5	High

3. Tricuspid Annular Plane Systolic Excursion (TAPSE) is a parameter that describes RV apical-to-base shortening, which correlates closely with RV ejection fraction. A small study by Deswarte and colleagues[39] resulted in a 100% specificity and sensitivity when there is a 40% increase in TAPSE with a more than 30% increase in pulomnary artery systolic pressure (PASP) during dobutamine infusion.

In the setting of a failing RV, interventions include inotropes, sildenafil, nitric oxide, avoidance of auto-peep and acidosis, and LVAD speed optimization. If efforts are still unsuccessful, including a cardiac index less than 2.0 L/min/m^2 and CVP greater than 20 mm Hg, consideration for temporary RVAD implantation should be given (**Table 5**).

In the study by Sandner and colleagues,[6] age was the only independent predictor of post-LVAD mortality (hazard ratio [HR] 1.4, 95% confidence interval [CI] 1.1-1.8, *p* value 0.003). This was speculated to be from higher post-LVAD renal failure and underlying comorbidities. Also, the older than 60 age group had a higher incidence of mortality from sepsis.

In the study by Adamson and colleagues,[11] there was no significant difference in terms of bleeding, infection, stroke, survival, and quality of life when comparing patients younger than 70 to patients 70 years or older. The investigators concluded that age was not a factor alone in deciding who should receive an LVAD. Looking at the data, however, there were differences in baseline characteristics of the 2 groups, with the prealbumin of those older than 70 significantly higher (P = .030), more of them were on an angiotensin-converting enzyme inhibitor (P = .015), and with CRT (P = .06).

In the analysis by Allen and colleagues,[14] patients older than 60 were evaluated from the United Network for Organ Sharing database. It found that there was higher 1-year mortality in patients who underwent LVAD BTT than those who went directly to OHT or inotropic bridge. Using multivariable analysis, increasing age per year past 60, creatinine level, and obesity (body mass index ≥30) were among other covariates that increased the hazard of first-year death. There was a 6.4% higher mortality of OHT with BTT over inotropy as bridge to OHT, possibly due to the risks of undergoing 2 separate open-heart surgeries. The investigators concluded that patients older than 60 have a lower short-term survival when undergoing OHT after BTT LVAD and that consideration should be given to direct transplantation or use of inotropic bridge, especially if there are other comorbidities present.

The study by Cowger and colleagues[15] devised a risk score (HMII risk score) derived from a CF-LVAD cohort, which was then applied to a validation cohort to develop an HMII risk score. It concluded that preoperative variables of age, serum albumin, creatinine, INR, and implant center experience offered improved risk discrimination and were predictive of survival after LVAD.

The study by Rosenbaum and colleagues[12] took 64 consecutive patients 65 years or older with a mean SHFM score of 2.14, and risk stratified them by age, SHFM score, implantation intention, and renal function. There was no significant difference in Kaplan-Meier survival among these variables.

In the study by Shah and colleagues[13] looked at 1149 CF-LVADs between May 2004 and May 2015, in which patients were stratified between younger than 70 or 70 years or older. The HR for early perioperative mortality was higher in elderly individuals, but there was no long-term difference in survival, P = .18. Its conclusion was, based on multivariate Cox regression analysis, age of 70 or older was not a predictor of mortality (HR 0.93, 95% CI 0.69–1.25, P = .62).

These observations underline 2 issues: first, age confers an intrinsic risk for morbidity and mortality, but many variables are important in the equation of risk. These results challenge the concept of looking at just age. Second, further efforts are needed to prevent complications in patients on a CF-LVAD.

LEFT VENTRICULAR ASSIST DEVICE SELECTION CRITERIA AND TIMING IN ELDERLY PATIENTS

Patient selection and timing of surgery are again important in lowering postoperative morbidity and mortality. Delaying LVAD implantation may

Table 5
Studies of CF-LVAD and age

Author/ Institution	Date of Data Accumulation	Device and Study Type	Patient Population, n	Age	Survival Perioperatively	Survival at 6 mo	Survival at 1 y	Survival at 2 y	Results
Sandner et al,[6] 2009/ University of Vienna	11/98–7/07	CF-LVAD	86	<60 y/o (56) vs ≥60 y/o (30)	Not specified	BTT 74% <60 y/o, BTT 37.5% ≥60 y/o	HT 87% <60 y/o, HT 90% >60 y/o	Not specified	Age only independent predictor; BTT careful selection in >60.
Adamson et al,[11] 2011/San Diego	2005–2010	HMII	55	<70 (25) ≥70 (30)	<70: 96% ≥70: 97% (30 d)	Not specified	<70 (93.3%) ≥70 (88%)	<70 (77%) ≥70 (71)	No significant difference in survival and QOL.
Allen et al,[14] 2012/Johns Hopkins	2005–2010	HMII	264 BTT 1142 OHT 1148 Inotropic bridge	≥60	30 d BTT 93.5% OHT 96.7% Inotropic bridge 96.6%	90 d: BTT 93.5% OHT 93.6% Inotropic bridge 94%	BTT 82.9 OHT 87.7 Inotropic bridge 89.3%	BTT 82% OHT 85.6% Inotropic bridge 80.7%	LVAD lower survival in 30 d and 1 y vs OHT.
Cowger et al,[15] 2013/ multicenter, University of Michigan and others	2005–2010	HMII	1122	58 ± 14	Not specified	86% ± 1% (90-d)	75% ± 2%	65% ± 2%	Derivation cohort to derive HMII risk score.
Rosenbaum et al,[12] 2014/ University of Minnesota	2005–2012	HMII 75% ventricular assist device 19% HW 6%	64	≥65 (65–82)	Not specified	85%	74%	55%	No significant differences in survival stratified by age.
Shah et al,[13] 2015	May 2004–May 2015	CF-LVAD	1149	<70 (986) ≥70 (163)	≥70 87% <70 92%	≥70 80% <70 88%	≥70 75% <70 84%	Not specified	No significant long-term difference in survival except GI bleeding.

Abbreviations: BTT, bridge to transplant; CF-LVAD, continuous flow left ventricular assist device; GI, gastrointestinal; HT, heart transplant; HW, heart ware; OHT, orthotopic heart transplantation; QOL, quality of life; y/o, years old.

result in worsening of the patient's medical condition, and development of biventricular failure can increase the operative risk. Alternatively, delaying LVAD implantation may allow optimization of nutrition status, physical conditioning, and renal function. Inotropy for medical optimization before LVAD has been proposed.[15] The indications for durable VAD overlap between the most common implant indications: (1) BTT, (2) bridge to decision (BTD), (3) DT, and (4) bridge to recovery. BTD, the most common indication listed in INTERMACS, may be used when a medical problem is not clear at the time of LVAD implant. For example, a patient who undergoes an LVAD implantation as DT with marginal renal function may recover and become a transplant candidate.[40]

Destination Therapy

The selection criteria for LVAD implantation as DT was adopted from inclusion criteria from 2 landmark trials, REMATCH and HeartMate II, and is without any reference to specific age limits. This is also the criteria for reimbursement from Centers for Medicare and Medicaid Services (CMS).[7] It includes all of the following:

1. Patients are not candidates for heart transplantation
2. Significant functional limitations consistent with chronic end-stage NYHA IV symptoms for 45 of the preceding 60 days despite the use of optimal medical therapy (OMT), or dependence on IABP for 7 days or 14 days of intravenous (IV) inotrope
3. LV ejection fraction less than 25%
4. A peak exercise oxygen consumption (peak Vo_2) of 14 mL/kg per minute or less, unless unable to perform the test or IABP-dependent or inotrope-dependent.

Bridge to Transplant

The upper age for heart transplantation is 70 to 72 and is therefore the inherent upper age for durable LVAD as BTT, although there is no established time frame to which LVADs are implanted. However, for inotrope-dependent patients, those who will have a long wait for OHT, such as those with ABO blood type O, high levels of HLA antibodies, or large body size, should strongly be considered for a durable LVAD. With data from the International Society for Heart and Lung Transplantation registry showing that 33% or more of patients with LVAD as BTT undergo transplantation,[41] age, especially at the upper end of the scale, may eventually become a factor, as there may be a longer support time owing to the lack of available donor hearts.

Preoperative Assessment

1. Nutritional assessment. Malnutrition is common in HF. Weight loss is found in up to 50% of patients with HF.[42] Cardiac cachexia results in higher perioperative mortality than in patients with noncachectic CHF when undergoing cardiac surgery.[42] It is therefore important that patients undergo a comprehensive assessment to determine any degree of malnutrition. Most widely used is the Subjective Global Assessment scale, which also helps determine when nutritional therapy should be started.[43]
2. Psychosocial assessment. Careful assessment of the psychosocial support system before LVAD placement is also important. One must determine the presence, commitment, and age of the 24-hour support (spouse or caregiver), who takes responsibility and can be around in case of a device malfunction.[44] Also, the home environment needs to be assessed for safety. A plan of care will need to be determined postoperatively to make sure the patient will be able to care for himself or herself including eyesight, hearing, dexterity, dentition, and compliance with prior medications. We must also look at the desire of the patient to live, as LVAD implantation is a high-risk surgery and his or her motivation is a critical factor to a successful outcome.
3. Neurologic assessment. Because the device would need to be operated safely, a neurologic assessment should be done to evaluate for degenerative central nervous system disease, history of stroke, cognitive function, psychiatric disorders, and substance abuse and to rule out dementia.
4. Informed consent. All patients and significant others should be given all appropriate information about the surgery, as well as expectations after surgery.

RISK STRATIFICATION FOR LEFT VENTRICULAR ASSIST DEVICE SUPPORT IN ELDERLY INDIVIDUALS

Age is an important risk factor for LVAD, especially because 80% of patients with HF are older than 65.[45] In heart transplantation, an age of 72 is a relative contraindication, but in DT or BTT LVAD, the upper patient age limit has not been defined. Age is not necessarily an independent variable. Patients older than 70 years often have multiple comorbidities, including noncardiac factors that negatively impact their survival.[46] There are no controlled large-scale studies involving the use of LVADs in elderly individuals. Also, patients 80 years and older are poorly represented in these data. Looking at the published case series summarized in **Table 3**, most come from small, single-center series, and patterns emerge from the preoperative variables: significant risks include renal and liver dysfunction, and prior gastrointestinal bleeding. Certainly, there is not one factor that confers prohibitive risk, but when looking at elderly patients, attempts should be made to minimize these risks. The best approach is to identify these risks and optimize them before implantation.

One-Year to 2-Year Risk

In selecting the appropriate patient, the 2013 American College of Cardiology/American Heart Association (ACC/AHA) guidelines suggest candidates have "a high predicted 1- to 2- year mortality...as suggested by clinical prognostic score," but they did not designate a risk model to estimate mortality nor did they define "high" as to a specific percentage. The prior 2009 AHA/ACC guidelines did identify appropriate patients for LVAD having more than 50% annual mortality. Assuming this still applies, then $\leq$50% would be alive in 1 year, and $\leq$25% would be alive at 2 years. Several well-validated models can then be used, including SHFM and HMII risk score (HM2RS).

Given that survival after LVAD in most high-risk patients with LVAD is relatively poor, HF specialists often question whether a specific patient would benefit from a high-risk implantation surgery. The major contribution of SHFM is that it can predict 1-year to 2-year survival after LVAD implantation by using a well-validated and easy-to-use, multimarker risk assessment model. The HM2RS has also been validated for 1-year to 2-year survival using age, creatinine, albumin, INR, and center volume. Both SHFM and HMRS incorporate age into their equations.

If the 1-year to 2-year mortality post-LVAD is very high according to SHFM or HMRS, then it would be appropriate to not proceed with LVAD implantation, as that would likely only worsen morbidity, not improve quality of life, and potentially increase the risk for death. These patients might be better suited for palliative inotropy, which has an actuarial 1-year survival as low as 6.0% and as high as 47.6%, with no surgical risks, but an increased risk for arrhythmia and infection from the venous access line. Conversely, if the patient has an anticipated survival of more than 1 to 2 years, it would be reasonable to offer LVAD to these patients to improve survival and quality of life. However, it is understandable that despite the procedural risks involved, many patients with end-stage HF may still want to undergo last-resort therapies. In such high-risk patients, at the very least, the SHFM and HM2RS could significantly aid discussions about prognostic expectations for anticipated short-term survival after a relatively high-risk LVAD implantation surgery. Palliative care consultation also is considered an essential aspect of the pre-LVAD planning in elderly individuals. It is necessary to have a clear conversation about goals of care with the patient, the patient's family, and caregivers should the patient suffer morbidities, such as stroke, ventilator dependence, liver failure, and renal failure requiring hemodialysis. Understanding the wishes of the patient before they happen help guide the family and health care agents in making difficult decisions about end of life.

Operative Risk

The highest risk is in the postoperative period, with 33% of early mortality after LVAD placement being due to hemorrhage, coagulopathy, and cerebrovascular accident.[37] There are 2 models that specifically assess outcomes after LVAD placement: DTRS and INTERMACS score. The DTRS, although derived from a cohort of first-generation HeartMate LVADs, still should be applicable in the immediate implantation period. It uses variables such as AST, albumin, blood urea nitrogen, and platelets. For example, having abnormal liver and renal function, as well as lower serum albumin, can identify, through multivariate analysis, who is too ill to undergo LVAD surgery.[27] The INTERMACS score also can assess risk based on INTERMACS level, and it can be used for immediate postoperative risk, but it fell short of discerning 90-day, 1-year, and 2-year mortality when put on the test. Frailty and immobility are additional, validated, important risk factors in the elderly.[28]

Selection and Risk Scores with Focus on the Right Ventricle

The RV then should be evaluated because of its association with morbidity and mortality. right ventricular systolic fractional shortening (RVSFS), although it did not use age as a predictor, can determine the chance that the RV will fail after LVAD implantation. The RVFRS also uses creatinine and bilirubin, which may represent congestion and hypoperfusion in those with RV dysfunction. Fitzpatrick score can also be used to predict who will need an RVAD after LVAD implantation with an 80% sensitivity and specificity.

Timing Based on Acuity

Interagency registry for mechanically assisted circulatory support level I

Patients in this level are challenging because they are at a higher risk for mortality for LVAD implantation, with a perioperative mortality (relative risk of 1.55).[4] Patients tend to have end-organ dysfunction due to the cardiogenic shock and an inflammatory state. Hence, these patients should be supported by temporary MCS devices, such as IABP, percutaneous axial-flow devices (Impella, Abiomed, Danvers, Massachusetts, USA), veno-arterial extracorporeal membrane oxygenation, percutaneous or surgical centrifugal devices (Tandem Heart, Tandem Life, Pittsburgh, Pennsylvania, USA; Centrimag, Thoratec, Pleasanton, California, USA). If they suffer irreversible end-organ damage (eg, hepatic, renal, neurologic), they are at a higher risk and are suboptimal candidates for durable MCS. Once they are stable, they can be considered for durable MCS.

Interagency registry for mechanically assisted circulatory support levels 2 and 3

INTERMACS levels 2 and 3 patients probably represent the most appropriate use of LVADs. These patients are inotrope-dependent and represent nearly 66% of all implanted LVADs. The outcome of continuous IV inotropic support is poorer based on the REMATCH, Intrepid, and COSI trials, with 1-year survival of 25%, 11%, and 6% respectively, compared with the 80% 1-year CF-LVAD survival.

Interagency registry for mechanically assisted circulatory support 4 to 6

It is the non–inotrope-dependent INTERMACS 4 to 6 (7 is not an indication because it is not equivalent to a class IIIB or IV) that are not clear-cut. The ROADMAP trial was a study to determine how these less-ill patients (not yet on inotropes) would do if an LVAD was implanted at these INTERMACS levels. Six of the 15 OMT patients who underwent delayed LVAD implantation deteriorated from baseline, moving them from level 4 to 6 to 2 to 3, as well as a worsening of NYHA class, albumin, 6-minute walk distance (6MWD), and SHFM score. In the intention-to-treat analysis, there was no difference in survival between the LVAD group (82% $\pm$ 4%) and OMM (81% $\pm$ 4%) at 1 year, indicating that patients in the OMM cohort did not pay a penalty for early or delayed use of an LVAD.[47] However, the OMM arm did not garner survival and health-related quality-of-life benefit, although higher hospitalizations were seen in the LVAD arm.

Unless quality of life is jeopardized, it appears from the study that the optimal time to implant an LVAD is level 2 to 3 or nearing the end of level 4 based on the ROADMAP trial. Moreover, the level 2 to 3 survival curve is nearly superimposable to that of levels 4 to 7.[4]

OUTCOMES AFTER LEFT VENTRICULAR ASSIST DEVICE

Survival

LVAD patient survival and outcomes continue to improve with time. Device technology advancement and application of patient selection criteria have improved survival post-LVAD implant. The 30-day perioperative survival has been reported at 95%,[48] and, based on the 2008 to 2014 INTERMACS, patients now enjoy a 1-year 80% and 2-year 70% survival with CF-LVAD.[4] Although INTERMACS is a valuable resource, it is multicenter with voluntary reporting and different management strategies and may report survival that may not be representative of all centers. A single-center experience from the University of Minnesota, using a standardized management protocol, reported a 3-year survival of 75% with CF-LVAD.[49]

Quality of Life

Virtually all LVAD studies assessing quality-of-life metrics, whether it be questionnaires, 6MWD, or NYHA class, have shown improvement after implantation. Including as early as the pulsatile-flow LVADs in the REMATCH trial, the physical-function and emotional-role component of the SF-36 (health status survey), the Beck Depression Inventory score, and the NYHA class were significantly improved in the LVAD group with the exception of the Minnesota Living with Heart Failure (MLWHF) questionnaires, which was not significant with a *P* value of 0.11.[8] The HeartMate II DT trial[23] demonstrated a 103% improvement in the Kansas City Cardiomyopathy questionnaire from a baseline score of 31 to a 6-month score of 61. The MLWHF questionnaire showed a 43% improvement from a baseline score of 71 to a 6-month score of 38 (lower score is better). There was also a significant increase in the 6MWD from 214 to 372 m at 6 months. Similarly, the ROADMAP trial showed significant improvement in the 6MWD, and heart-related quality-of-life and depression scores after 12 months in the LVAD arm compared with the optimal medical therapy arm.[47]

Complications Following an Left Ventricular Assist Device

Despite the improvement in survival and quality of life, LVAD therapy is not free of complications. **Fig. 3** illustrates that by year 3, only 10% are free of a first occurrence of a major event.

The most common complications are bleeding, LVAD thrombosis, strokes, and infections.

Bleeding

Gastrointestinal bleeding is the most common reported complication from CF-LVAD 30 days postoperatively. Reported annual incidence ranges between 6% and 13%.[50] Probable causes include background anticoagulation and antiplatelet requirement, absence of LVAD pulsatility leading to bleeding arterio-venous malformations (AVMs), and degradation of von Willebrand factors.[51]

Left ventricular assist device thrombosis

Estimated occurrences are 4.7% in 6 months, 7.5% in 1 year, and 12.3% in 2 years.[52] LVAD thrombosis is suspected when there is clinical evidence of HF, an elevated lactate dehydrogenase, and an increase in power. It can be confirmed with noninvasive and invasive studies showing the pump's inability to unload the left ventricle.

Strokes

The INTERMACS registry of 5300 patients with CF-LVAD found an estimated 1-month, 3-month, and 1-year incidence of strokes of 1%, 3%, and 11%, respectively.[48] Similarly, the University of Minnesota group reported a stroke rate of 10.4% in 1 year (13.9% in 2 years).[53] In general, a patient receiving an LVAD has an altered thrombotic profile different from that of the general population. Blood contact with CF-LVAD biomaterials increases the risk for coagulopathy leading to hypercoagulation, fibrinolysis, and platelet abnormalities.[54]

Infections

Incidence of sepsis in CF-LVAD recipients varies from 3% to as high as 36% in CF registries with more than 100 patients.[50] All devices require a driveline that penetrates the skin. This can act as a nidus for infection, leading to driveline infection and sepsis. Infection is associated with inflammatory states that can further promote higher rates of ischemic strokes and other prothrombotic complications.[55]

Summary of Outcomes after a Left Ventricular Assist Device

With improvements in LVAD technology and patient selection, reported survival has been as high as 75% in 3 years. This has left optimists wondering whether there will be a potential for transplantation versus LVAD trials someday. Although LVAD therapy does not come without risks, with only 10% experiencing freedom from a major complication by year 3, LVAD recipients do spend most of their time outside of the hospital enjoying a good quality of life.

CASE CORRELATION

The patient selection can then be applied to a real case: a 74-year-old woman with an ischemic cardiomyopathy, prior Left Main stent, ejection fraction of 22%, status post implantable cardioverter defibrillator (ICD), NYHA class IV, requiring IABP and milrinone drip at 0.25 μg/kg per minute. Cardiac index 1.9 L/min/m^2, RVSWI 0.24 mm Hg L/m^2, hemoglobin 8.5, hematocrit 28.4, platelet 126, lymphocytes 10%, sodium of 130, blood urea nitrogen 77, creatinine of 1.71, INR 1.01, uric acid 6.7 mg/dL, total cholesterol 140, AST 33, total bilirubin of 0.5, albumin of 3.2, weight 92 lb (43.8 kg), blood pressure 96/58, medications: furosemide 40 mg IV twice a day, rosuvastatin 10 mg, allopurinol. She is admitted in the coronary care unit of a VAD center with an implantation volume greater than 15 per year. Using the DTRS to

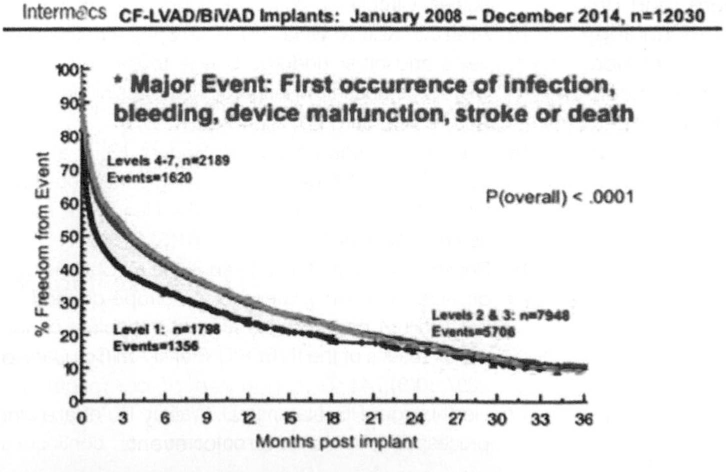

Fig. 3. Freedom from complications of infection, bleeding, device malfunction, stroke, or death stratified by INTERMACS levels. (*Data from* Kirklin JK, Naftel DC, Pagani FD, et al. Seventh INTERMACS annual report: 15,000 patients and counting. J Heart Lung Transplant 2015;34(12):1495–504.)

assess her early postoperative mortality after VAD implantation, her DTRS score is 23 (>19 is very high risk). For the overall outcome score, the SHFM score calculates a 27% 1-year and 8% 2-year survival; adding a VAD would increase 1-year to 51%, 2-year to 26%. Her 1-year and 2-year survival using the HMRS would be 2.13, which is a medium risk with an 84% to 89% 90-day and 72% 1-year survival. I would then calculate the right ventricular risk score to risk stratify the RV. Her RVFRS is 4.0, which is intermediate risk for RV failure, with the Fitzpatrick score resulting in 76 (>50 has a 80% sensitivity and specificity for the need of an RVAD). Armed with these data, the patient and providers will have a better idea of her risk for negative postoperative outcome and may guide them to try to optimize her preoperatively by improving her nutritional status and weight. A careful preoperative assessment would also inform the patient and family as to the risks, and allow a conversation of alternative for stage D HF, including palliative inotropy and hospice.

SUMMARY

LVADs continue to advance and have become an effective therapy for a growing and aging population in the background of limited donor supply. LVADs assist in unloading the LV, increasing cardiac output and improving end-organ perfusion. Recipients now enjoy a 1-year survival of 80%, and improvement in NYHA class, symptoms, and quality of life. Elderly individuals are a challenging population with divergent and sparse data, and age is just 1 risk factor. Selecting the proper patient involves assessment of indications, risk factors, scores for overall outcomes, assessment for RV failure, and optimal timing of implantation. However, LVAD complications remain an Achilles heel of LVAD implants, with a 5% to 10% perioperative mortality and complications of bleeding, thrombosis, stroke, infection, RV failure, and device failure. As LVAD engineering technology evolves, so will the risk-prediction scores. Hence, more large-scale prospective data from multicenters will continually be required to aid in patient selection, reduce complications, and improve long-term outcomes.

REFERENCES

1. Health, U.D.o. and H. Services, Profile of older Americans. 2014. Available at: http://www.aoa. acl.gov/Aging_Statistics. Profile/2014/docs/2014-Profile. pdf. Accessed November 10, 2016
2. Roger VL. Epidemiology of heart failure. Circ Res 2013;113(6):646–59.
3. Ammar KA, Jacobsen SJ, Mahoney DW, et al. Prevalence and prognostic significance of heart failure stages: application of the American College of Cardiology/American Heart Association heart failure staging criteria in the community. Circulation 2007;115(12):1563–70.
4. Kirklin JK, Naftel DC, Pagani FD, et al. Seventh INTERMACS annual report: 15,000 patients and counting. J Heart Lung Transplant 2015;34(12):1495–504.
5. Hogness JR, VanAntwerp M. The artificial heart: prototypes, policies, and patients. Washington DC, USA: National Academies Press; 1991.
6. Sandner SE, Naftel DC, Pagani FD, et al. Age and outcome after continuous-flow left ventricular assist device implantation as bridge to transplantation. J Heart Lung Transplant 2009;28(4):367–72.
7. Kochaneck K.D.e.a. National Vital Statistics Reports. Available at: www.cms.govmedicare-coverage-data basedetailsnca-decision-memo.aspxNCAId=268.pdf. Accessed June 30, 2016.
8. Rose EA, Gelijns AC, Moskowitz AJ, et al. Long-term use of a left ventricular assist device for end-stage heart failure. N Engl J Med 2001;345(20):1435–43.
9. Sorabella RA, Yerebakan H, Walters R, et al. Comparison of outcomes after heart replacement therapy in patients over 65 years old. Ann Thorac Surg 2015;99(2):582–8.
10. Mancini D, Lietz K. Selection of cardiac transplantation candidates in 2010. Circulation 2010;122(2):173–83.
11. Adamson RM, Stahovich M, Chilcott S, et al. Clinical strategies and outcomes in advanced heart failure patients older than 70 years of age receiving the HeartMate II left ventricular assist device: a community hospital experience. J Am Coll Cardiol 2011;57(25):2487–95.
12. Rosenbaum AN, John R, Liao KK, et al. Survival in elderly patients supported with continuous flow left ventricular assist device as bridge to transplantation or destination therapy. J Card Fail 2014;20(3):161–7.
13. Shah P, Pagani FD, Desai SS, et al. Elderly patients receiving durable LVAD support: insights and outcomes. Circulation 2015;132(Suppl 3):A13556.
14. Allen JG, Kilic A, Weiss ES, et al. Should patients 60 years and older undergo bridge to transplantation with continuous-flow left ventricular assist devices? Ann Thorac Surg 2012;94(6):2017–24.
15. Cowger J, Sundareswaran K, Rogers JG, et al. Predicting survival in patients receiving continuous flow left ventricular assist devices: the HeartMate II risk score. J Am Coll Cardiol 2013;61(3):313–21.
16. Rogers JG, Butler J, Lansman SL, et al. Chronic mechanical circulatory support for inotrope-dependent heart failure patients who are not transplant candidates: results of the INTrEPID Trial. J Am Coll Cardiol 2007;50(8):741–7.
17. Hershberger RE, Nauman D, Walker TL, et al. Care processes and clinical outcomes of continuous

outpatient support with inotropes (COSI) in patients with refractory end-stage heart failure. J Card Fail 2003;9(3):180–7.
18. Hashim T, Sanam K, Revilla-Martinez M, et al. Clinical characteristics and outcomes of intravenous inotropic therapy in advanced heart failure. Circ Heart Fail 2015;8(5):880–6.
19. Stewart G, Teuteberg JJ, Kittleman M, et al. INTERMACS profiling identifies risk of death or VAD among medically-managed advanced heart failure patients. J Heart Lung Transplant 2013;32(4):S133.
20. McCarthy PM. HeartMate implantable left ventricular assist device: bridge to transplantation and future applications. Ann Thorac Surg 1995;59(2 Suppl): S46–51.
21. Holman WL, Kormos RL, Naftel DC, et al. Predictors of death and transplant in patients with a mechanical circulatory support device: a multi-institutional study. J Heart Lung Transplant 2009;28(1):44–50.
22. Lee LS, Shekar PS. Current state-of-the-art of device therapy for advanced heart failure. Croat Med J 2014;55(6):577–86.
23. Slaughter MS, Rogers JG, Milano CA, et al. Advanced heart failure treated with continuous-flow left ventricular assist device. N Engl J Med 2009; 361(23):2241–51.
24. Oz MC, Goldstein DJ, Pepino P, et al. Screening scale predicts patients successfully receiving long-term implantable left ventricular assist devices. Circulation 1995;92(9):169–73.
25. Rao V, Oz MC, Flannery MA, et al. Revised screening scale to predict survival after insertion of a left ventricular assist device. J Thorac Cardiovasc Surg 2003;125(4):855–62.
26. Knaus WA, Draper EA, Wagner DR, et al. APACHE II: a severity of disease classification system. Crit Care Med 1985;13(10):818–29.
27. Lietz K, Long JW, Kfoury AG, et al. Outcomes of left ventricular assist device implantation as destination therapy in the post-REMATCH era: implications for patient selection. Circulation 2007;116(5):497–505.
28. Kirklin JK, Naftel DC, Stevenson LW, et al. INTERMACS database for durable devices for circulatory support: first annual report. J Heart Lung Transplant 2008;27(10):1065–72.
29. Alba AC, Rao V, Ivanov J, et al. Usefulness of the INTERMACS scale to predict outcomes after mechanical assist device implantation. J Heart Lung Transplant 2009;28(8):827–33.
30. Pfeffer MA, Skali H. PRAISE (prospective randomized amlodipine survival evaluation) and criticism. JACC Heart Fail 2013;1(4):315–7.
31. Levy WC, Mozaffarian D, Linker DT, et al. Can the Seattle Heart Failure Model be used to risk-stratify heart failure patients for potential left ventricular assist device therapy? J Heart Lung Transplant 2009;28(3):231–6.
32. Levy WC, Mozaffarian D, Linker DT, et al. The Seattle Heart Failure Model: prediction of survival in heart failure. Circulation 2006;113(11):1424–33.
33. Schaffer JM, Allen JG, Weiss ES, et al. Evaluation of risk indices in continuous-flow left ventricular assist device patients. Ann Thorac Surg 2009;88(6):1889–96.
34. Kormos RL. The right heart failure dilemma in the era of left ventricular assist devices. J Heart Lung Transplant 2014;33(2):134–5.
35. Patlolla B, Beygui R, Haddad F. Right-ventricular failure following left ventricle assist device implantation. Curr Opin Cardiol 2013;28(2):223–33.
36. Kalogeropoulos A, Siwamogsatham S, Weinberger JF, et al. Clinical scores and echocardiography for right ventricular failure risk prediction after implantation of continuous-flow left ventricular assist devices. J Heart Lung Transplant 2013;32(4):S273.
37. Matthews JC, Koelling TM, Pagani FD, et al. The right ventricular failure risk score: a pre-operative tool for assessing the risk of right ventricular failure in left ventricular assist device candidates. J Am Coll Cardiol 2008;51(22):2163–72.
38. Fitzpatrick JR, Fredeick JR, Hsu VM, et al. Risk score derived from pre-operative data analysis predicts the need for biventricular mechanical circulatory support. J Heart Lung Transplant 2008;27(12):1286–92.
39. Deswarte G, Kirsch M, Lesault PF, et al. Right ventricular reserve and outcome after continuous-flow left ventricular assist device implantation. J Heart Lung Transplant 2010;29(10):1196–8.
40. Miller LW, Guglin M. Patient selection for ventricular assist devices: a moving target. J Am Coll Cardiol 2013;61(12):1209–21.
41. Nativi JN, Drakos SG, Kucheryavaya AY, et al. Changing outcomes in patients bridged to heart transplantation with continuous- versus pulsatile-flow ventricular assist devices: an analysis of the registry of the International Society for Heart and Lung Transplantation. J Heart Lung Transplant 2011;30(8):854–61.
42. Anker SD, Ponikowski P, Varney S, et al. Wasting as independent risk factor for mortality in chronic heart failure. Lancet 1997;349(9058):1050–3.
43. Holdy K, Dembitsky W, Eaton LL, et al. Nutrition assessment and management of left ventricular assist device patients. J Heart Lung Transplant 2005;24(10):1690–6.
44. Chapman E, Parameshwar J, Jenkins D, et al. Psychosocial issues for patients with ventricular assist devices: a qualitative pilot study. Am J Crit Care 2007;16(1):72–81.
45. Roge VL, Go AS, Llyod-Jones DM, et al. Heart disease and stroke statistics–2012 update: a report from the American Heart Association. Circulation 2012;125(1):e2–220.
46. Huynh BC, Rovner A, Rich MW. Long-term survival in elderly patients hospitalized for heart failure:

14-year follow-up from a prospective randomized trial. Arch Intern Med 2006;166(17):1892–8.
47. Estep JD, Starling RC, Horstmanshof DA, et al. Risk assessment and comparative effectiveness of left ventricular assist device and medical management in ambulatory heart failure patients: results from the ROADMAP study. J Am Coll Cardiol 2015; 66(16):1747–61.
48. Kirkli JK, Naftel DC, Kormos RL, et al. Fifth INTERMACS annual report: risk factor analysis from more than 6,000 mechanical circulatory support patients. J Heart Lung Transplant 2013;32(2):141–56.
49. John R, Holley C, Eckman P, et al. A decade of experience with continuous-flow left ventricular assist devices. Semin Thorac Cardiovasc Surg 2016;28(2):363–75.
50. McIlvennan CK, Magid KH, Ambardekar AV, et al. Clinical outcomes after continuous-flow left ventricular assist device: a systematic review. Circ Heart Fail 2014;7(6):1003–13.
51. Crow S, John R, Boyle A, et al. Gastrointestinal bleeding rates in recipients of nonpulsatile and pulsatile left ventricular assist devices. J Thorac Cardiovasc Surg 2009;137(1):208–15.
52. Starling RC, Moazami N, Silvestry SC, et al. Unexpected abrupt increase in left ventricular assist device thrombosis. N Engl J Med 2014;370(1): 33–40.
53. Harvey L, Holley C, Roy SS, et al. Stroke after left ventricular assist device implantation: outcomes in the continuous-flow era. Ann Thorac Surg 2015; 100(2):535–41.
54. John R, Panch S, Hrabe J, et al. Activation of endothelial and coagulation systems in left ventricular assist device recipients. Ann Thorac Surg 2009; 88(4):1171–9.
55. Park SJ, Milano CA, Tatooles AJ, et al. Outcomes in advanced heart failure patients with left ventricular assist devices for destination therapy. Circ Heart Fail 2012;5(2):241–8.

End-of-Life Care in the Treatment of Heart Failure in Older Adults

John Arthur McClung, MD

KEYWORDS

• Terminal care • Heart failure • Ethical issues • Palliative care • Device therapy

KEY POINTS

- Prognostic uncertainty makes end-stage heart failure a more challenging entity than cancer that requires a more nuanced approach to therapeutic planning.
- Improved communication requires a more robust effort to frankly discuss the disease entity, its therapeutic challenges, patient preferences, and palliative care as early as possible.
- Device therapy and cardiopulmonary resuscitation provide their own complexity when discussing end-of-life issues.
- Palliative sedation requires careful planning and appropriate safeguards to be effective.
- Not all aspects of the dying process can be palliated.

The American Geriatrics Society position statement on the care of dying patients opens by stating that, "providing excellent, humane care to patients near the end of life, when curative means are either no longer possible or, no longer desired by the patient, is an essential part of medicine."[1] Although the essential nature of this discipline certainly cannot be denied, much of the prior literature dedicated to this topic has revolved around terminal care provided to patients with neoplastic diagnoses. Advanced heart failure presents its own unique challenges to the clinician who desires to make the recommendations of the American Geriatrics Society a tangible reality, the specifics of which have only recently begun to receive the attention that they deserve.[2–4] This is clearly appropriate because the proportion of patients referred to hospice with a diagnosis of heart disease has increased during the course of the past two decades. The American Geriatrics Society position statement itself is now more than 20 year old and has not been modified despite the major changes in health care delivery that have occurred since that time. This article focuses on updated specific clinical recommendations and an analysis of some of the ethical issues involved in the provision of care to elderly patients in the terminal stages of heart failure.

HOW DO WE KNOW WE HAVE ARRIVED?

The ability of physicians to accurately predict mortality has been demonstrated to be questionable in advanced heart failure and in cases of advanced malignancy.[5–7] Attempts to ascertain variables predictive of mortality in patients with heart failure have proven to be significantly difficult. An exhaustive review of the literature conducted in 1998 found few consistently predictive variables. Factors accounting for this included small sample size, differing patient populations, selective acquisition of variables, interrelationship of variables, differing measurement technologies, duration of follow-up, poor reproducibility, and

This is an updated version of an article that appeared in *Heart Failure Clinics*, Volume 3, Issue 4.
Division of Cardiology, Westchester Medical Center, New York Medical College, 100 Woods Road, Valhalla, NY 10595, USA
E-mail address: john.mcclungMD@wmchealth.org

Heart Failure Clin 13 (2017) 633–644
http://dx.doi.org/10.1016/j.hfc.2017.02.014
1551-7136/17/

problems with data handling.[8] Measures that seem to have consistent independent prognostic value include New York Heart Association symptom class, echocardiographic left ventricular dimensions, radionuclide ejection fraction, and ischemic cause. Hyponatremia has been previously documented to be associated with an extremely negative prognosis; however, it is unclear whether or not this remains as significant an indicator in patients treated with angiotensin-converting enzyme (ACE) inhibitors.[8,9] The Seattle Heart Failure Model, a more robust model for the prediction of mortality in advanced heart failure, incorporates multiple indicators including age, gender, New York Heart Association class, ejection fraction, cause, medication use, laboratory data, and device use that has been demonstrated to provide remarkably accurate 1-, 2-, and 3-year survival rates.[10] Notwithstanding its significantly improved overall accuracy, it remains a less than optimal guide for dealing with individual patients, particularly in patients with devices, in African Americans, and in patients referred for nonurgent transplantation.[11,12] Two simpler prognostic scoring systems have been developed consisting of seven and four items, respectively; however, when applied to individual patients are presumed to suffer from the same difficulties.[13,14]

Patients with heart failure present with the additional challenge of sudden death, which makes the generation of prediction models even more difficult. Up to 60% of heart failure patients die suddenly; however, prediction of who is most likely to suffer sudden death remains controversial.[15,16] Attempts to more precisely determine who is expected to die suddenly include studies of the prognostic efficacy of B-type natriuretic peptide (BNP) and a risk factor assessment that includes ejection fraction, left ventricular end-diastolic diameter, BNP level, presence of nonsustained ventricular tachycardia, and diabetes mellitus.[17,18] Accurate assessment of sudden death incidence is rendered all the more difficult by the increased prevalence of automatic indwelling cardioverter defibrillator insertion in patients with reduced ejection fraction, which concurrently enhances data collection about the incidence of dysrhythmia in patients with heart failure and decreases the overall mortality caused by dysrhythmia.[19,20] Further uncertainty is introduced by the use of a left ventricular assist device (LVAD) as destination therapy (see later).

The persistence of this prognostic uncertainty renders a discussion of patient preference difficult at best. Prior work done in patients with cancer diagnoses suggests that even a 10% probability of not surviving the next 6 months leads patients to consider different treatment options.[21] In part because of prognostic uncertainty, patients dying with heart failure have been documented to have a poorer understanding of their condition and less involvement in the decision-making process regarding their care.[22] A study of 274 dying patients, 26% of which had cardiovascular disease, found that some treatment was withheld or withdrawn in 84% of patients; however, only 35% of these patients were able to participate in the decision-making process.[23] Incorporation of quality of life measures into a prognostic index has demonstrated that a poor quality of life is more likely to be predicted by a low quality of life index, increasing age, and histories of diabetes, stroke, or dysrhythmia, whereas all-cause mortality is more likely to be predicted by BNP, the presence of a β-blocker at discharge, blood-urea-nitrogen, and a low serum sodium.[24]

Patients dying of heart failure who do not die suddenly deteriorate gradually; however, this gradual process is interrupted by acute episodes that frequently require hospitalization (**Fig. 1**).[25] This process is further complicated by LVAD therapy (**Fig. 2**).[26] The clinical hallmark of patients not presenting with sudden death is a combination of dyspnea and low output symptoms. Other commonly reported symptoms include pain in 78% of patients, depressed mood in 59%, insomnia in 45%, anxiety in 30%, anorexia in 43%, constipation in 37%, and nausea and vomiting in 32%.[27]

Hence, patients dying of heart failure do so suddenly; suffer a chronic, slow deterioration punctuated by acute episodes; or both. In either case, the physician misses many opportunities to explore patient preferences in this population unless these preferences are addressed early in course of the disease.

IMPROVING COMMUNICATION

Interviews conducted in Great Britain with patients dying of heart failure and their caregivers identified several problems unique to the treatment of this patient population.[22] Patients tended not to recall receiving any written information about their condition and often did not see an association between symptoms, such as dyspnea and edema, and their cardiac status. Similarly, patients and caregivers did not feel particularly involved in the decision-making process regarding the illness. This is further compounded by data from the United States suggesting that what prognostic information exists is frequently

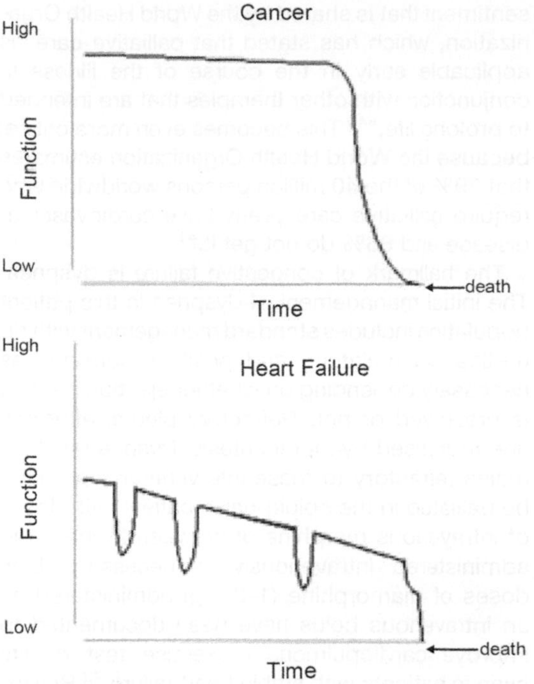

Fig. 1. Typical trajectory of disease for patients with cancer and heart failure. (*Top*) Patients with cancer have a long period of preserved function followed by a precipitous drop that starts within a few months before death. (*Bottom*) Patients with heart failure have an overall gradual decline in function punctuated by periods of exacerbations with acute drops in function followed by a return to near their previous level. (*From* McClung JA. End-of-life care in the treatment of advanced heart failure in the elderly. Cardiol Rev 2013;21(1):10; with permission.)

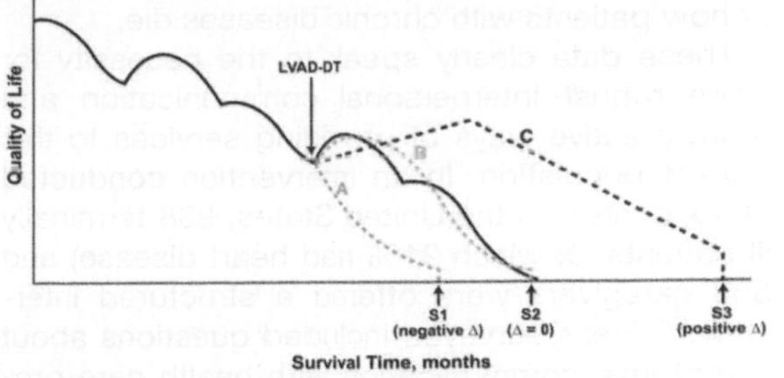

Fig. 2. End-of-life trajectory and quality-of-life (QOL) adjusted survival with LVAD as a destination therapy (DT). LVAD-DT has three possible effects (*dotted lines*) on QOL and end-of-life trajectory, compared with those of medically treated patients (*solid line*). (*A*) Premature decline in QOL with shortened survival time because of postoperative complications and high in-hospital mortality rate (range, 14%–27%) within 90 days after device implantation. Survival time (S1) is shortened by several months compared with survival in the medically treated patient. The LVAD is electively inactivated at the end of life resulting in abrupt death. (*B*) No substantial change in QOL or survival time (S2) compared with that of the medically treated patient. The LVAD is electively inactivated at the end of life resulting in abrupt death. (*C*) The LVAD-DT alleviates limitations of physical functioning related to left heart failure, with an initial enhancement of QOL. A gradual decline in QOL appears over a lengthened survival time (S3) because of high combined rates of late serious complications, such as infections, sepsis, neurologic disabilities, and device malfunction or failure beyond 90 days of device implantation. Average patient survival time after LVAD-DT can be lengthened by about 12 to 24 months, compared with that of the medically treated patient. The LVAD is electively inactivated at the end of life resulting in abrupt death. (*From* Rizzieri AG, Verheijde JL, Rady MY, et al. Ethical challenges with the left ventricular assist device as a destination therapy. Philos Ethics Humanit Med 2008;3:20; with permission.)

misinterpreted by surrogate decision makers.[28] Medication regimens are seen as difficult and burdensome despite their frequent effectiveness. The concurrent presence of comorbidity in this generally elderly population adds to the burden of the primary condition. Care is often seen as fragmented with an absence of the kinds of resources frequently available to patients with cancer.

Although identification of these problems is helpful, solutions are not necessarily obvious. Initially published more than two decades ago, the Study to Understand Prognoses and Preferences for Outcomes and Risks of Treatments (SUPPORT), which evaluated the care of hospitalized patients with life-threatening diagnoses, documented that only 47% of physicians were aware of their patients' wishes regarding cardiopulmonary resuscitation (CPR), that 50% of patients reported severe pain at least half of the time, and that 38% of patients spent 10 or more days in intensive care.[29] A subsequent intervention that provided written prognostic reports and written synopses of patient preferences regarding resuscitation and pain control for the physicians and a skilled nurse practitioner who monitored the patients' progress resulted in no measurable difference in any of the indices related to communication or outcome.[30] A post hoc analysis of 236 hospitalized patients dying of heart failure in the SUPPORT and Hospitalized Elderly Longitudinal Project (HELP) databases documented breathlessness in 65% of patients and severe pain in 42% during the last 3 days of life, whereas 40% received a major therapeutic intervention during the same time period.[31] To date, SUPPORT remains the only attempt at a rigorous assessment of how patients with chronic diseases die.

These data clearly speak to the necessity for more robust interpersonal communication and more creative ways of providing services to this patient population. In an intervention conducted at six centers in the United States, 988 terminally ill patients (of which 21% had heart disease) and 893 caregivers were offered a structured interview.[32] Areas surveyed included questions about symptoms, communication with health care providers, spiritual and personal meaning of dying, care needs, end-of-life plans, economic burdens, preferences regarding end-of-life care, and opinions about euthanasia and physician-assisted suicide among others. Each respondent was also asked how stressful and how helpful the interview had been. Of the patients responding, 88.7% reported little or no stress associated with the interview, whereas 46.5% thought the interview was somewhat or very helpful. Of the caregivers responding, 89.7% reported little or no stress associated with the interview, whereas 53.4% thought it was somewhat or very helpful. This suggests that the SUPPORT investigators did not go far enough in designing the intervention that was ultimately studied. The use of a more structured interview format with patients and family members might serve to initially improve communication between these individuals and their caregivers and set the stage for more focused and interactive palliative care. Examples of such a structured interview for patients with heart failure have already been presented in the literature.[33,34]

PALLIATIVE CARE IN HEART FAILURE

The previously described uncertainty regarding the trajectory of terminal heart failure can induce what has been termed "prognostic paralysis" regarding the initiation of discussion about palliative care and its actual implementation.[35] One commentator has suggested that patients with heart failure should be considered candidates for palliative care if a clinician answers "no" to the question, "Would I be surprised if my patient were to die in the next 12 months?"[36] Another suggested algorithm would initiate palliative intervention during or shortly after recovery from an acute exacerbation of heart failure.[37] Other potential triggers for discussion of palliative intervention include the lack of response to ACE inhibition and the initial discharge of an automatic indwelling cardioverter defibrillator.[38,39] What seems clear from the experience of many is that palliative care needs to be considered much earlier in the course of the disease process than is currently the case, a sentiment that is shared by the World Health Organization, which has stated that palliative care "is applicable early in the course of the illness in conjunction with other therapies that are intended to prolong life."[40] This becomes even more critical because the World Health Organization estimates that 39% of the 40 million persons worldwide who require palliative care yearly have cardiovascular disease and 86% do not get it.[41]

The hallmark of congestive failure is dyspnea. The initial management of dyspnea in this patient population includes standard management with diuretics, vasodilators, and positive inotropes as necessary depending on whether ejection fraction is preserved or not. Refractory pleural effusions are addressed by thoracentesis. Dyspnea that remains refractory to these interventions can often be palliated in the opioid-naive patient with doses of intravenous morphine of between 2 and 5 mg administered intravenously as necessary. Low doses of diamorphine (1–2 mg) administered as an intravenous bolus have been documented to improve cardiopulmonary exercise test results even in patients with stable heart failure.[42] Benzodiazipines can be considered as second-line agents only.[43] The use of supplemental oxygen and appropriate room ventilation is also helpful in patients with dyspnea with documented hypoxia.[44]

Pain is reported in nearly 80% of patients dying of heart failure, although 41% of patients dying of heart failure in the SUPPORT database had moderate to severe pain during the last 3 days of life.[45] Half these reported moderate to severe pain during the last 6 months of life. Pain has been reported in up to 89% of patients with class IV heart failure.[46] Treatment of pain with nonsteroidal anti-inflammatory agents in the setting of heart failure is contraindicated secondary to their propensity to retain sodium, to induce gastrointestinal bleeding, to antagonize the effect of ACE inhibitors, and to decrease renal function.[47] Doses of opioids similar to those effective for dyspnea are often effective for pain control in this population. This is often accompanied by the need to reassure patients and families that properly dosed and monitored opioid therapy is a safe and effective means of controlling discomfort.

Fatigue is often a result of low output and responds to therapy with positive inotropic agents except in the very end stage of heart failure. In class IV patients, continuous positive inotropic therapy is associated with a reduction in hospitalizations, but a concurrent increase in mortality.[48] Chronic nocturnal oxygen supplementation has been of some use in improving functional capacity for patients with severe heart failure.[49] Fatigue may also be related to coexistent depression, which is usually treated pharmacologically with selective serotonin reuptake inhibitors; however, the only randomized controlled trial of these agents in patients with advanced heart failure demonstrated no reduction in depression scores at 12 weeks of follow-up.[50] Also, use of these agents in the absence of appropriate psychological, spiritual, and social support is often compromised by noncompliance.

Treatment of comorbidities may also be helpful. The use of continuous positive airway pressure in patients with sleep apnea secondary to heart failure has been demonstrated to have no effect on survival; however, reductions in apnea and norepinephrine levels have been documented, as well as increases in nocturnal oxygen saturation, ejection fraction, and distance walked in 6 minutes.[51] Treatment of anemia in patients with New York Heart Association class II to IV heart failure with darbepoetin alfa has been demonstrated to improve walking distance and quality of life indicators[52]; however, caution is advised regarding the dose and the target hematocrit as a result of data demonstrating an increase in stroke risk associated with its use in patients with diabetes mellitus and chronic kidney disease.[53] Additional comorbidities frequently documented in this patient population that require intervention include chronic obstructive pulmonary disease, arthropathies, and diabetes mellitus.[54] The initiation of dialysis in elderly patients with multiple comorbidities has been demonstrated to increase the likelihood of dying in hospital, while contributing nothing to survival.[55]

Patients with heart failure may benefit from group visits in which palliative care issues are addressed. A randomized study of 321 elderly patients, 33% of whom had heart disease, demonstrated that patients who received monthly group visits with their primary physician and a nurse that included health education, prevention strategies, opportunities for socialization, and mutual support had fewer emergency department visits, fewer visits to subspecialists, and fewer repeat hospital admissions compared with a control population.[56] The Heart Failure Society of America provides monographs on several related topics including advance care planning and feelings about heart failure that can serve as discussion aids.[57,58]

Patients with end-stage heart failure suffer from a wide variety of other problems including the distress of living with a chronic, fatal condition; the disruption of social life, personal goals, income, faith, and daily function; and an increasing dependence on others with a reciprocal loss of self-esteem.[59] Sixty percent of patients in one observational review believed that one or more of their problems were inadequately addressed.[54] Identification of these issues was easily facilitated by asking the simple question, "What are your three most troublesome problems?"

Persons dying of heart failure have also been documented to have several spiritual needs that are characterized by feelings of hopelessness, isolation, and altered self-image.[60] Among their concerns are the meaning of life, physical needs and practical problems of living at home and in social settings, feelings of abandonment by the health care system, loss of dignity, changes in relationships, increasing dependence, and wishes for death. Responses to problems such as these include discussion of life goals and life closure issues, discussion of the meaning of the illness and its attendant suffering, discussion of coping ability, and the involvement of pastoral care services.[59]

In many instances support services may be best facilitated by a dedicated palliative care team that has significant experience with dying patients.[61] It is now common for hospice services to accept patients with heart failure for the provision of integrated services in inpatient and outpatient settings.[62]

DEVICE THERAPY

The increasingly common use of device therapy has significantly reduced the morbidity and mortality associated with heart failure. Notwithstanding, these devices pose significant problems for the end-stage patient who may wish to minimize or reduce the intensity of his or her care. The right of a patient with intact decision making capacity to refuse any and all medical interventions has a long and established history in bioethics and common law.[63,64] This right applies equally to the withholding and withdrawing of therapy and clearly extends to deactivation of pacemakers and defibrillators, each of which constitutes a highly technical medical intervention. In recognition of this, discussion of device inactivation for patients with heart failure at the end of life was codified as a Class 1 recommendation in the 2005 update of the American College of Cardiology/American Heart Association guidelines for the management of chronic heart failure.[65] For patients who lack capacity, all jurisdictions have procedures for identification of an appropriate surrogate decision maker or documentation of previously expressed health care wishes.[66] Hospitalized patients in the United States are required by law to have information recorded regarding the presence or absence of patient's advance directives at the time of admission and are also required to offer the opportunity for the patient to create one.[67] Notwithstanding this requirement, a survey of the next of kin of 100 patients dying with indwelling cardioverter defibrillators revealed that possible deactivation of the devices had been discussed antemortem in only 27 cases, and eight patients were defibrillated by their device only minutes before death.[68] A survey of physicians themselves revealed that 60% of cardiologists, 88% of gerontologists, and 95% of internists and family practitioners had discussed deactivation in two or fewer cases during the course of their careers.[69] This is unfortunate given that deactivation of an implanted defibrillator has been equated to the withdrawal of other technically complex medical interventions, such as hemodialysis, a situation in which consensus has emerged that discontinuation at the request of a patient or recognized surrogate is the appropriate moral response.[70]

Unlike the use of cardioverter defibrillators, cardiac pacing, even with biventricular resynchronization, has not been clearly shown to prolong life.[71] Only one randomized, intention-to-treat trial has documented a significant reduction in all-cause mortality associated with cardiac resynchronization compared with medical therapy alone, whereas another randomized comparison of medical therapy with both resynchronization and resynchronization with an indwelling defibrillator has demonstrated a modest reduction in death caused by pump failure with cardiac resynchronization alone; however, the overall effect was negligible because of the increased prevalence of sudden death in the absence of coexistent implantable cardioverter-defibrillator therapy.[72,73] Current guidelines do not support implantable cardioverter-defibrillator implantation in patients with chronic, severe refractory heart failure with no reasonable expectation for improvement or in patients with a life expectancy of less than 1 year.[74]

Regardless of its effect on life expectancy, there is no question that a primary benefit of cardiac pacing in the patient with heart failure is symptom relief. As a result, it is to be expected that informed requests for deactivation of cardiac pacing will be less frequent than those for deactivation of a defibrillator. Patients and surrogates who request biventricular pacemaker deactivation need to be appropriately counseled regarding the potential negative effect this decision may have on the quality of the patient's remaining life. Additional adjustments in timing to optimize AV and VV delay using echocardiography are occasionally helpful for relieving the symptoms of end-stage heart failuro.[75] Should a patient or surrogate still prefer that the device be inactivated, it is important to emphasize that it can always be reactivated should the extent of symptomatic deterioration be unacceptable. It is important to recognize that pacemaker therapy, including resynchronization, has been withdrawn in a series of case reports from the Mayo Clinic in patients who were clearly end stage with no obvious exacerbation of already existent severe symptoms.[76] The informed wishes of patients and surrogates who wish that device therapy be terminated need to be taken seriously and honored. Physicians who find this at odds with their own moral reasoning are not obligated to personally deactivate a device, but are obliged to inform the patient or surrogate of their objection and facilitate a transfer of care to a physician willing to accede to this request.[76]

Finally, the emergence of LVAD as destination therapy is adding yet another dimension to the definition of impending death in patients with advanced heart failure.[77] VAD therapy holds out the promise of significant improvement in cardiovascular function with resultant reduction in overall frailty and improvement in quality of life. Notwithstanding, the current generation of devices is associated with a risk for infection, hemorrhage, stroke, or other neurologic event in anywhere from 18% to 36% and a nearly 100% risk of rehospitalization during 2 years of follow-up.[78] The frequency and severity of these complications increase significantly in the presence of associated comorbidities, so that an informed decision as to whether to pursue this option requires extensive discussion (see **Fig. 2**).

CARDIOPULMONARY RESUSCITATION

Cardiopulmonary arrest, as an isolated episode, is not uncommon in patients with heart failure and does not, in and of itself, portend end-stage disease.[79] This may account for the observation that only 23% of patients with heart failure in the SUPPORT database initially preferred not to be resuscitated in the event of an arrest.[80] It probably also underpins the high percentage of patients (14%) who changed their preference in favor of resuscitation during the course of their hospitalization. Those who did not want to be resuscitated were older, in higher income brackets, had lower activity status in the 2 weeks before admission, and perceived their prognosis to be worse than those who opted in favor of resuscitation. Although the numbers are too small for accurate comparison, a preference not to be resuscitated seems to have some degree of prognostic significance in and of itself. Of 19 patients subjected to CPR who had expressed a preference for it, 10 were discharged alive. Of six patients subjected to

CPR who had expressed a preference against it, only one survived to discharge.[80] One of the reasons that the numbers are not more robust is that the event rate in hospital in this patient population was only 4% with most sudden death in patients with heart failure occurring out of the hospital.[79]

All of this simply confirms that the prognosis for patients with heart failure remains variable and rapidly changeable such that decisions regarding resuscitation status, just as all medical decisions for these patients, need to be revisited frequently as clinical status changes.

For those patients who have not expressed a prior objection, data suggest that family members prefer to be present during a resuscitative effort if possible, and that the presence of family members in this context is not usually disruptive.[81,82] A study of out-of-hospital cardiac arrests has concluded that the presence of a family member during CPR of an adult patient is associated with positive results on psychological evaluations and did not interfere with medical efforts, increase stress in the health care team, or result in medicolegal conflicts.[83] As a result, recommendations that family members be offered the opportunity to be present during a resuscitative effort are now included the current American Heart Association Guidelines for Cardiopulmonary Resuscitation and Emergency Cardiovascular Care.[82]

PALLIATIVE SEDATION

Patients at the end stages of pump failure not uncommonly present with hallucinations, delirium, myoclonic jerks, and sometimes seizures that frequently exceed the capability of nonpharmacologic measures for control. Hallucinations and delirium are pharmacologically managed in many situations with small doses of haloperidol, olanzapine, or risperidone.[84] For those patients in whom delirium is not controlled and for those who present with myoclonus and frank seizures, sedative therapy may be necessary. Commonly used medications for this purpose include midazolam, lorazepam, and propofol.[84,85] Use of these agents in this context has been termed palliative sedation.

The use of palliative sedation has given rise to a large volume of literature as a result of its threefold consequences of relief of suffering, removal of consciousness, and its potential to shorten life, particularly in patients with heart failure who commonly suffer from a combination of hypotension and reduced cardiac output. The appropriate use of palliative sedation has been justified based on two commonly used ethical principles: proportionality and double effect. Proportionality requires that positive benefit of an intervention needs to outweigh its potentially negative effects.

Double effect also recognizes that a single action can have positive and foreseen negative effects; however, its application is more involved, and uses proportionality as only one of its requisite components. For an action to be justified, it requires that four conditions be met: (1) that the agent intend the positive effect, (2) that the action itself not be morally wrong independent of its consequences, (3) that the positive effect cannot be accomplished solely by means of the negative effect, and (4) that there be proportionality between the intended and unintended effects.[85]

In the case of palliative sedation, the intention is understood to be the relief of symptoms rather than a hastening of mortality. Second, sedation itself is not considered immoral independent of its consequences. Third, the positive effect of symptom relief is achieved directly by sedation and not only in and of itself by the foreseen negative effect of a potentially shortened lifespan. Finally, the positive benefit of symptom relief is considered to outweigh the potentially negative effects of additional hypotension and further fall in cardiac output.

Several commentators have argued that this kind of reasoning overly depends on the intention of the agent, a factor that is difficult to observe let alone measure.[86] The difficulty of assessing adherence to the rule of double effect is suggested by a survey of physicians and nurses caring for 44 terminally ill patients in two hospitals in whom life support was being withdrawn.[87] Fully a third of physicians responding identified the relief of pain and hastening of death as their primary intentions in prescribing palliative sedation. By contrast, proponents of the rule argue in response that the simple fact that persons can have more than one intention does not invalidate the rule. It is also possible that the physicians who intend to hasten death do not consider this intention wrong. Under these circumstances, they do not need to appeal to the rule for justification of their actions because their decision is based on the assumption that the hastening of death is not fundamentally wrong.[88,89]

Opponents of the use of the rule of double effect also argue that physicians are and should be held accountable for all foreseeable consequences of their actions rather than simply for those that they intend.[90] As such, some authors argue that the principle of proportionality alone may be a more appropriate justification for the use of palliative sedation.[85]

Rendering the ethical landscape more murky still is something known as the principle of collaboration that holds that cooperation in wrongdoing is itself immoral. This is understood to include advising, assisting, or tempting others to engage in wrongful acts.[91] All of this can create a morally ambiguous environment for a physician who is morally opposed to euthanasia but is required to try to counsel patients or surrogates about potential treatment options when the intent of either the patient or the surrogate is primarily to shorten life.

Given this ambiguity, several safeguards are necessary when considering the use of palliative sedation. It is important that all other means of symptom control have been exhausted before its institution and that appropriate consultations with palliative care and pain management specialists have been obtained. Second, it is important that the patient or responsible surrogate is fully informed as to the rationale for palliative sedation and concurs with its use. Third, it is critical that other caregivers on the unit be clearly instructed as to how to proceed with appropriate protocols in place.[85]

CAVEATS OF PALLIATIVE CARE

One perhaps unexpected response to the gradual growth of palliative care initiatives has been the concept of what one author has called "palliative care triumphalism."[92] Although a somewhat pejorative label, it refers to the observation that the carefully managed palliative efforts of dedicated professionals, including the use of palliative sedation, run the risk of ignoring that death represents a chaotic disintegration of life that is fundamentally not controllable. To attempt to control it may, at some level, represent a fundamental denial of an existential fact of the end of life. One palliative care practitioner has said that, "despite all we might say and all we might do, the process of dying includes suffering and painful separations and unfinished business. Death cannot be tamed. Death is unknown. Death is other. Death is death."[93]

This observation dovetails into previously identified components of a "good death" as perceived by multiple observers including physicians, nurses, social workers, chaplains, hospice volunteers, patients, and recently bereaved family members.[94] Only one of the components was pain and symptom management. The other five were clear decision making, preparation for death, completion, contributing to others, and affirmation of the whole person. Implicit in these six components must be the understanding that some of them will come into conflict with others and that this, in and of itself, is not necessarily to be avoided or otherwise palliated.

This understanding was summarized during the last century in the following fashion: "Often the most effective intervention that we can offer is time spent with patients and family, listening to concerns and acknowledging their value and touching – a physician's role that is hard to teach and harder to learn in medical education dominated by subspecialist- and procedure-oriented medical centers. We can, at a minimum, heed the powerful lessons taught by experiences with illness and death in our colleagues and loved ones."[95]

SUMMARY

The terminal stages of heart failure present challenges to the patient and the clinician that are at least the equal of terminal cancer, but with facets that are unique to cardiovascular disease. Among these unique characteristics are prognostic uncertainty, episodes of acute decompensation followed by rapid improvement, and the relative frequency of device therapy. It is clear from the published literature that communication between patients, their family members, and caregivers remains suboptimal and needs to be enhanced through more creative endeavors than have been reported to date. This includes a more in-depth discussion of the clinical course of heart failure at an early stage of the illness. Palliative intervention for patients with heart failure, including hospice, is clinically indicated for patients presenting with progressively increasing pump failure. Deactivation of device therapy in end-stage patients is often appropriate and needs to be discussed with patients and appropriate surrogates. Similarly, resuscitation status needs to be reviewed on a regular basis given that preferences regarding resuscitation tend to change frequently in patients with heart failure. Palliative sedation is an option for patients with otherwise uncontrollable symptoms in the throes of end-stage disease; however, its use must be carefully scrutinized to avoid its employment in inappropriate situations.

A consensus conference held in 2004 identified five questions regarding of end-of-life care for patients with heart failure that are in need of further research data.[96] (1) How best can the physical and psychosocial burdens of advanced heart failure on patients and families be decreased? (2) Which patients will benefit from which interventions and how best can they be counseled? (3) Which interventions improve quality of life and best achieve the outcomes desired by patients and family? (4) How can care be coordinated between sites of care and barriers to evidence-based practice reduced? (5) How can prognosis and treatment options be communicated better? These five questions effectively summarize some of the gaps that are currently present in the care of patients with end-stage heart failure. The American Heart Association in concert with the Heart Failure Society of America and the American Association of Heart Failure Nurses has issued a scientific statement on decision making in advanced heart failure that attempts to deal with some of these questions.[97]

The profession and society at large need to reacquaint themselves with the existential reality of death. Confronting this reality for what it is in ourselves, our loved ones, and our patients and their families helps to ensure that patients are served to the best of our ability, in their living and in their dying.

REFERENCES

1. AGS Ethics Committee. American Geriatrics Society Position Statement: the care of dying patients. J Am Geriatr Soc 1995;43:577–8.
2. Goodlin SJ. End-of-life care in heart failure. Curr Cardiol Rep 2009;11:184–91.
3. Howlett J, Morin L, Fortin M, et al. End-of-life planning in heart failure: it should be the end of the beginning. Can J Cardiol 2010;26:135–41.
4. Lewis EF. End of life care in advanced heart failure. Curr Treat Options Cardiovasc Med 2011;13:79–89.
5. Lamont EB, Christakis NA. Prognostic disclosure to patients with cancer near the end of life. Ann Intern Med 2001;134:1096–105.
6. Lamont EB, Christakis NA. Complexities in prognostication in advanced cancer. JAMA 2003;290:98–104.
7. Yamokoski LM, Hasselblad V, Moser DK, et al. Prediction of rehospitalization and death in severe heart failure by physicians and nurses of the ESCAPE trial. J Card Fail 2007;13:8–13.
8. Cowburn PJ, Cleland JGF, Coats AJS, et al. Risk stratification in chronic heart failure. Eur Heart J 1998;19:696–710.
9. Lee WH, Packer M. Prognostic importance of serum sodium concentration and its modification by converting enzyme inhibition in patients with severe chronic heart failure. Circulation 1986;73:257–67.
10. Levy WC, Mozaffarian D, Linker DT, et al. The Seattle Heart Failure Model: prediction of survival in heart failure. Circulation 2006;113:1424–33.
11. Kalogeropoulos AP, Kalogeropoulos AP, Georgiopoulou VV, et al. Utility of the Seattle Heart Failure Model in patients with advanced heart failure. J Am Coll Cardiol 2009;53:334–42.
12. Gorodeski EZ, Chu EC, Chow CH, et al. Application of the Seattle Heart Failure Model in ambulatory patients presented to an advanced heart failure therapeutics committee. Circ Heart Fail 2010;3:706–14.
13. Huynh BC, Rovner A, Rich MW. Long-term survival in elderly patients hospitalized for heart failure: 14-year follow-up from a prospective randomized trial. Arch Intern Med 2006;166:1892–8.
14. Huynh BC, Rovner A, Rich MW. Identification of older patients with heart failure who may be candidates for hospice care: development of a simple four-item risk score. J Am Geriatr Soc 2008;56:1111–5.
15. Cohn JN, Johnson G, Ziesche S, et al. A comparison of enalapril with hydralazine-isosorbide dinitrate in the treatment of chronic congestive heart failure. N Engl J Med 1991;325:303–10.
16. Maisel A. B-type natriuretic peptide levels: diagnostic and prognostic in congestive heart failure. Circulation 2002;105:2328–31.
17. Berger R, Huelsman M, Strecker K, et al. B-type natriuretic peptide predicts sudden death in patients with chronic heart failure. Circulation 2002;105: 2392–7.
18. Watanabe J, Shinozaki T, Shiba N, et al. Accumulation of risk markers predicts the incidence of sudden death in patients with chronic heart failure. Eur J Heart Fail 2006;8(3):237–42.
19. Bardy GH, Lee KL, Mark DB, et al. Amiodarone or an implantable cardioverter-defibrillator for congestive heart failure. N Engl J Med 2005;352:225–37.
20. Daubert JP, Zareba W, Hall WJ, et al. Predictive value of ventricular arrhythmia inducibility for subsequent ventricular tachycardia or ventricular fibrillation in multicenter automatic defibrillator implantation trial (MADIT) II patients. J Am Coll Cardiol 2006;47:98–107.
21. Weeks JC, Cook EF, O'Day SJ, et al. Relationship between cancer patients' predictions of prognosis and their treatment preferences. JAMA 1998;279: 1709–14.
22. Murray SA, Boyd K, Kendall M, et al. Dying of lung cancer or cardiac failure: prospective qualitative interview study of patients and their carers in the community. BMJ 2002;325:929–33.
23. Faber-Langendoen K. A multi-institutional study of care given to patients dying in hospitals: ethical and practice implications. Arch Intern Med 1996; 156:2130–6.
24. Allen LA, Gheorghiade M, Reid KJ, et al. Identifying patients hospitalized with heart failure at risk for unfavorable future quality of life. Circ Cardiovasc Qual Outcomes 2011;4:389–98.
25. Goldstein NE, Lynn J. Trajectory of end-stage heart failure: the influence of technology and implications for policy change. Perspect Biol Med 2006;49(1): 10–9.
26. Rizzieri AG, Verheijde JL, Rady MY, et al. Ethical challenges with the left ventricular assist device as a destination therapy. Philos Ethics Humanit Med 2008;3:20.
27. McCarthy M, Lay M, Addington-Hall J. Dying from heart disease. J R Coll Physicians Lond 1996;30: 325–8.

28. Zier LS, Sottile PD, Hong SY, et al. Surrogate decision makers' interpretation of prognostic information: a mixed-methods study. Ann Intern Med 2012;156:360–6.
29. Covinsky K, Goldman L, Cook E, et al. The impact of serious illness on patients' families. JAMA 1994;272:1839–44.
30. The SUPPORT Principal Investigators. A controlled trial to improve care for seriously ill hospitalized patients: The study to understand prognoses and preferences for outcomes and risks of treatments (SUPPORT). JAMA 1995;274:1591–8.
31. Lynn J, Teno JM, Phillips RS, et al. Perceptions of family members of the dying experience of older and seriously ill patients. Ann Intern Med 1997;126:97–106.
32. Emanuel EJ, Fairclough DL, Wolfe P, et al. Talking with terminally ill patients and their caregivers about death, dying, and bereavement: Is it stressful? Is it helpful? Arch Intern Med 2004;164:1999–2004.
33. Adler ED, Goldfinger JZ, Kalman J, et al. Palliative care in the treatment of advanced heart failure. Circulation 2009;120:2597-606.
34. Goodlin SJ. Palliative care in congestive heart failure. J Am Coll Cardiol 2009;54:386–96.
35. Stewart S, McMurray JJV. Palliative care for heart failure: time to move beyond treating and curing to improving the end of life. BMJ 2002;325:915–6.
36. Murray SA, Boyd K, Sheikh A. Palliative care in chronic illness: we need to move from prognostic paralysis to active total care. BMJ 2005;330:611–2.
37. Hauptman PJ, Havranek EP. Integrating palliative care into heart failure care. Arch Intern Med 2005;165:374–8.
38. Kittleson M, Hurwitz S, Shah MR, et al. Development of circulatory-renal limitations to angiotensin-converting enzyme inhibitors identifies patients with severe heart failure and early mortality. J Am Coll Cardiol 2003;41:2029–35.
39. Mishkin JD, Saxonhouse SJ, Woo GW, et al. Appropriate evaluation and treatment of heart failure patients after implantable cardioverter-defibrillator discharge: time to go beyond the initial shock. J Am Coll Cardiol 2009;54:1993–2000.
40. World Health Organization. Palliative Care [Fact Sheet number 402]. 2015. Available at: http://www.who.int/mediacentre/factsheets/fs402/en/. Accessed December 1, 2016.
41. Connor SR, Bermedo MCS, editors. Global atlas of palliative care at the end of life. London: Worldwide Palliative Care Alliance; 2014. p. 5.
42. Williams SG, Wright DJ, Marshall P, et al. Safety and potential benefits of low dose diamorphine during exercise in patients with chronic heart failure. Heart 2003;89:1085–6.
43. Simon ST, Higginson IJ, Booth S, et al. Benzodiazepines for the relief of breathlessness in advanced malignant and non-malignant diseases in adults. Cochrane Database Syst Rev 2010;(1):CD007354.
44. Clemens KE, Quednau I, Klaschik E. Use of oxygen and opioids in the palliation of dyspnea in hypoxic and non-hypoxic palliative care patients: a prospective study. Support Care Cancer 2009;17:367–77.
45. Levenson JW, McCarthy EP, Lynn J, et al. The last six months of life for patients with congestive heart failure. J Am Geriatr Soc 2000;48(5 Suppl):S101–9.
46. Evangelista LS, Sackett E, Dracup K. Pain and heart failure: unrecognized and untreated. Eur J Cardiovasc Nurs 2009;8:169–73.
47. Bleumink GS, Feenstra J, Sturkenboom MC, et al. Nonsteroidal anti-inflammatory drugs and heart failure. Drugs 2003;63:525–34.
48. Hauptman PJ, Mikolajczak P, George A, et al. Chronic inotropic therapy in end-stage heart failure. Am Heart J 2006;152:1096.e1-8.
49. Broström A, Hubbert L, Jakobsson P, et al. Effects of long-term nocturnal oxygen treatment in patients with severe heart failure. J Cardiovasc Nurs 2005;20:385–96.
50. O'Connor CM, Jiang W, Kuchibhatla M, et al. Safety and efficacy of sertraline for depression in patients with heart failure: results of the SADHART-CHF (Sertraline Against Depression and Heart Disease in Chronic Heart Failure) trial. J Am Coll Cardiol 2010;56:692–9.
51. Bradley TD, Logan AG, Kimoff J, et al. Continuous positive airway pressure for central sleep apnea and heart failure. N Engl J Med 2005;353:2025–33.
52. VanVeldhuisen DJ, Dickstein K, Cohen-Solal A, et al. Randomized, double-blind, placebo-controlled study to evaluate the effect of two dosing regimens of darbepoetin alfa on hemoglobin response and symptoms in patients with heart failure and anemia. J Am Coll Cardiol 2006;47(Suppl A):61A.
53. Pfeffer MA, Burdmann EA, Chen CY, et al. A trial of darbepoetin alfa in type 2 diabetes and chronic kidney disease. N Engl J Med 2009;361:2019–32.
54. Ward C. The need for palliative care in the management of heart failure. Heart 2002;87:294–8.
55. Smith C, Da Silva-Gane M, Chandna S, et al. Choosing not to dialyse: evaluation of planned non-dialytic management in a cohort of patients with end-stage renal failure. Nephron Clin Pract 2003;95:c40–6.
56. Beck A, Scott J, Williams P, et al. A randomized trial of group outpatient visits for chronically ill older HMO members: the cooperative health care clinic. J Am Geriatr Soc 1997;45:543–9.
57. Advance Care Planning (Module 9). St Paul: Heart Failure Society of America; 2005. Available at: http://www.hfsa.org/wp-content/uploads/2014/10/module9.pdf. Accessed December 1, 2016.

58. Managing Feelings About Heart Failure (Module 6). St Paul: Heart Failure Society of America; 2006. Available at: http://www.hfsa.org/wp-content/uploads/2014/10/module6.pdf. Accessed December 1, 2016.
59. Albert NM, Davis M, Young J. Improving the care of patients dying of heart failure. Cleve Clin J Med 2002;69:321–8.
60. Murray SA, Kendall M, Boyd K, et al. Exploring the spiritual needs of people dying of lung cancer or heart failure: a prospective qualitative interview study of patients and their carers. Palliat Med 2004;18:39–45.
61. Bailey FA, Burgio KL, Woodby LL, et al. Improving processes of hospital care during the last hours of life. Arch Intern Med 2005;165:1722–7.
62. Gibbs JSR, McCoy ASM, Gibbs LME, et al. Living with and dying from heart failure: the role of palliative care. Heart 2002;88(Suppl II):II36–9.
63. Gostin LO. Deciding life and death in the courtroom: from *Quinlan* to *Cruzan, Glucksberg*, and *Vacco* – a brief history and analysis of constitutional protection of the "right to die". JAMA 1997;278:1523–8.
64. Snyder L. Ethics manual: sixth edition. Ann Intern Med 2012;156:73–104.
65. Hunt SA, Abraham WT, Chin MH, et al. ACC/AHA 2005 guideline update for the diagnosis and management of chronic heart failure in the adult: summary article. Circulation 2005;112:1825–52.
66. Gillick MR. Advance care planning. N Engl J Med 2004;350:7–8.
67. Greco PJ, Schulman KA, Lavizzo-Mourey R, et al. The Patient Self-Determination Act and the future of advance directives. Ann Intern Med 1991;115:639–43.
68. Goldstein NE, Lampert R, Bradley E, et al. Management of implantable cardioverter defibrillators in end-of-life care. Ann Intern Med 2004;141:835–8.
69. Hauptman PJ, Swindle J, Hussain Z, et al. Physician attitudes toward end-stage heart failure: a national survey. Am J Med 2008;121:127–35.
70. Berger JT. The ethics of deactivating implanted cardioverter defibrillators. Ann Intern Med 2005;142:631–4.
71. Braun TC, Hagen NA, Hatfield RE, et al. Cardiac pacemakers and implantable defibrillators in terminal care. J Pain Symptom Manage 1999;18:126–31.
72. Cleland J, Daubert JC, Erdmann E, et al. The effect of cardiac resynchronization on morbidity and mortality in heart failure. N Engl J Med 2005;352:1539–49.
73. Carson P, Anand I, O'Connor C, et al. Mode of death in advanced heart failure: the comparison of medical, pacing, and defibrillation therapies in heart failure (COMPANION) trial. J Am Coll Cardiol 2005;46:2329–34.
74. Heart Failure Society of America, Lindenfeld J, Albert NM, et al. HFSA 2010 comprehensive heart failure practice guideline. J Card Fail 2010;16:e1–194.
75. Bax JJ, Abraham T, Barold S, et al. Cardiac resynchronization therapy. Part 2: issues during and after device implantation and unresolved questions. J Am Coll Cardiol 2005;46:2168–82.
76. Mueller PS, Hook CC, Hayes DL. Ethical analysis of withdrawal of pacemaker or implantable cardioverter-defibrillator support at the end of life. Mayo Clin Proc 2003;78:959–63.
77. Vitale CA, Chandekar R, Rodgers PE, et al. A call for guidance in the use of left ventricular assist devices in older adults. J Am Geriatr Soc 2012;60:145–50.
78. Slaughter MS, Rogers JG, Milano CA, et al. Advanced heart failure treated with continuous-flow left ventricular assist device. N Engl J Med 2009;361:2241–51.
79. Stevenson LW. Rites and responsibility for resuscitation in heart failure: tread gently on the thin places. Circulation 1998;98:619–22.
80. Krumholz HM, Phillips RS, Hamel MB, et al. Resuscitation preferences among patients with severe congestive heart failure: Results from the SUPPORT project. Circulation 1998;98:648–55.
81. Tsai E. Should family members be present during cardiopulmonary resuscitation? N Engl J Med 2002;346:1019–21.
82. Morrison LJ, Kierzek G, Diekema DS, et al. Part 3: ethics: 2010 American Heart Association Guidelines for Cardiopulmonary Resuscitation and Emergency Cardiovascular Care. Circulation 2010;122(Suppl 3):S665–75.
83. Jabre P, Belpomme V, Azoulay E, et al. Family presence during cardiopulmonary resuscitation. N Engl J Med 2013;368:1008–18.
84. Casarett D, Inouye S. Diagnosis and management of delirium near the end of life. Ann Intern Med 2001;135:32–40.
85. Lo B, Rubenfeld G. Palliative sedation in dying patients: "We turn to it when everything else hasn't worked". JAMA 2005;294:1810–6.
86. Quill TE, Dresser R, Brock DW. The rule of double effect: a critique of its role in end-of-life decision making. N Engl J Med 1997;337:1768–71.
87. Wilson WC, Smedira NG, Fink C, et al. Ordering and administration of sedatives and analgesics during the withholding and withdrawal of life support from critically ill patients. JAMA 1992;267:949–53.
88. Sulmasy DP, Pellegrino ED. The rule of double effect: clearing up the double talk. Arch Intern Med 1999;159:545–50.

89. Sulmasy DP. Double effect: intention is the solution, not the problem. J Law Med Ethics 2000;28(1):26–9.
90. Brody H. Causing, intending, and assisting death. J Clin Ethics 1993;4:112–8.
91. Jansen LA, Sulmasy DP. Sedation, alimentation, hydration, and equivocation: careful conversation about care at the end of life. Ann Intern Med 2002;136:845–9.
92. Barnard D. The skull at the banquet. In: Jansen L, editor. Death in the clinic. Lanham (MD): Rowman & Littlefield; 2006. p. 66–80.
93. Kearney M. Mortally wounded: stories of soul pain, death, and healing. New York: Scribner; 1996. p. 131.
94. Steinhauser KE, Clipp EC, McNeilly M, et al. In search of a good death: observations of patients, families, and providers. Ann Intern Med 2000;132:825–32.
95. McCue JD. The naturalness of dying. JAMA 1995;273:1039–42.
96. Goodlin SJ, Hauptman PJ, Arnold R, et al. Consensus statement: palliative and supportive care in advanced heart failure. J Card Fail 2004;10:200–9.
97. Allen LA, Stevenson LW, Grady KL, et al. Decision making in advanced heart failure: a scientific statement from the American Heart Association. Circulation 2012;125:1928–52.

Printed and bound by CPI Group (UK) Ltd, Croydon, CR0 4YY
03/10/2024
01040302-0003